WAR TRAUMA IN VETERANS AND THEIR FAMILIES

Diagnosis and Management of PTSD, TBI and Comorbidities of Combat Trauma

From Pharmacotherapy to a 12-Step Self-Help Program for Combat Veterans

Edited by

JAMSHID A. MARVASTI, M.D.

(With 17 Other Contributors)

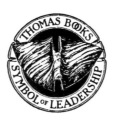

CHARLES C THOMAS • PUBLISHER, LTD.
Springfield • Illinois • U.S.A.

Published and Distributed Throughout the World by

CHARLES C THOMAS • PUBLISHER, LTD.
2600 South First Street
Springfield, Illinois 62704

ISBN 978-0-398-08724-1 (hard)
ISBN 978-0-398-08725-8 (ebook)

Library of Congress Catalog Card Number: 2011038999

Printed in the United States of America
CR-R-3

Library of Congress Cataloging-in-Publication Data

War trauma in veterans and their families : diagnosis and management of
PTSD, TBI, and comorbidities of combat trauma : from pharmacotherapy
to a 12-step self-help program for combat veterans / edited by Jamshid A.
Marvasti.
    p. cm. -- (American series in behavioral science and law)
    "Publication number 1114."
    Includes bibliographical references and index.
    ISBN 978-0-398-08724-1 (hard) -- ISBN 978-0-398-08725-8 (ebook)
1. War neuroses. 2. Post-traumatic stress disorder. 3. Brain damage. 4.
Veterans--Mental health. I. Marvasti, Jamshid A.

RC550.W367 2012
616.85'212--dc23

2011038999

CONTRIBUTORS

Attorney Robert J. Caffrey, J.D., M.A., Maj. (ret.) operates a private psychological counseling practice with a focus on men's issues and work with returning veterans. A fourteen-year veteran of the United States Army Reserve, he was deployed to Haiti (1995) and Bosnia (1996) as a peacekeeper and served in combat in Iraq in eastern Baghdad (2003–2004). His military awards include the Bronze Star, the Meritorious Service Medal, the Army Commendation medal with one oak leaf cluster, and the Combat Action Badge. He has trained in the martial arts for more than twenty years and holds a fourth-degree black belt in Shaolin Kempo Karate. Attorney Caffrey holds bachelor of arts degrees in history and sociology from the University of Notre Dame, a juris doctorate from Case Western Reserve University, and a master's in counseling psychology from Lesley University.

Karen L. Carney, R.N., L.C.S.W., F.T. is the bereavement program director for the D'Esopo Resource Center and Safe Place to Grieve Foundation, Inc., in Wethersfield, CT. She is the author and illustrator of several books for children and has authored a number of articles for professional publications. Ms. Carney has been developing programs for traumatized and bereaved persons of all ages for more than twenty years. She was nationally recognized for clinical excellence by the American Cancer Society, as recipient of the Lane W. Adams award, and was awarded the highest credential, fellow in thanatology, from the Association for Death Education and Counseling.

Christopher J. Doucot, M.A. is a cofounder of the St. Martin de Porres Catholic Worker community in Hartford, CT. Mr. Doucot holds a bachelor's degree from the College of the Holy Cross and a master of arts from the Yale Divinity School. He teaches about race, class, gender and religion, and nonviolence at Central Connecticut State University. Mr. Doucot has participated in or led more than ten peace campaigns in Bosnia, Iraq, Israel/Palestine, Darfur, and Afghanistan.

Valerie L. Dripchak, Ph.D., L.C.S.W. is a professor in the graduate school of Health and Human Services at Southern Connecticut State University in New Haven, CT. She received her doctorate degree from Fordham University in New York. Dr. Dripchak is a licensed clinician and has provided psychotherapeutic services to traumatized individuals and families for the past thirty years. She has developed graduate and postmaster's curricula for practitioners to become better skilled in the treatment of trauma and has presented more than thirty workshops on the topic of trauma at national and regional conferences. Dr. Dripchak has authored more than twenty publications and has received awards for her writing and excellence in clinical practice with children and adolescents.

Kenneth A. Fuchsman, Ed.D, a Vietnam veteran, has been affiliated with the Uuniversity of Connecticut since 1977 as an administrator, counselor, and faculty member, as well as executive director of general studies. He is currently assistant extension professor, teaching in both the individualized and the interdisciplinary major and the bachelor of general studies programs. Dr. Fuchsman's areas of specialty include the history of psychoanalysis, trauma and war, and interdisciplinary studies. Dr. Fuchsman is a research associate of the Psychohistory Forum and a frequent contributor to *Clio's Psyche* journal, and also serves on its editorial board.

Sidney Gitlin, Ph.D. grew up in a working-class family. He survived WW II, became a successful psychologist, and remains a loyal Air Force veteran. While in the service he was the pilot of a bomber, and during his active duty in Europe he experienced the losses of many of his fellow crew members. His vivid memories of war and its lasting horrors have challenged him and made him question its purpose. In 2011, he published his war memoir, which he dedicated to "the guys who didn't come back."

Robert Lerrigo, M.D. completed his bachelor of science degree at Stanford University and his medical degree from the University of California in San Francisco. His areas of interest include global healthcare systems, infectious disease, and molecular oncology. He is also an active advocate of rebuilding health-care infrastructures within nations in crisis affected by civil or natural disasters.

Ali Alim-Marvasti, M.B., B.Chir., M.A. graduated with double first-class honors from the University of Cambridge, England in undergraduate medical sciences (2006). He spent his final undergraduate year at the Massachusetts Institute of Technology, studying a combination of brain and cognitive sciences, psychology, neuropathology, fMRI, and special relativi-

WAR TRAUMA IN VETERANS AND THEIR FAMILIES

Publication Number 1114

AMERICAN SERIES
IN
BEHAVIORAL SCIENCE AND LAW

Edited by

RALPH SLOVENKO, B.E., LL.B., M.A., Ph.D.

Professor of Law and Psychiatry
Wayne State University
Law School
Detroit, Michigan

This book is dedicated to those brave veterans who returned from combat and disclosed the whole truth about the human cost of war and to those warriors who broke the silence of their souls and reported the brutality and inhumanity of their combat experiences.

"In the end, we will remember not the words of our enemies, but the silence of our friends."

Martin Luther King, Jr.

ty. He subsequently returned to Cambridge and completed his studies in clinical medicine (2009). He has worked in London NHS hospitals, where he was a senior house officer in neurosurgery. Dr. Alim-Marvasti is currently training in internal medicine in the United Kingdon, with an interest in neurology.

Jennifer Bordonaro Mastrocola, M.D. is a graduate of the University of Connecticut School of Medicine, where she received the dean's award for overall academic achievement. While in medical school, she was a member of the urban service track and was honored as an inductee into the gold humanism honor society. Her experience with PTSD in soldiers is partly a result of her work with paramedics returning from Iraq, but she also has a closer connection through her brother-in-law's military service experiences in Afghanistan. Dr. Mastrocola is a resident in family medicine at the University of Wisconsin School of Medicine and Public Health in Madison, WI.

Seth Mastrocola (First Lieutenant) began his military career in October 2004 as an enlisted member of the 304th Transportation Company in Springfield, MA. In the same year, he enrolled in the Connecticut National Guard simultaneous membership program between the 143rd Military Police Company (West Hartford) and the University of Connecticut reserve officer training corps (ROTC). Since receiving his commission, he served as the medical operations officer for the 1-102nd Infantry Regiment in Afghanistan during the year of 2010 to 2011. He currently serves as the medical operations officer on the Fourteenth Civil Support Team and is matriculated in the master of science, clinical mental health counseling program at Southern Connecticut State University.

Khairul Nual, was born in Bangladesh and raised in New York City. He is a student, majoring in psychology, at the University of Connecticut. He has assisted in research in myocardial infarction and is interested in the clinical aspects of the field of psychology. He is active in his community and involved in interfaith dialogues.

Claire C. Olivier received her bachelor of arts degree from Connecticut College in New London, CT. She is currently enrolled in a master's program in social welfare at the University of California at Berkeley, with a focus on community mental health. A trauma survivor, Ms. Olivier is exploring psychodynamic education for friends and family of trauma survivors. She is involved in an internship at a mental health agency in the San Francisco Bay area. Ms. Olivier contributed to Dr. Marvasti's book, *Psycho-Political Aspects of Suicide Warriors, Terrorism and Martyrdom* (2008).

Mary Paquette, Ph.D., R.N. is an assistant professor of nursing in California State University Northridge's R.N.-B.S.N. and accelerated bachelor of nursing program. She has extensive training and experience in crisis intervention, trauma, death and dying, violence prevention, and psychiatric/mental health nursing. She has maintained a private psychotherapy practice since 1984 and has given numerous presentations. Dr. Paquette has authored a number of publications on violence prevention, anger management and PTSD.

William J. Pilkington, S.T.M., M.A., Ed.D., C.T. is a pastoral counselor for a home hospice organization and adjunct faculty with the department of sociology at Central Connecticut State University, where he teaches courses in death and dying. Dr. Pilkington has more than thirty years of experience in pastoral care of those experiencing trauma and bereavement. He served as chaplain in the emergency department of a level 1 trauma center, and his pastoral care hospice experience has brought him into contact with many veterans of WWII, Korea and Vietnam. He is certified in thanatology by the Association for Death Education and Counseling.

Joseph E. Podolski, D.O. is a graduate of the University of New England College of Osteopathic Medicine. He completed his adult psychiatry residency at the Institute of Living in Hartford, CT and his fellowship in forensic psychiatry at the Medical College of Wisconsin.

Shazia Rahim Anwar, M.D. is a graduate of Dow Medical College in Karachi, Pakistan. She currently lives in Illinois, where she is devoted to helping her community, especially children. Her work with a group providing family support services is a reflection of this commitment. Dr. Anwar is currently studying to become a family counselor, focusing on the psychosocial well-being of our youth.

Alan R. Teo, M.D. completed his undergraduate education at Stanford University and went on to medical school and residency at the University of California, San Francisco. He has clinical and research experience in cultural psychiatry and anxiety disorders, in particular as they occur within the population of East Asia. Other scholarly interests include medical education and mental health services research. He has published more than ten peer-reviewed publications. He is currently completing a clinical research fellowship as a Robert Wood Johnson foundation clinical scholar at the University of Michigan.

PREFACE

Our mission in writing this book is to look beyond the politics of war in order to explore the extent of the ongoing and long-term human cost of war and military occupation. This book addresses the suffering of our troops and their families and our responsibility as a society, first to acknowledge and diagnose this suffering, and then to care for those who are affected by it. While it is not intended to take a moralistic or philosophical stance, the editor feels it is important to demonstrate the scale of human agony and loss inherent to war.

We Americans seem to be divided in our response to the present-day military conflicts in the Middle East and North Africa. On one extreme are those who are wholeheartedly supportive of the war and U.S. military invasions abroad. This group believes in America's inherent "goodness" and holds fast to American exceptionalism, arguing that military intervention is beneficial for the liberation and transformation of the world. On the other end of this spectrum are those who are considered peace oriented and who often see the long wars in the Middle East as based more on profit than principle. Some have accused the government and mainstream media of collaborating to sell the concept of war to an unwitting nation.

The largest segment of our population remains the group whose viewpoints lie somewhere in the middle of these two poles, often those who have ambiguous feelings surrounding the wars and U.S. involvement overseas. Some may be unaware of the long-term impact of war on our troops, their families, and society at large. Others may be openly against violence and aggression, but unwilling to challenge the status quo or even unsure of how to initiate change.

Our warriors are an extension of our society, and, therefore, they fall into the same three categories. Some remain steadfastly devoted to the military and the government's interests in war. Others may become conscientious objectors or advocates for peace, perhaps shifting their views of what it means to be "patriotic." Still others are conflicted in their feelings about war, and especially in the roles they may have played in Iraq or Afghanistan.

Scientific research reveals that multiple deployments and our troops' 24/7 involvement in combat where there is no clear front-line is causing serious emotional disorder and physical exhaustion, which contributes to war trauma and combat stress injury. This editor suggests that one way to decrease the suffering of our veterans is *to reinstate the draft*, even if that means "political suicide" for any policymaker who advocates for such a change. Furthermore, it is unethical and immoral when those who created the war do not send their children, grandchildren, nephews and nieces to fight in it. If war is indeed patriotic and necessary for the survival of our country, then citizens from all socioeconomic classes must take the risk of losing lives, limbs, and developing combat trauma and PTSD. We must all bear the burden of war equally.

Some Americans feel that the current wars are being fought by America's poor and not by the children of millionaires/billionaires and other VIPs. Under conditions of a draft, perhaps more of our leaders would hesitate before supporting a protracted war. Others feel that the draft is not a solution, because even with a draft in place, those in power or with special influence are able to find a way to escape their obligations, as evidenced during and after the Vietnam War.

The U.S. media has provided Americans with vast amounts of information about the basics of the Iraq and Afghanistan wars. Terms such as WMD and IED have become part of daily discourse. We are aware that our servicemen and servicewomen face grave physical danger while patrolling war zones amid 130-degree temperatures while carrying 120-pound loads on their backs. We may, however, be less aware of the psychological strain felt by these men and women as they face multiple deployments in combat zones where civilian casualties and the deaths of comrades are common occurrences. The editor applies a general label to the resultant crisis for combat veterans as psychologically *battered soldier syndrome*.

This editor also sides with those who advocate *giving the Purple Heart to veterans with war trauma*. Combat veterans who commit suicide as a result of their experiences are also victims of war and deserve to receive the Purple Heart, just as those who are killed on the battlefield. When a wounded warrior returns home and becomes home*less*, it is a tragedy for the nation and a shame for the government. In this sense, does our society present these military personnel with a "broken heart," rather than a Purple Heart?

The following poem, written by a WWII veteran, illustrates some of the limitations of rehabilitation from war trauma in a metaphoric way, confirming General Sherman's statement, "War is hell." (Source: Lee, K. A., Vaillant, G., Torrey, W., & Elder, G. 1995, April 4, A 50-year prospective study of the psychological sequelae of World War II combat. *American Journal of Psychiatry, 152*, 516–522.

Wheat fell headless in the field
Till Death did reap enough.
We seek to bury the revealed
No earth is deep enough.
You cannot wash the stain from minds
No one can weep enough.
Nor shut the past behind the blinds
No night has sleep enough.

DESCRIPTION OF THE BOOK

This book is divided into two sections. The first, "Clinical Issues of War Trauma," contains chapters on signs and symptoms, diagnosis, and pharmacotherapy of war trauma. The second section, "Witnesses to War," is comprised of four first-hand accounts of experiences in combat zones, during and after conflict.

The chapters of this book were written by professionals from different disciplines and with different ideologies. Some have had first-hand involvement in combat, from the Vietnam War to the wars in Iraq and Afghanistan. A chapter by a Ph.D. psychologist describes his experience as a bomber pilot during WWII; he still suffers from PTSD. Other contributors include a young lieutenant and medical officer deployed to Afghanistan; a professor of social work who is the daughter, sister, and wife of a veteran; and a therapist/lawyer who is a retired major of U.S. Army Reserves and was assigned to peacekeeping duties in Bosnia and Haiti, in addition to serving several months in the Iraq War.

The editor included his 12-Step Self-Help Principles for Combat Veterans with PTSD in the Appendix to the book. A Glossary by a physician follows the Appendix for the convenience of readers.

PART I: CLINICAL ISSUES OF WAR TRAUMA

Chapter 1
Impact of War and Combat on Veterans

In this chapter, Dr. Marvasti, a trauma specialist and Dr. Fuchsman, a Vietnam veteran and university faculty member, discuss the negative psychological impact of war on the warrior. They explain that war may have long-lasting effects and emphasize the stages of emotional reaction to combat. In summation, Dr. Fuchsman, says that, just as we see in cigarette packaging, there should be a warning in military advertisements: "The military can be hazardous to your health."

Also included is an exploration of the impact of participation or exposure to atrocities and the killing of enemy combatants, plus adverse impact on self-image and core beliefs of soldiers. Postcombat changes in thinking patterns and content and emotions such as grief and guilt are described.

Chapter 2
Blast-Wave Injuries and TBI:
Epidemiology, Pathophysiology, and Symptomatology

In this chapter, two physicians (J. Marvasti and A. Alim-Marvasti) explore the signs and symptoms and pathophysiology of combat-related TBI. They explain that TBI has psychological symptoms, (e.g. anxiety, depression, mood disorder, sluggishness, fatigue, etc.), nonpsychological symptoms, (e.g. headache, nausea, ataxia, tinnitus, dizziness, blurred vision, slurred speech, etc.), and mixed-category symptoms (e.g. amnesia and impaired attention/concentration capacity).

These two physicians advise that any soldiers with mild TBI should not be placed in combat situations where the risk of secondary trauma increases.

Chapter 3
PTSD in Veterans: Signs and Symptoms

In this chapter, Dr. Marvasti and Dr. Anwar explore the symptomatology of PTSD and suggests that although some soldiers should be clinically diagnosed with PTSD, one or two of the symptoms required for an official DSM-IV diagnosis may be absent. There may be a need for new, less-limited criteria for the diagnosis of PTSD.

Every veteran with war trauma presents with unique symptoms in an individual way according to his or her psychology and biology. Leo Tolstoy is quoted, "All happy families resemble one another, each unhappy family is unhappy in its own way."

Chapter 4
Spiritual Distress as a Component of PTSD: The Need for
Spiritual Healing

Mary Paquette Ph.D., R.N., discusses spiritual and psychological distress as an aspect of war trauma. She points out that although DSM-IV-TR does not recognize spiritual distress as a PTSD symptom, treatment should nevertheless address ways of relieving it. The military has trained soldiers in how to kill. This training does not prevent the trauma involved in killing, however, which has moral and ethical ramifications.

Chapter 5
Prozac Army:
Medicated Military in Combat, a Controversial Subject

Dr. Marvasti explains his review of clinical literature in regard to (a) the number of veterans on medication (which is excessive, in his opinion) and (b) the efficacy of medication versus the setbacks of side effects. He describes "a medicated army" whose population is divided into two categories; those who need medication to fight and remain hypervigilant and those who need it to reduce mental anguish and achieve a feeling of normalcy. Never in the history of war has such a large quantity of medication been prescribed to its combatants. Marvasti expresses his concern for the practice of administering medication and sending traumatized soldiers to combat, which is not a cure but merely postpones the effects of war trauma. The side-effects of medications may have caused mission failure, suicide, homicide, and violence among veterans of war.

Ultimately, he writes, the best treatment for war trauma is prevention. If PTSD, depression, and suicide are caused by multiple deployments, exhaustion, witnessing of civilian casualties, and exposure to atrocity, then the only way to truly avoid war trauma is to minimize these circumstances.

Chapter 6
Pharmacotherapy for PTSD: Antidepressant Medications

In this chapter, the efficacy, indications, and side effects of antidepressant medications are explored in regard to war trauma and PTSD. The use of antidepressant medications in various classes is discussed, including SSRIs, SNRIs, TCAs, and MAOIs.

Dr. Marvasti refers to literature that indicates that military personnel who are engaged in special high-risk duties (such as aviation and handling of nuclear weapons) are restricted from taking some of these medications while performing their jobs.

Chapter 7
Mood Stabilizers and Antiadrenergics

In this chapter, Dr. Marvasti explores current research on use of mood stabilizers such as divalproex, topiramate, lamotrigine, and so on, and antiadrenergics (alpha- and beta-blockers). These medications are being used on veterans with war trauma for alleviation of some of the symptoms, including mood swings, explosiveness, violence, and sleep disorder. He discusses combat considerations and explains that mood stabilizers and antiseizure medications may not be appropriate for combat veterans, since some require regular monitoring of blood levels.

Chapter 8
Pharmacotherapy for PTSD: Tranquilizers, Hypnotics, and Neuroleptic Medications

Here, Dr. Marvasti discusses the efficacy, indication, and side effects of tranquilizers (e.g. benzodiazepines), hypnotics (e.g., zolpidem), and neuroleptic antipsychotic medications. Because benzodiazepines may lead to dependency and addiction and also have side effects including amnesia, impaired cognitive/motor function, impaired judgment, drowsiness, ataxia, and rebound anxiety, they are not recommended for any veteran who is in a combat situation. Nonbenzodiazepine sedative or hypnotic medications for insomnia are explored, and their mechanism of action is discussed. These medications include trazodone, prazosin, and doxepin. The author also explains that some classes of drugs, such as beta-blockers, SSRI antidepressants, ACE inhibitors, and antipsychotics, may cause nightmares as a side effect.

Chapter 9
Pharmacotherapy for Alcohol Problems as a Comorbidity of PTSD

In this chapter, Dr. Marvasti and Khairul Nual focus on the impact of alcohol on veterans and discuss alcohol disorder as a possible comorbidity of PTSD and war trauma. As research indicates, PTSD-diagnosed soldiers who consume alcohol are more prone to having anxiety, mood disorders, disruptive behavior, and chronic physical illness. Also, medications used in the treatment of alcohol problems are discussed in detail including, disulfiram naltrexone, acamprosate, and topiramate.

Chapter 10
Fighting for Your Life: Clinical Issues in War Trauma Bereavement

The basic function of any system is considered to be survival, and so it is with grief and bereavement. Survival methods are innate as well as learned.

In this chapter, Karen L. Carney and William J. Pilkington explain the steps involved in acquiring survival techniques. Three main styles of grief expression are described. The authors also examine complicated grief and identify ten risk factors. They offer methods for treating this difficult condition.

The case history of one WWII soldier is presented; his job was to place explosives in caves where the enemy was thought to be hiding. As the man grew older, he was conflicted about his role in the war. While serving, he had considered himself a good soldier, yet all along he knew that women and children also hid in the caves and that he was therefore responsible for the deaths of many innocents. The history describes his expectation, as he neared the end of his life, to be punished after his death for his sins.

Chapter 11
Forensic Aspect of Combat Trauma and PTSD: Special Veterans' Court, Malingering, and Criminal Conduct

A forensic psychiatrist (Dr. Podolski) and a trauma specialist (Dr. Marvasti) explore the issue of malingering and symptom exaggeration in PTSD litigation and compensation procedures. They discuss the connection between PTSD in combat veterans and their criminal activities after they have returned from war, including discussion of veterans in the criminal system and the advantages and disadvantages of having a special treatment court for veterans.

This chapter also reviews the statements of defense attorneys representing combat trauma veterans accused of criminal activity at home. They claim that their clients were not criminals before deployment but rather were "programmed there to be killers" by the military and not then "deprogrammed" upon their return home.

Chapter 12
VETERANS' EXPERIENCES OF WAR

In this chapter, Dr. Dripchak reports on the results of the qualitative research project that she undertook in 2010 under the auspices of Southern CT State University in New Haven, CT. The men and women included in this study were living in the northeast part of the United States at the time when they were interviewed and had served in combats from World War II to the present.

Chapter 13
The Battle After The War:
Cultural Challenges for Those Coming Home

In this chapter, Claire Chantal Olivier writes about cultural challenges for veterans who return home with combat trauma. She discusses ways in which they are affected by our culture and society and asks such questions as, "Do heroes have nightmares?" Other subjects such as the dilemma of invisibility and difficulties of working with the VA health system are discussed. She also touches on the subject of "warriors for peace," which explains how a number of war veterans become human rights advocates, religious believers, or peace activists.

Chapter 14
The Effect of Parental Deployment on Children
in Military Families

Recent research revealed the surprising discovery that rates of PTSD in family members of war veterans were higher than those in the veterans themselves. This reflects the burden placed on not only the spouses of the deployed but also their children, who may interpret deployment as the loss of a parent and experience increased emotional distress as a result. In this chapter, Dr. Nina Dadlez focuses on children's adjustment, by age group, to the deployment of their parents as she reviews the overall impact on military families. She documents increased psychological morbidity and emotional and behavioral problems in children whose parents have been deployed to war.

Chapter 15
Families of Veterans: The Forgotten War Front

Here, Dr. Dripchak refers to the military adage, "If the military had wanted you to have a family, they would have issued you one," as she reviews the ways in which sending military personnel into combat impacts their family members. She discusses the sacrifices family members are required to make for war, even though they did not themselves volunteer for military duty. In general, life in the military is not compatible with family life.

Chapter 16
Veteran's Suicide: Prevalence, Contributing Factors, and Prevention

Amidst the highly publicized spike in veterans' suicides, the effect of combat trauma is being investigated more than ever before in our country's history. In this chapter, Dr. Marvasti, a trauma specialist, and Dr. Fuchsman, a Vietnam veteran, explore the connections between suicide and combat trauma, PTSD, TBI, side effects of medication, and substance abuse. Distinctions are made between several stages and/or categories of suicide, including suicidal ideation, attempt, parasuicidal behavior, and "inviting suicide."

There is also an overview of the ethical conflicts for combat clinicians who must choose between supporting the warrior or supporting the war. For example, should they evacuate a traumatized (suicidal) soldier or make an attempt at rehabilitation on site? One decision may save the soldier but decrease the fighting capacity of the unit. Dr. Marvasti emphasizes that a clinician must remain a clinician at all times, even in a combat zone, and cannot ignore this responsibility in order to conserve the fighting force. That consideration is the duty of the military command and politicians who initiated the war.

Chapter 17
PTSD in Asian Cultures: Can We Learn From How Other Societies Handle Trauma in Natural Disaster?

Drs. Teo and Lerrigo discuss the emerging field of disaster mental health and how it may serve to inform individuals in coping with combat trauma. They do this by looking to the disaster-prone areas of the Asia-Pacific region. They then attempt to correlate these events in ways that make them applicable to the situation of war and combat trauma. Trauma events that are considered "man-made" have been thought to have a different impact on mental health outcomes when compared to natural disasters; however, these authors focus on the numerous similarities between the two.

PART II: WITNESSES TO WAR

Chapter 18
Warrior Values in Modern Times: My Experience in the Iraq War

In this chapter, Robert Caffrey describes some of his experiences in the war in Iraq, particularly how they relate to what he terms "warrior values." These five core ideals, which he feels are the backbone of warrior conduct, are summarized as discernment, restraint, mercy, adaptability, and honor. Caffrey discusses each of these values in terms of concrete examples from his own experiences as a major (now retired) in the U.S. Army Reserves.

Caffrey also makes the distinction between warriors and policy makers and notes that not all policy makers live up to warrior values when they are engaged in the decision making process that affects us all. He calls attention to the difficulty we encounter when our enemies seem to be fighting without regard to these warrior values, quoting Nietzsche, who warned, "If we do what they do, no matter how justified we believe we are, we will ultimately become what they are." Caffrey cautions readers against the psychological perils of engaging in war without a moral code and expresses his belief that to do so is to dishonor the foundation of warriorhood.

Chapter 19
My Experiences as a Medical Operations Officer in Afghanistan

In this chapter, First Lieutenant Seth Mastrocola discusses his experience in the Afghanistan war as a medical operations officer. Mastrocola recounts one of his most difficult experiences, when one of his soldiers committed suicide by placing a live grenade under his own body. He describes the medics' unsuccessful attempt to revive the young man and the lingering question, "Could I have done more?"

Chapter 20
Guided Missiles and Misguided Leaders: Civilians in War Zones as Observed By a Christian Activist

In this chapter Chris Doucot summarizes some of his observations of the suffering of Iraqi civilians, especially children. Doucot has witnessed the horrors of war first hand, having traveled to Iraq, Afghanistan, Palestine, and

Darfur as a Christian peace activist. He quotes Howard Zinn who said, "Every war is a war against children." Doucot shares what he learned from children who have been gravely injured in U.S. missile attacks, as well as the parents of these children. He reminds us that "In a democracy, we bear responsibility for the actions of our government."

Chapter 21
Far From Being a Hero: My Life as a WWII Pilot

This chapter is the personal account of retired psychologist Dr. Sidney Gitlin, who flew a bomber plane during WWII. He admits to having nightmares and other symptoms of PTSD, and describes what his life is like after sixty years of being flooded with "memories and anxiety reactions to past memories of friends and crew."

Dr. Gitlin shares some of his most difficult experiences, such as when he watched a plane blow up upon landing at the home base. He also describes his discomfort at seeing segregated African-American troops and explains his surprise when, at a movie night, the German prisoners "were seated with all of us, and the African-Americans were segregated to the balcony." His sadness is evident in his comment that when WWII ended he wondered why it could not have been stopped sooner.

J.A.M.

ACKNOWLEDGMENTS

A project such as the creation of this book could not be accomplished without the professional dedication of a number of individuals whom I owe and am thankful for, in addition to the contributing authors.

First, Dori Smith was most helpful in inspiring me to write and in providing me with resources and materials from the beginning to the end of this project. My thanks, also, to Janet Dauphin for her editorial talent and for assisting me in my research. In addition, Talat Azimi, Sharron Freeman, and Mana Zarinejad were helpful in organizing and correcting several chapters. My gratitude to Mary Ellen Procko for her organizational skills. References were organized, checked, and rechecked multiple times by Alexandra Saldana, Laila Marvasti, Kayvon Ghoreshi, and Daria Marvasti, to whom I am very grateful.

My deepest gratitude to the Manchester Memorial Hospital library staff: Jeanine Cyr Gluck and Shelley Zinkerman, for providing resources, articles, and books that were needed to research up-to-date findings.

CONTENTS

PART II: WITNESSES TO WAR

WAR TRAUMA IN VETERANS AND THEIR FAMILIES

Part I

CLINICAL ISSUES OF WAR TRAUMA

Chapter 1

IMPACT OF WAR AND COMBAT ON VETERANS

Jamshid A. Marvasti and Kenneth A. Fuchsman

INTRODUCTION

Death and the risk of bodily injury are known entities in regard to the dangers of combat. What is less obvious is the threat that serving as a soldier can pose to one's mental well-being. One of the great paradoxes of human existence is that much of human civilization alternates between cooperation and conflict, diplomacy and combat (Fuchsman, 2008). As historian John Keegan claims, "Warfare reaches into the most secret places of the human heart" (Keegan, 1993). Gwynne Dyer asserts that "War may be an inescapable part of our genetic heritage" (Dyer, 2004). Yet, for all the possible ways that victory in war has helped cultures survive and prosper, it has come with serious emotional and physical consequences for many immersed in its brutalities.

For many of the veterans who make it back from combat, the aftermath of war and military service and the transition from combat to civilian life can also be hazardous. Absent from the military guidelines are some realities that any veteran entering combat should know: (a) combat exposure may cause posttraumatic stress disorder (PTSD); (b) PTSD is a neurobiological and hormonal imbalance in the human being; (c) untreated PTSD almost always gets worse; (d) those experiencing PTSD may resort to self-soothing and self-medicating through alcohol and street drugs; (e) combat PTSD frequently has comorbidities, such as depression, suicidal behavior, interpersonal difficulties, intimacy disorder, and rage reaction.

Young veterans in combat may get to know chaos, evil, and death in an intimate way, often witnessing each of these multiple times (Nash, 2007).

Lifton (1988) referred to the radical intrusion of the reality of death into the mind of these young veterans as "death's imprint." Because of its suddenness, its protracted nature, and its association with the terror of premature unacceptable dying, Lifton explained, death's imprint may be very difficult for young warriors to assimilate or to remove. There are almost no circumstances, other than combat, when men and women in their teens and early twenties face the reality of their own mortality so brutally (Lifton, 1988). The alternation between the fear of being attacked and the furious readiness to kill others is at the heart of war and, likewise, at the dark edge of what it means to be human.

STAGES OF EMOTIONAL REACTION TO COMBAT

Mental disorders due to war trauma tend to develop in three sequential phases following exposure to severe psychological anguish:

1. **Immediate phase**–during or immediately following traumatic events. Problems such as brief psychotic disorder, substance abuse, exacerbation of preexisting mental illness, acute stress disorder, and adjustment disorder may arise at this point (Cozza et al., 2004).
2. **Delayed phase**–usually occurs within two weeks after exposure to trauma. Among the difficulties arising in this phase are substance abuse, early PTSD, somatoform disorders, depressive disorders, psychotic disorders, and anxiety disorders (Cozza et al., 2004). According to a report by the government-sponsored Mental Health Advisory Team (MHAT), 28 percent of soldiers and Marines in high combat in Iraq experienced acute stress or PTSD (MHAT-IV, 2006).
3. **Chronic phase**–occurs months to years after the traumatic event. In this phase, clinicians may see substance abuse or dependence, mood disorders, psychotic disorders, and PTSD. Homelessness among veterans is a frequent finding and is considered an event of the chronic phase. Veterans make up 11 percent of the general population over age 18, yet in 2007 they accounted for roughly 26 percent of the homeless (Cunningham, Henry & Lyons, 2007). According to the Veterans Administration, 35 percent of all homeless individuals are veterans (male and female). Fifty-five percent of homeless veterans are African-American or Hispanic. Additionally, 45 percent suffer from mental illness (including PTSD), and 70 percent of homeless veterans have addiction problems (Bradley, 2009).

The Grant Study of Adult Development at Harvard followed the lives of a selected group of men from the classes of 1939 through 1941 over the course of 50 years, including those who served in World War II (WWII). In

1995, data were analyzed from the participants in the study to see how "pre-morbid variables" influenced the development of, or protected combat veterans from, the onset of PTSD. The authors of this study state that of the "four potential pre-morbid predictors of PTSD symptoms (poor childhood, psychological issues in college, physical symptoms with stress, and combat exposure) only combat exposure made a significant statistical contribution to development of PTSD symptoms." Notably, in the Grant Study, "men with high combat exposure continued to report more symptoms of PTSD forty years later" (Lee, Vaillant, Torrey & Elder 1995, p. 520).

It is often in the period after the threats to life and limb are diminished that pent-up stress comes out. A 1999 veterans health study discovered that 31 percent of veterans had depressive symptoms, which is higher than rate of depression in the general public (Mundell, 2007). Of male Vietnam veterans, 44.5 percent reported at least one significant postwar problem with readjustment. More than a decade after the 1975 fall of Vietnam, one in four of those who had served in Vietnam still had at least one serious adjustment problem. For those male Vietnam veterans with PTSD, at least one of their children is more likely to have behavioral problems than the offspring of male Vietnam veterans without PTSD (Kulka et al., 1990). Have the sufferings of the fathers been passed on to their children?

IMPACT OF EXPOSURE/PARTICIPATION IN ATROCITIES AND KILLING ENEMY COMBATANTS

As the MHAT reports (2006), the level of PTSD in soldiers and Marines may depend on the intensity of combat they experienced and the length of time they spent in a combat zone. Those who served more than one tour were more likely to have PTSD than those with comparable exposure to danger who served shorter tours of duty (MHAT-IV, 2006). Additionally, it is not only experiencing high levels of combat that matters, but also what kind of combat a soldier experienced. Psychiatrist Judith Herman writes (1992), "It was the participation in meaningless acts of malicious destruction that rendered men most vulnerable to lasting psychological damage." She continues, "Years after their return from the war, the most symptomatic men were those who had witnessed or participated in abusive violence." Supporting these findings, another study of Vietnam veterans found that every one of the men who acknowledged participating in atrocities had posttraumatic stress disorder more than a decade after the end of the war (Herman, 1992). It is reported that among Vietnam veterans, 22 percent witnessed abusive violence (atrocities), and 9 percent personally participated in such activities (Laufer, Frey-Wouters & Gallops, 1985). Among veterans who participated in or witnessed atrocities, research revealed the presence of depression, guilt feelings, PTSD, self-destructive behavior and suicide (Maguen et al., 2010; MacNair, 2002). Laufer, Gallops, and Frey-Wouters (1984) reported that the loss of a friend in combat may lead to violent acting out such as killing unarmed civilians or prisoners of war (POWs), which may in turn result in more trauma and stress and guilt feelings.

In some cases, soldiers were eventually able to express that they indirectly or "unintentionally" committed unnecessary violence that resulted in civilian casualties. One may speculate that only "antisocial or sociopathic" individuals are *not* emotionally disturbed by committing war crimes. However, for some it takes many years to get in touch with the reality of their actions in the combat zone. For example, Joe, a gunner in an HMMVVV (Humvee), told his clinician about his experience driving with his unit in the streets of Baghdad. Someone shot a bullet at the caravan from one of the buildings. Joe and the other gunners, following their military protocol, immediately fired back with machine guns at windows in that building. When they went inside the building, they found women and children covered in blood. They could not find any weapons or the person who shot at them. Joe felt that the shot came from a different building than the one they had assumed. He reported (years after the event) that none of the soldiers involved had talked about the incident while in Iraq. "It seemed it didn't bother us, or we were in the adrenalin rush of battle." A couple of years after this incident, Joe is now talking about it with his therapist and has significant feelings of shame and guilt and self-destructive behavior. He is diagnosed as having PTSD, traumatic brain injury (TBI), depression, and drug addiction.

Some combat veterans have explained that the exact action of killing another human being is by itself traumatic and devastating (Matsakis, 2007). Killing unarmed civilians or POWs can have an even more traumatic impact on the perpetrators. For some military personnel the first few "kills" are the most difficult ones, but the passing of time eventually numbs them and killing becomes a routine part of their mission or profession. Some soldiers may even feel "high" and euphoric during hand-to- hand combat, and a small number become "addicted" to killing. As Matsakis (2007) explained, these veterans are often labeled as inhuman, not only by others but, unfortunately, also by themselves as well. Sometimes, to decrease their psychic pain, veterans may distance themselves from the killing events by dissociating or developing amnesia. Other times, alcohol and drugs are used to decrease the psychic pain and extend the numbing state. This process allows the veteran to continue fighting without emotional breakdown.

IMPACT OF COMBAT ON SELF-IMAGE

Soldiers who are suffering from combat PTSD may also have problems with self-image, self-esteem, self-ideal, and self-confidence. A young recruit may go to war with a fantasy of performing heroic actions in foreign lands, rescuing innocents from tyrants, bringing freedom to those living under dictatorship, closing torture chambers, and feeding hungry children, then returning home as a hero or freedom fighter, with a chest decorated with medals, a mind filled with satisfaction, and a soul proud of humanitarian accomplishments.

Sadly, more than a few return with wounded souls, scattered minds, and feelings that they have been betrayed and deceived or that they have participated in an unjust war. Perhaps they were exposed to atrocities, saw the torture chambers rebuilt and reopened, and witnessed hungry children receiving bullets, not food. A few of these veterans may feel that they sacrificed part of their life, time, and energy to protect a corrupt foreign government. They may have seen civilians massacred by their own missiles and innocent bystanders killed in "collateral damage."

As Matsakis (2007) has explained, some veterans have such a negativistic self-impression that they feel they are "more animalistic and brutal" than previous wars' veterans. The resulting sense of shame and self-hate can be intense. Veterans who experience self-hate and shame on an unconscious level may not be able to articulate these feelings to others (Matsakis, 2007), and counseling (clinical or spiritual) may not help because it relies on verbal communication. Profound self-hate may result in self-punishment and even suicide. Rage and homicidal urges that are always present during combat are suddenly transferred toward the self. Now the enemy is within. Soldiers may not believe they are committing suicide, because the self that they are killing is not their true self. Their self-ideal was to be a hero, rescuer, and freedom fighter, but war has changed their self-concept to that of a murderer. This is illustrated by a new term used by some disappointed military personnel, who have changed the label collateral damage to collateral murder (Kall, 2010).

Brian, an injured soldier with PTSD, explained that he went to war with strength, motivation, and love of humanity and now has returned home with PTSD and a devastated self-ideal and self-value. His "ego ideal" was to be a hero; instead, he is being chased in his dreams by souls of murdered unarmed civilians. He wakes up sweating, screaming, and panicky. He feels guilty because he did not live up to his image of himself as a freedom fighter and liberator—a hero.

Another soldier, Alex, dared to feel his pain, telling his counselor, "I am not the hero; the hero is the woman who had a bullet in her body while covering her baby from our aimless shooting, pointing at her child and begging us in Arabic not to harm her baby. After searching the three-floor building, we couldn't find any suspicious items. When we returned to the mother, she was dead, but the baby in her arms was crying and touching her face. Now, I wake up at night hearing the baby crying–to this day, whenever I hear a baby crying I get crazy."

Rewriting, Reshaping, and Distortion

When some combat veterans look back at their war experience they feel proud of their actions and have gained psychological strength from the horrors and trials they endured. Others wish they had acted more appropriately, wisely, bravely, and heroically. A small number may deal with their shortcomings during combat by rewriting the scenario and making themselves believe the opposite of what really happened. After recurrent and persistent episodes of rewriting and reshaping the events as they wished they had happened, they gradually believe in the new, fabricated stories as if they were fact. In these situations, reality is sacrificed, distorted, and reshaped as an ego defense mechanism for the sake of maintaining self-respect and avoiding psychic pain.

Distortion as a psychological defense in service of ego is another example of the impact of war on the veteran's pattern of thinking. Some veterans, especially those with injuries and loss of body parts or function, have wondered if their sacrifices were in vain. They may use distortion to maintain their opinion that their superiors did the right thing by invading a foreign land and deploying U.S. troops. They need to believe that the invasion was part of a "holy and just" war.

Change in Core Beliefs and Shattered Assumptions

War may change the participants' perceptions of their faith, ideology, and philosophy and their trust in the goodness of humanity. These changes in belief may result in an existential crisis that reshapes the basic concept of the warrior's world view. Shay (1994) explained that combat trauma "destroys the capacity for social trust" because it shatters the illusion that human beings are basically benevolent and good natured.

Many authors, such as Janoff-Bulman and Epstein, have talked about shattered assumptions in trauma victims. Often these shattered assumptions, which change our world view and make us vulnerable and insecure, are walled off. They are not well-integrated, challenged, or analyzed. Pretrauma assumptions tend to give an impression that the world is meaningful, fair, reasonable, predictable, rewarding, and orderly. The assumptions are that people get what they deserve and that a moral order exists in the universe. If people do good things, then they are rewarded, and bad things never happen to good people (Epstein, 1991; Janoff-Bulman, 1992; Scurfield, 1994).

The hell of war and its component of atrocity are capable of shattering these basic assumptions in traumatized veterans. They may develop profound despair, self-degradation, and vulnerability and consider the world to be disorganized, cruel, and without justice. These dramatic changes may eventually transfer to soldiers' partners and their children, who become unofficial casualties of war. Shay (1994), writing about Vietnam veterans, describes how the betrayal in war of the moral order–of our basic beliefs about what is right and wrong–can destroy the characters of these young fighters. Grossman (1995) maintained that for many young soldiers the very act of killing another human being can shatter core beliefs, especially beliefs in one's own basic goodness.

Impact of War on Thinking Patterns and Contents

War frequently involves dehumanizing the enemy, projecting evil onto the opponents, and making one's own side represent goodness. Although this type of splitting can be self-deceptive, it does serve a psychological function. This moral characterization of the other side justifies killing and maiming. Sadly, in peace and war, being a person often includes depersonalizing others (Fuchsman, 2008).

A mindset is defined as a set or series of thinking patterns that an individual develops as a reaction to internal and external events. War can affect the mindsets of veterans with or without PTSD. During combat there are mindsets that are learned and practiced by participants as self-protection and survival skills. At times these mindsets may be useful in civilian life, but at other times, they may be counterproductive and even dangerous. Some of the mindsets of war-related trauma, as explained in literature (Matsakis, 2007), are:

1. **All-or-nothing (now-or-never) thinking.** This mindset is a learned pattern during combat. In battle, almost all phenomena or events are split into "bad" or "good" –cowboy or Indian, feast or famine–with nothing in between. Neutrality is not accepted, and gray areas are not present; things are black or white. There is no such thing as saving one's life in moderation or killing the enemy just a little bit.
2. **"Friend or foe" thinking.** The concept of being with us or against us has been used in political conflicts throughout history to polarize individuals

and force them to choose sides. In 2001, President George W. Bush addressed a joint session of Congress, saying "Either you are with us, or you are with the terrorists." Dual issues of "friend or foe" thinking can cause conflicts in civilian life.

3. **Perfectionism.** This mindset of doing something perfectly or not doing it at all (shoot at the heart), combined with lack of tolerance for any mistake or shortcoming (in self or others) is an adaptive and beneficial survival skill in combat. When veterans return home, however, this pattern of thinking becomes maladaptive. A returning soldier expects perfection from others and cannot tolerate anyone in the moderate line.

Many family members of veterans have reported that they constantly need to remind the veterans that they are "not in the battlefield," and a mistake does not mean the death of a comrade or failure of a mission. One military wife described her family's response to her veteran husband's authoritative attitude at home, saying it caused her children to write slogans on the walls of their rooms, such as "This is not a barrack" and "We are not in Fallujah."

COMBAT STRESS REACTIONS

Combat stress reaction (CSR) is psychophysiological reaction of soldiers to the stress of combat. As clinical and research literature indicates, those who are overwhelmed by their anxiety during combat may develop multiple emotional and somatic symptoms, such as feelings of vulnerability, powerlessness, and the sensation of near-death experiences. They may experience intense rage and paranoid thinking, which may result in impulsive acts such as shooting suddenly and aimlessly. Somatic symptoms might include excessive tiredness, shakiness, loss of bladder and bowel control, and conversion reaction (e.g. blindness or paralysis without organic basis). Cognitive dysfunction may also be present in some soldiers, including confusion, memory problems, unreal feelings, dreamlike states, and dissociative disorder.

Confusion may reach a level where veterans do not know who or where they are. These symptoms may be collectively diagnosed as acute stress disorder, which may evolve into PTSD (Solomon, 2008). Bremner (2002) explains, "Our bodies have biological systems that respond to life-threatening danger, acting like fear alarm systems that are critical for survival." When danger is imminent, "a flood of hormones and chemical messengers is released into our brains and bloodstream almost instantly. This stress-responsive activation of biological systems helps us in doing whatever it takes to survive." Yet, functioning under high stress is not easy. "The short-term survival response can be at the expense of long-term function." This can include various kinds of neurological damage and trauma-related psychiatric disorders. "The same biological systems that help us survive life threats can also damage the brain and body" (Bremner, 2002, pp. 3–4).

Stresses of War on Veterans

Given the spectrum of emotions within human psychology, the horrors of war generate a diversity of responses. One side of war celebrates competition, the need to dominate, the desire to destroy and, as such, grandly empowers the warrior. On the other hand, those who are killed, maimed, or emotionally disabled are reminders of the awful tragedies inevitably accompanying the orgy of destruction that is called modern warfare (Fuchsman, 2008).

Lieutenant Colonel Dingmann, a military psychiatrist in the Iraq War estimated that 60 percent of the combat troop in Iraq had symptoms of acute stress disorder. He connected this high number to the "360-degree" battlefront encountered in Iraq. The intensity of combat in Iraq is more than what soldiers experienced in WWII. For example, infantrymen in WWII were exposed to an average of eighty-one days of combat during the course of the war. In the Iraq war, however, a veteran could amass that number of days of combat in three to four months (Young, Gillan, Dingmann, Casinalli & Taylor, 2008).

Focusing on the trauma of war, researchers have delineated several stressors that veterans in recent wars have experienced:

1. Extent and severity of combat exposure, which veterans defined as being fired upon; being exposed to the sights, sounds, and smells of human death; and seeing refugees and destroyed villages.
2. Life-threatening events and concerns about the possibility of exposure to biological weapons of mass destruction. During duty in Southwest Asia, veterans may have been exposed to disease and pathogens such as tuberculosis, malaria, anthrax, and tularemia, as well as a variety of viral and chemical agents used in warfare (Reeves, Parker & Konkle-Parker, 2005). Some veterans have developed long-term disabilities due to side effects of the medications that were given to prevent or treat these diseases.
3. Unknown and difficult living and working conditions, such as uncomfortable weather, poor living sites, lack of desirable food, and long working hours.
4. Concerns about how deployment would affect their family lives and careers. More than 50 percent of service members are married.

5. Uncertainty of length of deployment. Soldiers live with the constant possibility that the military will reassign them to the combat zone. (Some veterans have been deployed, or "recycled" up to eight times.)
6. Sexual and gender harassment, especially among female veterans. Around 16 percent of the active U.S. armed forces are female (Cozza et al., 2004).
7. Ethnocultural stressors for minority soldiers, especially those of Muslim parentage or faith (Litz & Orsillo, 2004). Ethnic minorities make up a significant portion of the armed forces, ranging from 24 percent in the Air Force to 40 percent in the Army (Cozza et al., 2004).
8. Fear of abuse, torture, or execution if captured. Soldiers serving in the Middle East wars fear the potential of abuse or execution and the possible mutilation and desecration of their bodies by enemy combatants.
9. Friendly fire, which results in the death of a comrade due to commission or omission by a comrade.
10. Disappointment, betrayal, and the discovery that they are fighting to support a possibly corrupt government.
11. Possible involvement in atrocities and exposure to civilian casualties (collateral damage).

Research Findings

Vasterling and colleagues (2006) studied 654 U.S. Army personnel who deployed to Iraq. Their research indicated that 55 percent witnessed a serious wounding or killing of a fellow soldier (American or ally) and 61 percent witnessed the wounding or killing of an enemy combatant. In this same study, 98 percent reported "seeing people begging for food," 77 percent saw homes or villages being destroyed, and 63 percent saw Americans or allies after they had been severely wounded or disfigured in combat (Begany, 2006; Vasterling et al., 2006). A study of more than 88,000 soldiers returning from war zones revealed that the impact of war may not appear until months after a veteran's reentrance to the United States. Soldiers show more mental distress after they have been home for six months than they do when first returned home. This research also indicates that national guard and reservist veterans are twice as likely to require mental health care as their regular army peers are (Levin, 2007; Milliken, Auchterlonie & Hoge, 2007). In general, 20 percent of the active duty soldiers and 40 percent of reservists needed psychiatric treatment.

A compulsory screening of Canadian land/sea/air force members who were deployed to Afghanistan revealed that four to six months after their return, 20 percent had psychiatric symptoms such as mood disorder, anxiety attacks, or alcohol use disorder (AUD) (Levin, 2007). The impact of combat on soldiers not only is psychological or medical but also can manifest in criminal activity, another side effect of war. Research reveals that more than 60 percent of combat veterans with PTSD have a history of at least one arrest after returning home from the wars in Iraq and Afghanistan. Studies in clinical literature indicate that PTSD in civilians is also a strong risk factor for both juvenile delinquency and adult crime. In addition, PTSD has played a very powerful role in steering women into prostitution and men into drug dealing and pathological gambling (Goulston, 2008).

GRIEF AND COMBAT

Another symptom of war trauma is grief. We think of grief as the normal reaction to the loss of a loved one through death. This definition can be expanded, however, to include a reaction to the loss of human ideals, such as ethics, honesty, belief system, honor, and dignity (Nash, 2007). Grief is not reversible, nor is it a choice. The losses that provoke grief are afflictions. Although each person mourns and grieves in his or her own way, there are certain common presentations that are thought of as typical symptoms of grief. Stroebe, Hansson, Stroebe & Schut (2001) describe these as the following:

1. Emotional symptoms, such as anger, hostility, depression, guilt, anxiety, and despair.
2. Behavioral symptoms, such as crying, isolation, and agitation.
3. Cognitive symptoms, such as memory loss, concentration problems, self-reproach, and preoccupation with the deceased.
4. Physical symptoms, such as fatigue, lack of energy, loss of appetite, and sleep disturbance. Sometimes the grieving soldier may demonstrate the symptoms or traits of the deceased person.

In addition, Jacobs (1999) reported that grief in reaction to loss can include some of the symptoms of PTSD or acute stress reaction, such as (a) dissociative symptoms causing the grieving individual to feel stunned, dazed, shocked, or numb; (b) intrusive, painful recollections about the deceased individual; (c) frequent attempts to avoid reminders of the deceased person; and (d) damage to belief systems, including loss of security and trust.

Nash (2007) explains that grief symptoms are common in soldiers who have lost comrades or valued leaders. Service members often do not experience the full impact of their grief until after they have returned to their base or U.S. fort and their adaptive numbness and denial have worn off.

Sometimes, the reality of combat losses may not begin to sink in until they are on an airplane flying home, surrounded by too many empty seats (Nash, 2007).

Combat Euphoria and a Life of Dysphoria

Combat arouses powerful emotions. Dread of death, the drive to survive, and possibly even a delight in killing arouse a whole spectrum of human emotions among soldiers in battle. There are two sides to the grim environment of war. For many soldiers, combat can bring a level of excitement that is unsurpassed. Scurfield reports that "some combatants experience feelings of euphoria and adrenalin rush, feelings of being more 'alive' in the midst of death-defying episodes" (2006, p. 35). Paradoxically, the deep satisfaction that some feel in the midst of combat can bring with it a lifetime of emotional scarring. Another appeal of combat is what Gray (1959) calls "the delight of destroying," which takes on an "ecstatic character." Killing others in battle may give one a sense of power; the death of an enemy can bring a sense of vitality.

"Part of the love of war," Vietnam veteran William Broyles writes, "stems from its being an experience of great intensity. War stops time; intensifies experience to the point of a terrible ecstasy" (1984, p. 56). Witnessing the men under his command "perform perfectly under heavy fire" in Vietnam made Marine Officer Philip Caputo feel "a drunken elation . . . I had never experienced anything like it before . . . an ache as profound as the ache of orgasm passed through me" (1977, p. 268).

There are limitations to the ecstasy of combat. Bringing life and death so close together can engender extraordinary stress. Psychiatrists J. W. Appel and G. W. Beebe in 1946 wrote "There is no such thing as 'getting used to combat.' Each moment of combat imposes a strain so great that men will break down in direct relation to the intensity and duration of their exposure. Thus, psychiatric casualties are as inevitable as gunshot and shrapnel wounds in warfare" (1946, xx). By their estimation, this psychic break down appears to occur after an average of 200 to 240 aggregate combat days (Appel & Beebe, 1946, p. 1470).

Wounded Veterans: From Euphoria to Dysphoria

For many wounded veterans there may initially be a sense of great relief, almost euphoria as they think, "Thank God I am alive." Wounded soldiers may receive a lot of attention from hospital personnel, their family members, and commanders, as well as from the media, political figures, and celebrities.

They may receive medals. Wounded veterans may also compare themselves to comrades who were killed or seriously injured in the same action and realize that they are luckier than others.

As Wain, Grammer, Stasinos and DeBoer (2006) stated, however this initial euphoria or relief may give way to a negative emotional reaction. Many wounded soldiers have pain that cannot be managed with pain medication. They may have been athletic before the injury and now find that they are permanently disabled. They become concerned about financial difficulties and relationship problems, which increases their vulnerability for the development of psychiatric symptoms. Some may have survivor guilt, be disappointed in the community's reaction, or feel dismay over being separated from their units. They may use unhealthy coping mechanisms for their depression and despair, such as becoming involved with alcohol and street drugs.

Psychologist and Army Reserve Lieutenant Colonel Kathy Platoni asserts that the experience of combat can cause a unique trauma in veterans, decreasing their tolerance for frustration. She states, "I can understand why somebody would come back feeling like, 'I made all of these sacrifices, I suffered all of these horrible things, and now fate or God or society or my girlfriend-whatever-is doing me wrong again' " (DeBrosse & Srivastava, 2010). Mary Tendall, a California psychologist and specialist in trauma in veterans, explains that "Soldiers have spent prolonged time in combat zones and developed a kind of hypervigilant attitude. A 'lock-and-load' mentality dominates their brain chemistry for years after they return." She goes on to say, "Their whole existence is coming from that primitive, reptilian-like place of survival within the brain, it is fight-flight-or-freeze." She added that any trigger, such as a nightmare, a disappointment, or even a minor provocation, can inject the traumatic past into the present reality. That may translate into a veteran's wanting to kill somebody who just pulled in front of him at a traffic light (DeBrosse & Srivastava, 2010).

POSTCOMBAT INVINCIBILITY, RISK-TAKING, AND REPETITION COMPULSION

Killgore and associates (2008) tried to classify potentials for increased risk-taking and unsafe behavior among veterans of war. They identified thirty-seven different combat experiences in the Iraq War, from which they evaluated 1252 U.S. Army soldiers immediately after returning home from combat deployment. Killgore and coworkers then re-evaluated the same group three months after their initial postdeployment survey. Their finding was that specific combat experiences (exposure to violent combat, killing another person, and contact with high levels of human trauma) were predictive of greater risk-taking propensity in veterans after returning home. Greater exposure to these combat experiences was also predictive of actual risk-related behaviors in the preceding month, including more frequent and greater quantities of alcohol use and excessive verbal and physical aggression toward others. The authors reported that exposure to violent combat, human trauma, and having direct responsibility for killing another person may alter the veteran's perceived threshold of invincibility and increase the propensity to engage in risky behavior upon arriving home. (Killgore et al., Oct.).

Freud was first to explain that trauma victims might have a compulsion to repeat their trauma. He felt that repetition of the trauma is done for the purpose of ego mastery. A number of veterans with PTSD get into high-risk or rescue-oriented jobs such as police work, fire protection, crisis intervention work, or emergency medical services as they try to transfer their experience in a meaningful way. High-risk behaviors such as skydiving, rock climbing, or reckless speeding, however, may also be common. Living "on the edge" creates an adrenalin rush that might ward off depression or feelings of boredom and helplessness, which one may experience due to trauma. An endorphin, a stress-triggered opiate in the brain, acts like a natural painkiller similar to morphine.

Repeating the trauma may create an oddly comfortable feeling of familiarity, predictability, and control; it does not generally resolve the original trauma, however. Some literature indicates that repeating the trauma may even help one to continue to avoid dealing with the original trauma (Daniels & Scurfield, 1994).

CONCLUSION

Those who serve in the military are much more likely to die by their own hand, be depressed, be homeless, and suffer from posttraumatic stress than civilians are. Those with PTSD are more likely to have children with behavioral problems. Emotional problems in veterans may present themselves upon their returning home. A recent combat veteran of Iraq said there is "a defining moment for any soldier, but once you cross that point and stop fearing death, how do you change back to a normal person? Once you get home, you don't want to give up that courage about death. You're back, and you're still fighting a war" (Buck, 2009). It is also the rage, the hatred, and the intensity of combat that are often brought home by soldiers, who are in one reality but still feeling that they are in another. Jason Haines, after returning from serving in Iraq, told a reporter, "I'm not afraid of going to war, I'm afraid of coming back home" (Somma, 2009).

The impact of being at war is long lasting and, for many, severe. Of course, one does not see these facts on any military recruitment poster or television commercial. As with cigarettes, there should be a warning included in these advertisements: ***The military can be hazardous to your health.*** Although there may not be any good reason for smoking, there can be justifications for war and for joining the service. Still, in too many instances, war has scarred people's lives across generations and will continue to do so.

REFERENCES

Appel, J.W., and Beebe, G. (1946, August 31). Preventive psychiatry: An epidemiologic approach. *Journal of the American Medical Association, 131*(18), 1468–1471.

Begany, T. (2006, October). The neuropsychological and mental health fallout of disasters. *NeuroPsychiatry Reviews, 7*(10). Retrieved June 12, 2011, from http://www.neuropsychiatryreviews.com/oct06/disasters.html

Bradley, M. (2009). A civilian's primer on understanding the combat veteran's experience. *Basic Understanding of the Veteran Experience.* Retrieved May 28, 2011, from http://www.omnibuswellness.org/documents/danville/CivilianPrimer-CombatVeteransExperience.doc

Bremner, J.D. (2002). *Does Stress Damage the Brain? Understanding Trauma-Related Disorders from a Mind-Body Perspective.* New York: W.W. Norton & Company.

Broyles, W. Jr. (1984, November). Why men love war. *Esquire,* S5–55.

Buck, R. (2009, February 22). New breed of counselors deals with veterans' PTSD. *Hartford Courant.* Retrieved June 12, 2011, from http://www.courant.com/news/health/hc-ptsd.artfeb22,0,295771,print.story

Caputo, P. (1977). *A Rumor of War.* New York: Holt, Rinehart & Winston.

Cozza, S.J., Benedek, D.M., Bradley, J.C., Grieger, T.A., Nam, T.S., and Waldrep, D.A. (2004). Topics specific to the psychiatric treatment of military personnel. In *Iraq War Clinician Guide* (2nd ed., pp. 4–20). White River Station, VT: National Center for Post-Traumatic Stress Disorder, Department of Veterans Affairs.

Cunningham, M., Henry M., and Lyons, W. (2007). *Vital Mission: Ending Homelessness Among Veterans.* Washington DC: Homelessness Research Institute. Retrieved June 12, 2011, from www.endhomelessness.org/files/1839_file_Vital_Mission_Final.pdf

Daniels, L.R.; and Scurfield, R.M. (1994). War-related post-traumatic stress disorder: Chemical addictions and nonchemical habituating behaviors. In M.B. Williams and J.F. Sommer (Eds.), *Handbook of Post-Traumatic Therapy* (pp. 205–220). Westport, CT: Greenwood Press.

DeBrosse, J., and Srivastava, M. (2010). For some, battle goes on long after the shooting stops. *Dayton Daily News.* http://www.daytondailynews.com/project/suicide/daily/1010suicide.html

Dyer, G. (2004). *War: The Lethal Custom.* New York: Carroll & Graf.

Epstein, S. (1991). The Self-Concept, the Traumatic Neurosis, and the Structure of Personality. In D. Ozer, J. M. Healy, Jr., and R. A. J. Stewart (Eds.), *Perspective on Personality* (Vol. 3). Greenwich, CT: JAI.

Fuchsman, K. (2008). Traumatized Soldiers. *Journal of Psychohistory, 36*(1), 72–84.

Goulston, M. (2008). *Post-Traumatic Stress Disorder for Dummies.* Hoboken, NJ: Wiley.

Gray, J.G. (1959). *The Warriors.* New York: Harper & Row.

Grossman, D. (1995). *On Killing: The Psychological Cost of Learning to Kill in War and in Society.* Boston, MA: Back Bay.

Herman, J.L. (1992). *Trauma and Recovery.* New York: Basic Books.

Jacobs, S. (1999). *Traumatic Grief: Diagnosis, Treatment, and Prevention.* New York: Brunner/Mazel.

Janoff-Bulman, R. (1992). *Shattered Assumptions: Towards a New Psychology of Trauma.* New York: Free Press.

Kall, R. (2010, April 9). Rob Kall Speaks to Veteran of "Collateral Murder" Company WikiLeaks Reported. *OpEdNews.* pp. 1–2. Retrieved April 9, 2011, from http://www. opednews.com/Podcast/Member-of-Same-Bravo-Compa-by-Rob-Kall-100409-149.html

Keegan, J. (1993). *A History of Warfare.* New York: Vintage Books.

Killgore, W.D.S., Cotting, D.I., Thomas, J.L., Cox, A.L., McGurk, D., Vo, A.H., Castro. C.A., and Hoge, C.W. (2008, October). Post-combat invincibility: Violent combat experiences are associated with increased risk-taking propensity following deployment. *Journal of Psychiatric Research, 42*(13), 1112–1121.

Kulka, R.A., Schlenger, W.E., Fairbank, J.A., Hough, R.L., and et al. (1990). *Trauma and the Vietnam War Generation: Report of Findings from the National Vietnam Veterans Readjustment Study.* New York: Brunner/Mazel.

Laufer, R.S., Frey-Wouters, E., and Gallops, M.S., (1985). Traumatic stressors in the Vietnam war and post-traumatic stress disorder. In C. Figley (Ed.), *Trauma and Its Wake.* New York: Brunner/Mazel.

Laufer, R.S., Gallops, M.S., and Frey-Wouters, E. (1984). War stress and post-war trauma. *Journal of Health and Social Behavior, 25*, 65–85.

Lee, K.A., Vaillant, G., Torrey, W.; and Elder, G. (1995, April 4). A 50-year prospective study of the psychological sequelae of World War II combat. *American Journal of Psychiatry, 152*, 516–522.

Levin, A. (2007, December 7). War's impact may not appear until months after return. *Psychiatric News, 42* (23), p. 4.

Lifton, R.J. (1988). Understanding the traumatized self: Imagery, symbolization, and transformation. In J.P. Wilson, Z. Harel, and B. Kahana (Eds.), *Human Adaptation to Extreme Stress.* New York: Plenum Press.

Litz, B., and Orsillo, S.M. (2004). The returning veteran of the Iraq War: background issues and assessment guidelines. In *Iraq War Clinician Guide* (2nd ed.). White River Station, VT: National Center for Post-Traumatic Stress Disorder.

MacNair, R.M. (2002). Perpetration-inducted traumatic stress in combat veterans. *Peace and Conflict: Journal of Peace Psychology, 8,* 63–72.

Maguen, S., Lucenko, B.A., Reger, M.A., Gahm, G.A., Litz, B.T., Seal, K.H., Knight, S.J., and Marmar, C.R. (2010). The impact of reported direct and indirect killing on mental health symptoms in Iraq War veterans. *Journal of Traumatic Stress, 23*(1), 86–90.

Matsakis, A. (2007). *Back from the Front: Combat Trauma, Love, and the Family.* Baltimore, MD: Sidran Institute Press.

Mental Health Advisory Team (MHAT) IV, (2006).

Milliken, C.S., Auchterlonie J.L., and Hoge C.W. (2007, November). Longitudinal assessment of mental health problems among active and reserve component soldiers returning from the Iraq war, *Journal of the American Medical Association, 298*(18), pp. 2141–2148.

Mundell, E.J. (2007, October 30). Younger veterans at greater suicide risk. *The Washington Post.* Retrieved June 12, 2011, from http://www.washingtonpost.com/wpdyn/content/article/2007/10/30/AR2007103001317pf.html

Nash, W.P. (2007) Combat/Operational Stress Adaptations and Injuries. In C. R. Figley & W. P. Nash (Eds.), *Combat Stress Injury: Theory, Research, and Management* (pp. 33–63). New York: Routledge.

Operation Iraqi Freedom 05-07 Final Report (pp. 21–23). Washington D.C.: Office of the Surgeon, Multinational Force-Iraq, and Office of the Surgeon General, United States Army Medical Command.

Reeves, R.R., Parker, J.D., & Konkle-Parker, D.J. (2005). War-related mental health problems of today's veterans: New clinical awareness. *Journal of Psychosocial Nursing and Mental Health Services, 43* (7), 18–28.

Scurfield, R.M (1994). War-related trauma: An integrative experiential cognitive and spiritual approach. In M.B. Williams and J.F. Sommer (Eds.), *Handbook of Post-Traumatic Therapy.* Westport, CT: Greenwood Press.

Scurfield, R.M. (2006). *War Trauma: Lessons unlearned from Vietnam to Iraq.* New York: Algora Publishing.

Shay, J. (1994). *Achilles in Vietnam: Combat trauma and the undoing of character.* New York: Simon and Schuster.

Solomon, Z. (2008). Combat stress reaction. In G. Reyes, J.D. Elhai, and J.D. Ford (Eds.), *The Encyclopedia of Psychological Trauma* (pp. 24–25). Hoboken, NJ: Wiley.

Somma, A.M. (2009, February 22). Lawmaker: Courts should take veterans' problems into account. *Hartford Courant.* Retrieved June 12, 2011, from groups. yahoo.com/group/davonline/message/11733.

Stroebe, M.S., Hansson, R.O., Stroebe, W., and Schut, H. (2001). Introduction: Concepts and issues in contemporary research on bereavement. In M.S. Stroebe, R.O. Hansson, W. Stoebe, and H. Schut (Eds.), *Handbook of Bereavement Research: Consequences, Coping, and Care.* Washington, DC: American Psychological Association.

Vasterling, J.J., Proctor, S.P., Amoroso, P., Kane, R., Gackstetter, G., Ryan, M.A., and et al. (2006). The Neurocognition Deployment Health Study: A prospective cohort study of army soldiers. *Military Medicine, 171,* 253–260.

Wain, H., Grammer, G.G., Stasinos, J., and DeBoer, C.M. (2006). Psychiatric intervention for medical and surgical patients following traumatic injuries. In E. Ritchie, M. Friedman, and P. Watson (Eds.), *Interventions Following Mass Violence and Disasters: Strategies for Mental Health Practice* (pp. 278–299). New York: Guilford Press.

Young, R.S.K., Gillan, E., Dingmann, P., Casinalli, P., and Taylor, C. (2008, January). Army health care operations in Iraq. *Connecticut Medicine, 72*(1), 13–17.

Chapter 2

BLAST-WAVE INJURIES AND TBI: EPIDEMIOLOGY, PATHOPHYSIOLOGY AND SYMPTOMATOLOGY

Jamshid A. Marvasti and Ali Alim-Marvasti

INTRODUCTION

The element of TBI in warfare has been well-documented throughout history, even as far back as the biblical story of Adam and Eve. Cain, motivated by sibling jealousy, purportedly delivered the blow that caused a fatal temporal lobe herniation in his brother Abel. Evidence of mild TBIs is documented in the writings of ancient Greece and Rome, as well as in the records of the American Revolution and Civil War. In fact, although not always recognized or diagnosed, post-concussive symptoms and their consequences have been noted in veterans of virtually all battles in recorded history (Cifu & Caruso, 2010).

Blast-wave injuries are the result of high-order explosives (HE) and can result, directly or indirectly, in TBI. In the current wars in the Middle East, the majority of blast-wave injuries are caused by improvised explosive devices (IEDs), vehicle-borne explosive devices (VBEDs), and rocket-propelled grenades (RPGs). U.S. veterans of the wars in the Middle East seem to have sustained and survived far greater injuries in terms of severity and number of wounds than seen in previous wars. In the Vietnam War, two soldiers were killed for every five wounded; in the Iraq War, this rate improved to one soldier killed for every sixteen wounded. Due to improvements in military vehicles, protective body armor, rapid evacuation of the wounded, advanced technological and medical devices and clinical care, the survival rate in the Iraq War was almost 90 percent (Lew et al., 2007).

Despite these improvements, TBI remains "the silent affliction," because its symptoms may take hours, days, weeks, or longer to manifest. This makes TBI more relevant as the survival rate increases in war veterans. The acuteness of the battlefield and coexistence of polytraumatic injuries prevent accurate and detailed evaluation of a soldier's neurological condition, especially in mild TBI (Sayer et al., 2009). A mild head injury may be neglected for years; its symptoms often unnoticed or mistaken for PTSD. Concussion is thought to result from the biochemical and physiological changes in neurons that arise as a result of TBI; sometimes resulting in loss of consciousness at the moment of trauma. Soldiers may be completely unconscious or remain awake but dazed and confused. The majority of these soldiers recover within seconds to minutes; they may have retrograde and/or anterograde amnesia surrounding the event, however (Dziedzic, 2008).

EPIDEMIOLOGY OF COMBAT TBI

TBI is an invisible wound that may leave a variety of neurological and psychiatric symptoms. Even mild TBI is troubling. Reports reveal that about 29,000 military personnel sustained TBIs in 2009, most of them classified as "mild." The majority of these resulted from combat injury and motor vehicle accidents (Levin, 2010). Previously, health officials from the military reported that as many as 360,000 returning troops had experienced at least transitory effects of blasts from roadside bombs or other explosive devices. The 360,000 is approximately 20 percent of all troops; half of those cases resolved by the time the troops returned to their homeland, however (Levin, 2009).

Approximately 28 percent of all field medical evacuations are due to TBI (Warden, 2006). During the Vietnam conflict, 24 percent of the troops hospitalized required medical care for head injuries. Some researchers believe the actual incidence of TBI in soldiers to be higher, because those with less severe injuries might not have sought help, or if they did seek help, TBI may not have been diagnosed. Additionally, if a diagnosis was made, the soldiers might have refused medical care or refused to be treated in a hospital, seeking treatment on an outpatient basis instead and thus being omitted from the study.

A difficulty in detecting mild TBI is that the signs and symptoms may be so subtle that they do not interfere in a soldier's performance to the level that would prompt him or her to seek help. Sometimes, the soldier may not even recall the traumatic event itself. If these subtle symptoms are left untreated, the individual may encounter further problems. Sometimes mild TBI presents very similarly to PTSD, with overlapping symptoms. There are also indications that PTSD may exacerbate the effects of other disorders, such as concussion (Hoge et al., 2008; Hopewell & Christopher, 2007).

A recent Rand report suggested a 19 percent rate of TBI in a survey of almost 2000 previously deployed service members (Tanielian & Jaycox, 2008). The rate of brain injury in the Vietnam War was 12 to 14 percent (Okie, 2005), which indicates that the present war may have a higher rate of TBI (McAllister, 2009).

Hoge and colleagues (2008) surveyed 2525 U.S. Army infantry soldiers who had been in Iraq for at least one year. Ninety-five percent were men, interviewed three to four months after their return from Iraq. About 5 percent reported injuries with loss of consciousness lasting from a few seconds to three minutes. Among them, 43.9 percent met the criteria for PTSD, a rate that is much higher than that among soldiers who reported concussion but remained conscious. Furthermore, soldiers who lost consciousness were significantly more likely to report poor general health, absenteeism from work, and higher numbers of visits to their doctors in the prior month than soldiers who did not lose consciousness. These authors hypothesized that loss of consciousness on the battleground may indicate a highly traumatic event–for example, a close call on one's life–that can lead to PTSD and depression. These mental disorders may then lead to a higher prevalence of physical health problems due to neuroendocrine dysregulation and autonomic central nervous system reactivity (Hoge et al., 2008).

COMBAT INJURIES AND TBI

Although helmets are designed to protect against sharp blast injury to the skull and brain, diffuse axonal injury (DAI) may still occur. It is the rapid acceleration/deceleration injury, especially rotary movements of the head due to explosions or motor vehicle accidents, which cause shearing and DAI. Approximately half of TBI victims who suffer a loss of consciousness will develop DAI. Likewise, armor may prevent a bullet from penetrating the body, but U.S. soldiers are seldom shot at. Instead, the majority of injuries and fatalities in the Iraq and Afghan Wars are sustained as a result of explosives (Scott et al., 2006).

The primary motor, somatosensory, and visual cortices are seldom damaged from contusion; however, the medial orbital frontal lobe and the anterior temporal lobe are much more vulnerable. This indicates that the areas of the brain that are concerned with social function and decision-making are more likely to be affected in TBI, and therefore, the neuropsychiatric sequelae surpass neurophysical side effects as the major cause of disability after TBI (Fleminger, 2010).

BLAST INJURY, TBI AND CONTUSION

Clinical literature indicates four components to the early phases of blast-wave trauma, categorized as primary, secondary, tertiary, and quaternary:

1. **Primary blast injury** refers to the initial shock wave that passes through the body. The effect of this injury on the brain is variable; it is a common cause of perforated tympanic membrane, however (Cifu & Caruso, 2010).

2. **Secondary blast injury** is injury due to fragments or other objects that are propelled and may cause a blunt closed head injury or penetrating brain injury. Thus, in addition to the pressure of the primary wave, blast victims may also be hit by shrapnel and other objects and debris propelled by the explosion (Levin, 2010).

3. **Tertiary blast injury** is a feature of a high-energy explosion in which the victim may be lifted off the ground and strike stationary objects such as vehicles or sides of buildings (Taber, Warden & Hurley, 2006). This may cause brain injuries that result in diffuse axonal damage, including focal axonal swelling. If swelling persists for several hours, it may cause axonal disconnection. The most common regions of the brain damaged in this type of injury are the corticomedullary junction, frontal and temporal lobe areas, internal capsule, deep gray matter, midbrain, and corpus callosum. A mismatch between demand for ATP, and oxygen extraction by the brain, may lead to metabolic and neurotransmitter dysfunction. This may lead to a cascade of events such as release of excitatory neurotransmitters, massive efflux of potassium, axonal swelling, and eventual axotomy (Moore, Hopewell & Grossman, 2009).

4. **Quaternary blast injury** encompasses the additional miscellany of injuries that may result from the explosion, including burns, respiratory injuries, and such crushing injuries as hypoxic or ischemic brain injury. In many incidents, there may be fire and inhalation of hot gases. Evidence from animal studies indicates that ionized gases that are propelled by an explosion may cause an electromagnetic pulse that disrupts calcium channels in brain parenchyma. These studies provide a model of the pathophysiology of concussion; however, it is not yet known how these findings can be applied to human beings (Halstead et al., 2010).

In animal studies, concussion shows an initial disruption of the neuronal membrane, resulting in the efflux of potassium to the extra-cellular space. This may cause a release of the excitatory amino acid, glutamine. Glutamine may then contribute to more loss of potassium, and eventually result in cell depolarization and suppression of neuronal activity. This cascade of consequences continues, eventually leading to the accumulation of lactate and reduction of cerebral blood flow. Large quantities of calcium collect in the cells, resulting eventually in the cell death. The concussed area of the brain converts to a hypo-metabolic state that may continue for up to four weeks following injury (Halstead, Walter & The Council on Sports Medicine and Fitness, 2010).

Warden (2006) and Okie (2005) have reported that penetrating injuries are the cause of blast-related TBI (penetrating secondary blast-wave trauma); they are outnumbered by closed brain injuries, however. The frequent cause of closed brain injuries is a pressure wave that develops due to exploding munitions.

PATHOPHYSIOLOGY OF TBI

The brain is made of soft tissue cushioned by cerebrospinal fluid and encased in the protective shell of the skull. When an individual sustains trauma, the impact can jar the brain, sometimes causing it to ricochet within the skull. Traumatic brain injuries can cause skull fractures, cerebral contusion, hemorrhage, and injury to the nerves.

TBI may be characterized as an acceleration/deceleration injury, in which the brain may slam into the skull in acceleration phase (coup) and then "bounce" off the opposite side in deceleration (contrecoup). It may also rotate inside the skull, causing further damage to the brain (Hitti, 2008). It is believed that altered consciousness in concussion is due to functional disruption of the reticular activating system, either by rotational force on the midbrain or cerebral perfusion changes as a result of the injury. In cerebral contusion, blood leaks into the extravascular space. Contusion may result in death of the cells and local loss of tissue (Elder et al., 2010).

Diffuse Axonal Injury

Rapid acceleration/deceleration movements of the head (especially with an angular-rotary component) cause stretching and shearing of axons due to inertia that may result in DAI. DAI is a common type of TBI that affects white matter and may be followed by generalized atrophy with ventricular enlargement. This change may take a few weeks or months to develop. DAI in the brainstem is usually responsible for the slurred speech and ataxia that are seen in some patients who are disabled after TBI.

DAI, however, does not always accompany concussion. In DAI, axons swell, and there may be tiny hemorrhages around the deep white matter. DAI is common in the corpus callosum (linking the right and left cerebral hemispheres) and the hippocampus. Brain function depends on axons or nerve fibers that may become edematous with TBI and DAI. For reasons yet unknown, dysfunction of these axons can be delayed and continue for decades following the TBI event, which may explain the lag that sometimes occurs between a TBI and symptom manifestation (Wartenberg and Mayer, 2007; French et al., 2011; Cifu and Caruso, 2010)).

Research suggests that in mild TBI there may be a lack of structural integrity in the axons of the corpus callosum. This change may result in reduced functional anisotropy (possibly due to misalignment or disruption of fibers, edema, or axonal degeneration). Following the trauma, there may be a cascade of cellular and vascular changes in the brain. This neurobiology involves ionic shifts, abnormal energy metabolism, decreased cerebral blood flow, and impaired neurotransmission. The majority of affected cells may have the capacity to repair themselves through a reversible series of metabolic events (Iverson et al., 2007; Zink et al., 2010). The ultimate outcome of brain cells depends on the extent of traumatic axonal injury, which can culminate in secondary axotomy. Not all injured cells, however, undergo secondary axotomy, and many may recover to a normal cellular function. In most cases of mild TBI, the brain is able to undergo dynamic restoration, and the person may return to normal functioning (French et al., 2011).

CLASSIFICATION OF TBI

TBI can be classified as primary or secondary as explained in clinical literature. Primary damage in TBI results from the initial injury. Its effects are immediate and include (a) contusion, (b) vascular injury, (c) hemorrhaging, and (d) axonal shearing (stretching and tearing of axons). Secondary injury is the indirect result of primary injury from endogenous evolution of cellular damage or from secondary systemic processes, such as hypotension or hypoxia. Endogenous secondary pathophysiology includes (a) ischemia, excitotoxicity, energy failure, and cell death cascades (e.g. necrosis and apoptosis); (b) edema; (c) traumatic axonal injury; and (d) inflammation (Kochanek, Clark & Jenkins, 2007). Magnetic resonance imaging (MRI) can sometimes identify abnormalities in brain tissue or outside the brain (i.e.

extra-axial space). This kind of injury may include, but is not limited to, hemorrhagic contusions, nonhemorrhagic contusions, hemorrhagic or nonhemorrhagic shearing injuries, herniations, and cerebral edema. Extra-axial manifestations include epidural hematomas, subdural hema- tomas, subarachnoid hemorrhaging, intraventricular hemorrhaging, and hydrocephalus (Barkley et al., 2007).

CUMULATIVE MILD TBI AND DEVELOPMENT OF DEMENTIA

It is well-documented that brain damage in TBI is cumulative, meaning that each incident leaves the veteran with more vulnerability to injury after subsequent blasts (Levin, 2010). Because the signs and symptoms of TBI may not be apparent immediately, soldiers with TBI are often exposed to multiple head trauma. There has been much attention given to concussion in sports, and strict guidelines have been developed concerning when an athlete can return to play. Despite this evidence, soldiers with mild TBI are often sent back into combat. One retired Marine estimates that he was involved in fifty to sixty explosions while part of an ordinance disposal unit. He explains, "My brain has been rattled" (Neergaard, 2009).

The Defense and Veterans Brain Injury Center (DVBIC, 2006) documents that, with numerous deployments and the nature of urban combat, veterans are at risk of sustaining more than one mild TBI or concussion in a short time frame. Multiple concussions (i.e. three or more) over the course of one's life may cause the potential for traumatic encephalopathy (Cifu & Caruso, 2010). Clinical literature indicates this disorder is progressive and may result in functional difficulty and even early death. It is caused by a combination of DAI and physiological changes in axons. Clinical features of this syndrome range from mild cognitive and memory impairment to severe dementia.

TBI patients may exhibit symptoms of dementia later in life, which may be very similar to the deterioration seen in Alzheimer's patients (Smith, 2010). The method of trauma and severity of the TBI is a factor in the degree of memory loss and the likelihood that the victim will be vulnerable to Alzheimer's disease. Although literature reveals that a number of individuals with TBI will experience some degree of progressive axonal damage, it is difficult to predict who will develop cognitive changes years later.

As clinical literature indicates, the synaptic strengths and connectivity of the remaining healthy axons may overcompensate for the losses sustained in TBI. The healthy axons increase the strength of their electrical communication and try to restore the normal speed of information processing. However,

this is usually a temporary phenomenon and may cause even more sensitivity to a second central nervous system trauma (Smith, 2010). Currently there
are no remedies for either short- or long-term damages. Along with increased susceptibility to further damage, it has been argued that soldiers who
sustain a TBI should not be sent back to combat (Smith, 2010).

SIGNS AND SYMPTOMS OF MILD TBI

Signs and symptoms of TBI may be categorized for our purposes into psychological and nonpsychological symptoms, with some overlap between the
two. Symptoms may depend on the severity and the location of the brain
damage. For example, frontal lobe damage may cause disinhibition, reduce
executive functioning, and affect areas that modulate fear, arousal, and emotion (Donavon-Westby & Ferraro, 1999). Damage to the hypothalamus is associated with intermittent explosive disorder (Tonkonogy & Geller, 1992). In
contrast, most mild traumatic brain injuries leading to concussions contribute
to a minute but generalized damage at the cellular level (axonal shearing,
physiological changes) that may subsequently become manifest as the long-
term neuropsychiatric symptoms of TBI (Taber et al., 2006).

An unnoticed mild TBI can present with non-specific physical symptoms
such as headache, sleep disorder, and fatigue. In more severe brain injury,
however, there are additional neurological and psychiatric symptoms (e.g.
paralysis, speech deficit, visual or hearing deficits) (Callaway, 2008). Severe
brain injury gives a typical clinical picture, including significant cognitive
impairment, especially in domains of attention, concentration, psychomotor
speed, memory, and executive function. The patient may also experience
fatigue and problems with motivation. TBI may result in skull fractures and
parenchymal or vascular injury. Parenchymal injury may cause concussion,
loss of or decreased consciousness, seizures, focal neurological deficit, nausea, vomiting, and amnesia of events surrounding the TBI (McAllister, 2010;
Riggio, 2010).

Signs and Symptoms of TBI in Three Categories

Psychological Symptoms
Confusion or a feeling of being dazed
Avolition or sluggishness
Fatigue
Insomnia or sleep disorder
Anxiety
Depression
PTSD or acute stress disorder
Nonpsychological Symptoms
Nausea and/or vomiting
Ataxia or clumsiness
Dizziness or loss of balance
Tinnitus
Photophobia or excessive sensitivity to light/noise
Blurred vision
Dysarthria or slurred speech
Seizures
Mixed Category Symptoms
Impaired attention/concentration
Behavioral or personality changes
Amnesia
Headache

Headache may be the most frequent complaint, and one needs to differentiate other causes of headache from TBI.

Agitation and Restless Behavior in Mild TBI

Excessive psychomotor activity, poor impulse control, irritability, and, in some cases, frank aggression may be seen in mild TBI. Initially, the victim may have some subtle behavioral problems such as irritability, decreased interpersonal communication skills, and inability to postpone gratification (Cifu & Caruso, 2010).

The etiology of this behavior is connected to damage in focal subcortical (limbic) and cortical (frontal and temporal lobe) structures. It is most commonly related to the frontal lobe, which is responsible for controlling behavior (Mysiw & Sandel, 1997). Temporal lobe epilepsy may present with increased agitation, dissociation, and restlessness. With regard to the differential diagnoses, one must consider that the agitation and restless behavior of TBI is also present in delirium, manic states, substance abuse, benzodiazepine withdrawal, seizures, hyperthyroidism, and side effects of psychiatric medications (Mysiw & Sandel, 1997).

Irritability and aggression are probably the most common behavioral consequences of TBI; however, at times it is difficult to diagnose or connect it to TBI if the patient has had this behavior before the trauma. Aggression on the part of the brain-injured patient is usually impulsive and quite out of proportion to the trigger and does not usually include cold, goal-directed aggression. When aggression due to TBI is severe, it may be described as episodic dyscontrol syndrome (EDS) (Fleminger, 2010). In these cases, prognosis for complete recovery is good during the acute period but decreases after eight weeks of dysfunction (Cifu & Caruso, 2010).

Attention Deficit Disorder (ADD) in Mild TBI

Attention deficit disorder (ADD) may become a permanent characteristic of mild TBI, symptoms of which include distractibility and difficulty concentrating. In clinical expression, the patient may show a slow reaction time but is accurate in his or her response; in more complex tasks (especially with competing stimuli), however one may see a detectable impairment that was not evident in simple acts. Tasks that were previously automatic, such as reading, typing, or riding a bicycle, may require rigorous concentration after a TBI.

For a definitive diagnosis, tests that require higher complexity are needed for the purpose of detecting the attention deficit in mild TBI. Most soldiers with TBI-induced ADD will show improvements within the first twelve to eighteen months (Cifu & Caruso, 2010).

Cognitive Deficits in Mild TBI

As medical literature indicates, these deficits include attention and concentration problems and impairment in learning, memory, and executive function. Executive function refers to cognitive control or cognitive process that guides the behavior of human beings. Memory disorder refers to deficits in encoding, consolidation, and retrieval. The term posttraumatic amnesia (PTA) refers to the time between the injury and the return of continuous, day-to-day memories. If PTA lasts less than one week, it indicates a good outcome; however, if it lasts longer than one month it may predict significant disability (Cifu & Caruso, 2010; McAllister, 2010).

The cause of cognitive dysfunction in TBI is primarily due to cortical lesions. In mild TBI, there may be spontaneous recovery of cognitive function; this is in contrast to moderate to severe TBI. Sometimes depression may mimic symptoms and signs of cognitive deficit (Cifu & Caruso, 2010).

Disinhibition in Mild TBI

Disinhibition may be present in mild TBI and is indicated by a decreased capacity to edit or manage impulsive responses as a result of damage to the frontal lobe. Clinical features of disinhibition are lack of control in motor, emotional, cognitive, instinctual, and perceptual aspects. For example, hypersexuality, hyperarousal, and aggressive explosive behavior are referred to as instinctual drives. This needs to be differentiated from acute intoxication, temporal lobe epilepsy, delirium, and mania.

With regard to prognosis, disinhibition is frequently seen early after moderate and severe TBI and usually improves within three to six months following the injury. If symptoms still persist after six months, however, medication and behavioral control strategies are indicated, because there is usually no spontaneous improvement (Cifu & Caruso, 2010; Kim, 2002).

Executive Function Disorder in TBI

Executive functioning is the ability to respond in an adaptive way to different situations. It requires cognition, comprehension, and sound judgment, all three of which may be disturbed by TBI. A component of executive functioning is response inhibition, or a capacity to inhibit an impulsive response that interferes with completing a task (Cifu & Caruso, 2010). The etiology of this impairment is generally an injury to the prefrontal cortex. Generally, abstract thinking, planning, and working memory are the tasks of the dorsal lateral prefrontal cortex. Motivation and attention processes are mediated by the medial prefrontal cortex. Damage to the orbital frontal cortex may cause disinhibition, emotional lability, and lack of sensitivity to the needs of other people (Levine, Robertson, Clare & Carter, 2000). Clinical features may become especially evident when the victim is involved with an unfamiliar situation. The individual may have difficulty with tasks that need divided or alternating attention, or experience difficulty recognizing and assessing others' reactions. Superficially, these patients may appear to be highly functioning individuals; however, they have difficulty in social and vocational aspects of life. They may have mutable job loss and marital problems. Other clinical features are apathy or abulia, disinhibition, emotional lability, avolition, and decrease in social activity.

If executive function disorder worsens following TBI, it may indicate an acute process such as edema of the brain or seizure disorder. In addition, one also needs to consider other disorders not connected to brain injury, such as behavioral and medication problems, severe pain, and, in civilian cases, litigation and secondary gain. (Cifu & Caruso, 2010; Levine et al., 2000). A study by Campbell and coworkers (2009) indicates that performance on neuropsychological measures of executive functioning and speed of verbal processing are altered in people with PTSD, TBI, and coexistent TBI and PTSD. Executive functions include

• Setting goals and priority; decision making
• Assessing strengths and weaknesses in self; judgment
• Planning and/or conducting activity
• Initiating activities and/or inhibiting behavior
• Measuring and checking performance or activity
• Evaluating results of performance
• Abstract thinking; social cognition
• Motivational processes; regulation of attention

(Cifu & Caruso, 2010; Riggio, 2010; Silver et al., 2002).

Emotional Lability in TBI

Emotional lability in TBI is indicated when individuals display a pathological and fluctuating intensity of emotion that is not harmonious or congruous with their actual mood. This condition is seen in at least 5 percent of patients with TBI. Although the etiology is unknown, there is an indication of widespread cerebral pathology including the corticobulbar tracts (Cifu & Caruso, 2010; McAllister, 2010).

Clinical features of emotional lability are an elevated readiness to laugh or cry. This excessive laughing or crying is not connected to feelings of happiness or sadness, and the patient has no control over the extent or duration of this response. Crying is more frequent than is laughter, and symptoms may be provoked by triggers. Emotional lability may be very mild, although it can sometimes cause social problems. Individuals are generally well-aware of this effect, but they feel that they may not be able to control these emotional impulses (Cifu and Caruso, 2010).

When differentiating diagnoses, one should consider that this symptom may also be present in cerebral vascular accidents, multiple sclerosis, motor neuron disease, epilepsy, dementia, chronic alcohol abuse, Park- inson's disease, and depression. If symptoms worsen, it may indicate the presence of the comorbidity of another disorder, such as depression. The prognosis in cases of emotional lability is generally good, although the severity of the injury is a contributing factor. Also, the presence of little or slow recovery by six months may indicate poor prognosis (Rao & Lyketsos, 2000).

THE PSYCHIATRIC SEQUELAE OF TBI

Bryant and colleagues (2010) investigated the extent of psychiatric disorders that develop post TBI. They evaluated more than 1000 traumatically injured patients, and then reevaluated them twelve months after the injury. Their findings revealed that 30 percent of the patients reported symptoms of a psychiatric disorder, and 22 percent were diagnosed with a new-onset psychiatric disorder that they had never experienced before. The most common new psychiatric illnesses were depression (9%), generalized anxiety disorder (9%), PTSD (6%), and agoraphobia (6%). They were able to conclude that a significant range of psychiatric symptoms and illnesses develop after traumatic injury and require identification and treatment by a clinician (Bryant and colleagues, 2010; Silver et al., 2002). Sometimes undiagnosed medical problems (e.g. a closed head injury) present themselves through emotional symptoms. By their nature, closed head injuries are difficult to diagnose without knowledge of the incident; however, such injuries have been found to have lasting effects, such as high anxiety, mood swings, and subsequent development of depression or PTSD.

As reported by Dr. Sunil Sabharwal (cited in Callaway, 2008), the lingering symptoms in mild TBI can be emotional, such as episodes of rage, explosiveness, impulsivity, and unpredictability. Many of the veterans who suffered TBI may demonstrate behavior that is impulsive and not premeditated. Thus, operant conditioning is of little benefit in such cases, and any kind of punishment or negative consequence or instruction may be unhelpful because most of the aggressive actions are impulsive and without premeditation (Callaway, 2008).

Personality Change in TBI

DSM-IV-TR (2000) diagnostic criteria for personality change due to traumatic brain injury

A. A persistent personality disturbance that represents a change from the individual's previous characteristic personality pattern. (In children, the disturbance involves a marked deviation from the normal development or a significant change in the child's usual behavior patterns lasting at least 1 year).
B. Evidence from the history, physical examination, or laboratory findings that the disturbance is the direct physiological consequence of a general medical condition.
C. The disturbance is not better accounted for by another mental disorder (including other mental disorders due to a general medical condition).
D. The disturbance does not occur exclusively during the course of a delirium and does not meet criteria for a dementia.
E. The disturbance causes clinically significant distress or impairment in social, occupational, or other important areas of functioning.

Specify type:
Labile type: if the predominant feature is affective lability.
Disinhibited type: if the predominant feature is poor impulse control as evidenced by sexual indiscretions, etc.
Aggressive type: if the predominant feature is aggressive behavior.
Apathetic type: if the predominant feature is marked apathy and indifference.
Paranoid type: if the predominant feature is suspiciousness or paranoid ideation.
Other type: if the predominant feature is not one of the above, e.g., personality change associated with a seizure disorder.
Combined type: if more than one feature predominates in the clinical picture.
Unspecified type

(Adapted from Silver et al., 2002)

As medical literature indicates, prominent behavioral patterns such as disorderliness, suspicion, argumentativeness, disruptiveness, anxiety, and tendency to isolate are more pronounced after brain injury. Because the prefrontal and frontal regions of the brain are very vulnerable to contusion, the injuries in this area are common and more likely to give rise to change in personality. This is referred to as "frontal lobe syndrome." Psychological disturbances associated with frontal lobe syndrome are labile affect, decreased attention to personal appearance and hygiene, boisterousness, increased risk-taking, and impaired judgment. Impaired judgment may include uncharacteristic lewdness, inability to appreciate the effect of one's behavior or remarks on others, loss of social graces (such as eating manners), unrestrained drinking of alcohol, indiscriminate selection of food, and decrease in concern for the future. These individuals appear shallow, indifferent, or apathetic. Because they exhibit a lack of concern for the consequences of their behavior, they may not respond to punishment. Additionally, impulsivity may cause them to act without thinking (Silver et al., 2002).

Orbital frontal syndrome, which is the result of damage to the orbital frontal section of the brain, is associated with behavioral excesses, such as impulsivity, disinhibition, distractibility, hyperactivity, and labile mood. Injury to the dorsolateral frontal cortex may result in slowness, apathy, and perseveration. Damage to the inferior orbital surface of the frontal lobe and anterior temporal lobes may cause outbursts of rage and violent behavior (Silver et al., 2002). In severe TBI, the patient is likely to be self-centered, thoughtless, and crude in social milieu and may present disinhibited behavior and inappropriate sexual gesture, agitation, and repetitive purposeless behavior with a labile mood. These individuals may be described as odd, childish, or moody (Fleminger, 2010).

CONTROVERSIAL DIAGNOSIS OF MILD TBI

An article by Hoge and associates, (2008) in the *New England Journal of Medicine* revealed not only that soldiers who suffered concussion in Iraq are at high risk of developing PTSD and depression, but also that it may be the depression and PTSD, and not the head injuries, that are the cause of ongoing cognitive and physical symptoms. This theory has become very controversial and is the subject of ongoing debate.

It may be surprising to find that symptoms generally associated with TBI and concussion, such as dizziness, headaches, memory problems, irritability, and impulsivity, could actually be related to PTSD and/or depression, rather than the traumatic injury. A number of clinicians report that a great number of the symptoms of TBI and PTSD are similar, and, at times, differentiating between PTSD and postconcussion syndrome may be in the eyes of the beholder. Symptoms such as headache, dizziness, and fatigue could be psychosomatic and related to PTSD and anxiety or depression; however, these could also be due to postconcussion syndrome. Some critics claim that the tendency of military officials is toward diagnosis of PTSD because treatment of TBI is considerably more costly for the Army and may include a lifelong disability payment.

Case History of Sergeant Ryan Kahlor

Sergeant Ryan Kahlor, a veteran with TBI, is worried that the Army may make it more difficult for soldiers to get appropriate medical care because "The military does not want to diagnose people with brain injury." He continued, "So what they will do is play it off as PTSD as the sole injury for everyone, because PTSD and traumatic brain injury have very similar symptoms" (Lee, 2008).

He explained that disability compensation is a lot higher for TBI than for PTSD. "What the military says is, 'you cannot be diagnosed as having a brain injury until you recover from PTSD.' It is kind of a paradox." He says he has documents stating he has signs of TBI, such as retinal detachment, seizures, inner ear expansion, and postconcussion syndrome, which gives him severe headaches. Even so, he has been unable to get an official diagnosis of TBI. He reported that "A doctor in Fort Irving looked at me and glanced at my file for ten minutes, then wrote in my records that he thought my symptoms, my claims, were psychosomatic, that I made them up myself." Kahlor said that this doctor saw him only once, then wanted to send him to med board to get him out of the Army as soon as possible and "palm me off to the VA system" (Lee, 2008).

MULTIDISCIPLINARY MANAGEMENT OF TBI

It is important to emphasize that any treatment and rehabilitation for TBI should be done in a specialized, polytrauma clinic equipped with neuropsychological testing, a neuropsychologist, and neurosurgeon. Specialists in different fields of medicine may be required to treat those who suffer from visual loss, sleep disorders, or headache. Patients may require cognitive therapy (to improve memory and concentration), occupational therapy (for tasks of daily living and job-related tasks), or physical therapy (for psychomotor impairment). Medication may be necessary for behavioral and emotional symptoms such as depression and anxiety. Many patients who have suffered multiorgan trauma are also at risk of developing PTSD, depression, and/or anxiety and may benefit from a resident psychiatrist (Callaway, 2008). Clinicians report that brain injury generally complicates the patient's rehabilitative process, possibly due to cognitive impairment. In this respect, as proposed by Dr. Sunil Sabharwal (cited by Callaway, 2008) evaluation and treatment of TBI should be a priority, because TBI may interfere concurrently with rehabilitation from other injuries. Facilities should have access to computerized tomography (CT) scan, MRI, and position emission tomography (PET) scan.

THE FUTURE OF NEUROREHABILITATION
OF VETERANS WITH TBI

Rehabilitation of veterans with TBI must occur in specialized units that have biotechnology orientation and devices. These therapies include corticostimulation to enhance motor recovery, deep brain stimulation, vagus nerve stimulation, and transcranial magnetic stimulation (Zafonte, 2006). Bioscaffolding techniques have been used for wound healing and offer promise in the area of neurorestoration for TBI patients. There is also some hope that stem cell research will eventually be helpful. The research in technology of creating neuroprosthetics is promising, and there is hope that it will eventually be possible to create injectable microstimulating neuroprosthetics that will enhance motor function in veterans (Zafonte, 2006).

FAMILIES OF VETERANS WITH MILD TBI

The families of veterans with mild TBI need to be educated and involved in therapy and rehabilitation of the veteran. It is imperative to alert them to the fact that the soldier with TBI may forget his or her appointments, may miss the bus, and may not be able to manage routine tasks. These veterans may need written or verbal instruction to carry out daily responsibilities. Education may need to be made simpler, and they may need to carry a notebook and write down assignments or appointments, as well as the names of people they are going to be involved with, because memory problems may be present (Callaway, 2008). Many of those who suffer from mild TBI are easily distracted, cannot concentrate, and have attention span problems. They may benefit from a structured daily routine. It is not unusual that a spouse must keep notes to guide the veteran, including messages on refrigerator doors, such as "Do not give milk to the dog."

CONCLUSION

With regard to prognosis, clinicians report that speed of recovery is variable and individualized. A minority of veterans may have persistent symptoms. Moderate and severe TBI are considered to cause chronic complications, and one should not expect a full recovery to be speedy, even with some of the best treatment and rehabilitation efforts. One must also remember that even a mild TBI can have a major impact on a person's performance, relationships, quality of life, and employability (Callaway, 2008). The outcome of the TBI is varied on the basis of the location of the injury, severity of injury, and also preinjury factors such as medical and psychiatric factors (De Silva et al., 2009).

Most of those patients who were exposed to mild TBI have symptoms in three broad areas: cognition (memory, attention, slowed thinking), somatic problems (headache, fatigue, disequilibrium), and emotional troubles (irritability, anxiety, and dysphoria) (Levin et al., 1987). Most individuals report improvement of these symptoms over several days to weeks after the trauma, and most are free from medical complaints within three to six months (McAllister, 2005). However if the symptoms remain, further evaluation should be done.

Clinical literature indicates that up to 15 percent of patients will have persistent or chronic problems after TBI. The cause of persistent or chronic symptoms in TBI is a controversial issue and has been challenged by different clinicians. One cause may be subtle diffuse axonal injury. Another factor may be development of a psychiatric disorder such as depression or PTSD. Recent research indicates that the presence of depression and PTSD in soldiers who have TBI may count for much of their distress (Hoge, Goldberg & Castro, 2009). In mild TBI, symptoms such as fatigue, tiredness, headache, dizziness, depression, or concentration or memory problems are nonspecific and can be seen in other disorders, such as those with muscular skeletal injury with no head injury, and in patients with chronic pain or chronic fatigue syndrome. In a few patients with long-standing postconcussional symptoms, there may be indication of somatization disorder. It is suggested that when symptoms develop soon after the brain injury, they are secondary to the direct effect of trauma to the head and brain. However, over time, psychological factors may interfere and prevent healthy recovery (Lishman, 1988).

REFERENCES

Barkley, J.M., Morales, D., Hayman, L.A., and Diaz-Marcham, P.J. (2007). Static neuroimaging in the evaluation of TBI. In Zasler, N.D., Katz, D.I., Zafonte, R.D. (Eds.). *Brain injury medicine: Principles and practice.* New York: Demos Medical Publications, pp. 129–148.

Bryant, R.A., O'Donnell, M.L., Creamer, M., McFarlane, A.C., Clark, C.R., and Silove, D. (2010, March). The psychiatric sequelae of traumatic injury. *American Journal of Psychiatry, 167*(3), 312–320.

Callaway, R. (2008, April). Medical consequences of the Iraq War. Part 2: Traumatic brain injury (TBI). *HealthCare Ledger*, 12–15.

Campbell, T.A., Nelson, L.A., Lumpkin, R., Yoash-Gantz, R.E., Pickett, T.C., and McCormick, C.L. (2009, August). Neuropsychological measures of processing speed and executive functioning in combat veterans with PTSD, TBI, and comorbid TBI/PTSD. *Psychiatric Annals Online, 39*(8) 797–803.

Cifu, D.X., and Caruso, D. (2010). *Traumatic Brain Injury.* New York: Demos Medical.

De Silva, M., Roberts, I., Perel, P., Edwards, P., Kenward, M., Fernandes, J., and et al. (2009). Patient outcome after traumatic brain injury in high-, middle- and low-income countries: Analysis of data on 8927 patients in 46 countries. *International Journal of Epidemiology, 38*(2), 452–458.

Donavon-Westby, M.D., and Ferraro, R.F. (1999). Frontal lobe deficits in domestic violence offenders. *Genetic, Social, and General Psychology Monographs, 125*, 75-102.

DVBIC. (2006)/ Defense and veterans brain injury center working group on the acute management of mild traumatic brain injury in military operational settings. *Clinical practice guideline and recommendations.* Washington, D.C.: Defense and Veterans Brain Injury Center.

Dziedzic, J. (2008, March 3). Mild TBI among US soldiers leads to PTSD and physical health problems. *NeuroPsychiatry Review, 9*(3) 1–2.

Elder, G.A., Mitsis, E.M., Ahlers, S.T., & Cristian, A. (2010). Blast-induced Mild Traumatic Brain Injury. *Psychiatr Clin N Am, 33*, 757–781.

Fleminger, S. (2010, March 9). Neuropsychiatric effects of traumatic brain injury. *Psychiatric Times, 27*(3), 45–45.

French, L.M., Iverson, G.L., and Bryant, R.A. (2011). Traumatic brain injury. In D.M. Benedek and G.H. Wynn (Eds). *Clinical Manual for Management of PTSD* (pp. 383–414). Washington, DC: American Psychiatric Publishing, Inc.

Halstead, M.E., Walter, K.D., and The Council on Sports Medicine and Fitness. (2010). Clinical report: Sport-related concussion in children and adolescents. *Pediatrics, 126*(3), 597–614.

Hitti, M. (2008 January 30). Soldiers' concussions, PTSD linked: Study shows concussions suffered in Iraq deployment may have link to posttraumatic stress disorder. *WebMD Health News.* Retrieved on October 27, 2011 from http://www.webmd.com/brain/news/20080130/soldiers-concussions-ptsd-linked.

Hoge, C.W., McGurk, D.M., Thomas, J.L., Cox, A., Engl, C. & Castro, C. (2008). Mild traumatic brain injury in U.S. soldiers returning from Iraq. *New England Journal of Medicine, 358*, 453-463.

Hoge, C.W., Goldberg, H.M., & Castro, C.A. (2009). Care of war veterans with mild traumatic brain injury–flawed perspectives. *New England Journal of Medicine, 360*, 1588–1591.

Hopewell, C.A., and Christopher, R. (2007). Military Personnel and Combat Trauma: *Operation Iraqi Freedom; Operation Enduring Freedom.* Sparks, NV: Professional, Clinical, and Forensic Assessments.

Iverson, G.L., Lange, R.T., Gaetz, M., Zasler, N.D. (2007). Mild TBI. In N. D. Zasler, D. I. Katz, & R. D. Zafonte (Eds.), *Brain Injury Medicine: Principles and Practice* (pp. 333– 371). New York: Demos Medical Publications.

Kim, E. (2002). Agitation, aggression, and disinhibition syndromes after traumatic brain injury. *Neurorehabilitation, 17*(4), 297–310.

Kochanek P.M., Clark R.S.B., Jenkins L.W.,(2007) TBI: pathobiology (pp 81-96), in N.D.Zasler; D.I. Katz;R.D. Zafonte (Eds) *Brain Injury Medicine: Principles and Practice.* New York, Demos Medical Publications.

Lee, Y. (2008). Study: PTSD, not brain injury, may cause vets' symptoms. *International CNN.com.* Retrieved March 20, 2011, from http://www.cnn.com/2008/HEALTH/01/30/brain.injury/index.html

Levin, A. (2009, May 15). Health officials criticize Pentagon's TBI criteria. *Psychiatric News.*

Levin, A. (2010, October 1). Blast-affected troops to get mandatory TBI evaluations. *Psychiatric News, 45*(19), 6.

Levin, H.S., Mattis, S., Ruff, R.M., Eisenberg, H.M., Marshall, L.F., Tabaddor, K., et al. (1987). Neurobehavioral outcome following minor head injury: A three-center study. *Journal of Neurosurgery, 66*(2), 234–243.

Levine, B., Robertson, I.H., Clare, L., Carter, G. (2000). Rehabilitation of executive function: An experimental-clinical validation of goal management training. *Journal of the International Neuropsychological Society, 6*(3), 299–312.

Lew, H.L., Cifu, D.X., Sigford, B., Scott, S., Sayer, N., and Jaffee, M.S. (2007). Team approach to diagnosis and management of traumatic brain injury and its comorbidities. *Journal of Rehabilitation Research and Development , 44*(7), vii–xi.

Lishman, W.A. (1988). Physiogenesis and psychogenesis in the post-concussional syndrome. *British Journal of Psychiatry, 153*, 460–469.

McAllister, T. (2005). Mild brain injury and postconcussive symptoms. In J. Silver, S. Yudofsky, and T. McAllister (Eds.), *Textbook of Traumatic Brain Injury* (2nd ed., pp. 279–308). Arlington, VA: American Psychiatric Press.

McAllister, T. (2009). Psychopharmacological issues in the treatment of TBI and PTSD, *The Clinical Neuropsychologist, 23*, 1338–1367.

McAllister, T.W. (2010, November). Psychiatric disorders and traumatic brain injury: What is the connection? *Psychiatric Annals, 40*(11), 533–539.

Moore, B.A., Hopewell, C.A., and Grossman, D. (2009). After the battle: Violence and the warrior. In S.M. Freeman, B.A. Moore, and A. Freeman (Eds.), *Living and Surviving in Harm's Way* (pp. 307–327). New York: Routledge.

Mysiw, W., and Sandel, M. (1997, February). The agitated the brain injured patient. Part 2: Pathophysiology and treatment. *Archives of Physical Medicine and Rehabilitation, 78*(2), 213–220.

Neergaard, L. (2009, November 12). *Scanning invisible damage of PTSD in veterans.* Reflector.com Retreived on November 12, 2011, from http://www.reflector.com/features/scanning-invisible-damage-of-ptsd-in-veterans-950739.html.

Okie, S. (2005). Traumatic brain injury in the war zone. *New England Journal of Medicine, 352*, 2043–2047.

Rao, V., and Lyketsos, C. (2000). Neuropsychiatric sequelae of TBI. *Psychosomatic, 41*, 95–103.

Riggio, S. (2010, December). Traumatic brain injury and its neurobehavioral sequelae. *Psychiatric Clinics of North America, 33*(4), 807–819.

Sayer, N.A., Cifu, D.X., McNamee, S., Chiros, C.E., Sigford, B.J., and Scott, S. (2009). Rehabilitation needs of combat-injured service members admitted to the

VA polytrauma rehabilitation center: The role of PM & R in the care of wounded warriors. *PM & R, 1*(1), 23–28.

Scott, S.G., Belanger, H.G., Vanderpoeg, R.D, Massemgale, J. and Scholtem, J. (2006). Mechanism of injury approach to evaluating patients with blast related polytrauma. *The Journal of the American Association, 106*, 265–270.

Silver, J.M., Hales, R.E., and Yudofsky, S.C. (2002). Neuropsychiatric aspects of traumatic brain injury. In S.C. Yudofsky and R.E. Hales (Eds.), *Neuropsychiatry and Clinical Neurosciences* (pp. 625–672). Washington, DC: American Psychiatric Publishing.

Smith, D. (2010, May/June). Can an old head injury suddenly cause detrimental effects much later in life? *Scientific American Mind,* 70.

Taber, K.H., Warden, D.L., and Hurley, R.A. (2006). Blast-related traumatic brain injury: What is known? *Journal of Neuropsychiatry and Clinical Neuroscience, 18*, 141–145.

Tanielian, T., and Jaycox, L.H. (Eds.). (2008). *Invisible Wounds of War: Psychological and Cognitive Injuries, Their Consequences, and Services to Assist Recovery.* Santa Monica, CA: Rand Corporation. Accessed July 11, 2010.

Tonkonogy, J.M., and Geller, J. L. (1992). Hypothalamic lesions and intermittent explosive disorder. *Neuropsychiatry and Clinical Neuroscience, 4*, 45–50.

Warden D. (2006). Military TBI during the Iraq and Afghanistan wars. *The Journal of Head Trauma Rehabilitation, 21*, 398–402.

Wartenberg, K.E. and Mayer, S.A. (2007). Trauma. In J.C.M. Brust (Ed.), *Current Diagnosis & Treatment in Neurology.* New York: McGraw-Hill.

Zafonte, R. (2006). Update on biotechnology for TBI rehabilitation. A look at the future. *The Journal of Head Trauma Rehabilitation, 21*(5), 403–407a.

Zink, B.J., Szmydynger-Chodobska, J., & Chodobski, A. (2010). Emerging concepts in the pathophysiology of traumatic brain injury. *Psychiatr Clin N Am,* 33, 741–756.

Chapter 3

PTSD IN VETERANS: SIGNS AND SYMPTOMS

Jamshid A. Marvasti and Shazia Rahim Anwar

INTRODUCTION

PTSD is considered by some professionals to be a normal response by normal people to an abnormal situation (Schiraldi, 2009). This rationale is based on the assertion that the development of PTSD is understandable, and even predictable, for those who are exposed to abnormal traumatic situations. PTSD occurs in less than 50 percent of those veterans who were exposed to trauma, however. This low percentage may be explained by the fact that people can develop PTSD at various stages, meaning they may experience several symptoms of PTSD at one time and later develop other symptoms. Additionally, there is no time restriction on PTSD. Various people may develop symptoms right after the traumatic event; for others it may take years.

Soldiers with severe PTSD report that they feel they are "losing their minds" or "going crazy." They feel that they are "doomed," and "different from everyone else." They report bruised souls and shattered or devastated minds. They may be very pessimistic and feel dead inside and torn apart (Scott & Stradling, 1992). The story of Humpty Dumpty may be a good analogy for what is at the crux of severe PTSD, because "all the king's horses and all the king's men couldn't put Humpty together again."

Soldiers and their families cannot expect a combat veteran to be capable of returning to the person he or she was before going to war. All people are constantly changing, whether they are adjusting to the death of a spouse or adjusting to living a civilian life versus one on the battlefield. According to Heraclitus, no man can step into the same river twice, for the second time it's not the same river, and he's not the same man. Therefore, expectations around what is possible with healing and recovery may need to be adjusted. A soldier cannot change what happened during war; however he or she can potentially integrate this experience into his or her life moving forward.

PTSD: SIGNS AND SYMPTOMS

Generally, PTSD symptoms develop in three categories: (1) Reexperiencing the trauma (nightmares, flashbacks, or intrusive thoughts); (2) dissociation, avoidance, and emotional numbing; and (3) increased autonomic arousal, including hyperarousal, hypervigilance, and exaggerated startle response.

REEXPERIENCING THE TRAUMATIC INCIDENT

Nightmares, Intrusive Dreams, and Insomnia

There are a variety of symptoms associated with sleep disorders among trauma victims, including dyssomnia (primary insomnia and primary hypersomnia) and parasomnia (nightmare disorder, sleep terror disorder, and substance-induced sleep disorder) (Housley & Beutler, 2007). Any PTSD patient may develop a sleep disorder, and sleep disorders are not limited to nightmares but also include difficulty falling asleep, early morning awakening, and anxiety over going to sleep (including the fear of going back to sleep after frightening nightmares) (Nisenoff, 2008). Such individuals may condition themselves to stay awake so they can avoid the anxiety produced by trauma-related nightmares. Schreuder, Kleijn, and Rooijmans (2000) evaluated a group of WW II combat veterans from the Netherlands forty years after the war had ended and found that they were still the victims of nightmares. Even more than four decades after the original event, these soldiers reported that they were often disturbed by intrusive recurrent dreams.

Analysis of polysomnograms revealed that patients with PTSD had more stage 1 sleep, less slow-wave sleep, and greater rapid eye movement (REM) density than those patients without PTSD (Kobayashi, Boarts & Delahanty, 2007).

Case History of Nightmare

Even though Rodney Vivian was the son of a WW II veteran and a psychiatric resident, he was unaware of certain concepts of trauma, such as those that result in changes to personality structure. He wrote a letter to the editor of *Psychiatric News* (Vivian, 2010), in which he describes how he learned that his own father likely had stress reaction, or PTSD, after his experiences in the Burmese jungle where he was a victim of atrocities. Back home in England after 1945, the man would scream the middle of the night and wrap his hands around his wife's neck. Terrified, she began to hide in the bathroom, especially during thunderstorms. His father had survived the war but was killed after carelessly driving his car into the path of a train. In 1999 Dr. Vivian spent the night at his aunt and uncle's home, also in England. He recalls that around 2 AM he was awakened by his uncle's scream. In the morning he asked his aunt if his uncle was having problems, and she replied, "No, not really–he wakes up every night since he returned from the war in 1945." She added, "All of the men who came back from the war do that–it's normal."

Sometimes the nightmares are so frequent that family members and partners are awakened multiple times at night and may themselves develop sleep disorders and fatigue. In extreme cases, living with veterans in this state may be a trauma in and of itself (Matsakis, 2007). At times veterans with nightmares will wake others to reassure themselves that they are safe and alive. Some veterans may drink a lot of coffee at night to avoid sleep altogether. Others may overindulge in alcohol, food, and drugs to numb themselves with the hope that during sleep they will be in a semicomatose state and not experience terrifying nightmares.

According to Wittman, Schredl, and Kramer (2007) about 50 percent of dreams and nightmares in PTSD individuals are replications of traumatic incidents. The content of these nightmares may be a duplication of their combat experiences or an exaggeration of their most fearful fantasy. Nightmares generally embody the worst-case scenario. For example, one soldier explained that he had nightmares of being trapped in a foxhole with enemy soldiers trying to drag him further down in the hole. Another soldier describes a dream of being wounded and put in a body bag and carried into a cellar. He says, "I am screaming at people that I am not dead, but they continue putting me there anyway." Some have nightmares about helplessness due to a malfunctioning weapon. Another describes dreaming of being chased and says, "I cannot run too fast, everything is in slow motion" (Ziarowsky & Broida, 1984). Sometimes nightmares begin to emerge or intensify when a veteran becomes sober after substance abuse or begins a program for healing from war recovery. It is not uncommon during psychotherapy for a provider to hear, "I was better off when I was not in therapy." When patients get in touch with their trauma, they often feel "worse" initially. At times, psychotherapy may trigger nightmares.

One soldier reported recurring nightmares about the ghosts of dead Iraqis who were trying to kill him. With time, the dreams became less frequent and less horrifying to him. After his mother developed Alzheimer's disease, however, his nightmares returned in full force. "Just seeing my mother waste away brought back my nightmares about hospitals in Iraq full of the dying, crying people" (Matsakis, 2007, p. 86).

Flashback

Flashbacks, like nightmares, are a form of intrusive thought and of re-experiencing the traumatic incident. A veteran who has flashbacks is, in some ways, reliving the events of the past, such as being on a battleground. A flashback has a visual element, although flashbacks could include all five sensory modalities: seeing, hearing, smelling, touching, and tasting. (Matsakis, 2007). In addition to these sensory modalities, soldiers may develop "kinesthetic flashback," in which they experience the sensation of movement, such as flying out of a car seat due to a wave of explosion. Some victims of PTSD, however, may eventually realize that the flashbacks are not reality, and some are able to identify the triggering elements that caused them. Many use avoidance techniques to decrease the likelihood of flashbacks and intrusive thoughts. For instance, they may refrain from watching war movies or news about military actions or attending fireworks displays, because they know any of these elements may stimulate an adverse reaction.

Sometimes flashbacks may be triggered by excessive tiredness, sleep disorder, or the stress of a present life situation (Peterson, Prout & Schwarz, 1991). Although some PTSD victims use street drugs to suppress flashbacks, there are indications that some of these drugs may, by themselves, cause flashbacks and intrusive thoughts.

Trigger elements may be external or internal. External triggers could include a fast-moving police vehicle, a person in uniform, or a car alarm. There may also be other kinds of sensory modalities, for example, if the veteran smells Middle Eastern food, it may trigger a traumatic memory of the war. Triggers may also be internal, that is, those thoughts that invade the mind of the veteran (Schiraldi, 2009). Sometimes, if the specific content of a flashback is about the enemy, a veteran can confuse family members for enemies. Partners of veterans with PTSD report that their mates alternate between recognizing them as loved ones and seeing them as enemy combatants. It is possible for a flashback to be the factor that initiates dissociation. In addition, epilepsy (seizures disorder) may start with flashback, dissociation, and several psychiatric symptoms; however, it may also include loss of consciousness, blackout, or loss of sphincter control, which may not be present in PTSD.

At times, a provider may grow frightened when a veteran begins to experience flashback because they have little training in how to handle this kind of extremely delicate situation (Blank, 1985). There is always a risk that a caregiver may become the subject of aggression by a veteran who is experiencing flashbacks.

Some combat veterans may hear the screams and moans of injured or distressed civilians or comrades during flashbacks. One military interrogator who claims to have used "rough and tough" procedures to obtain information from prisoners reports that he hears the screams of his victims whenever he is in a quiet place. He puts an air conditioner on to make white noise and block out his internal noise. Conversely, there are other veterans with PTSD who cannot tolerate a noisy environment, such as a children's playground, because it triggers memories of the generally noisy scene of combat.

Flashback Versus Psychotic Hallucination

Hallucination and flashback may display certain similarities; hallucination however, may be a sign of psychotic disorder. Under the stress of combat, a soldier with certain vulnerability may demonstrate psychotic breakdown. Clinicians must differentiate psychotic-like breakdowns from PTSD and schizophrenia. A family history of psychotic disorder or schizophrenia may be an important factor for differential diagnosis. Psychotic flashbacks or hallucinations generally include certain distinguishing characteristics. These may include elements of bizarreness or content that is unconnected to the trauma of war. The patient may also exhibit inappropriate affects. For example, a psychotic patient may talk about a frightening memory while smiling.

In psychotic hallucinations an individual may hear voices, explosions, and cries for help. Upon further questioning, he may attribute the voices to paranormal elements, such as in the case of one patient who explained that a voice was "being transmitted by aliens from the moon into my ear."

In veterans with PTSD, however, emotions relating to flashbacks are usually appropriate to the content. For example, a frightening flashback may be accompanied by fear. Following the flashback, the veteran may then shift to a numbing state with blunt affect, similar to a psychotic mood. In PTSD, the flashback, and any visual or auditory component of it, is generally related to a veteran's combat experiences. Some professionals consider the flashback to be a form of hallucination and may diagnose the veteran with some form of psychotic disorder. To differentiate PTSD from schizophrenia or psychotic disorder one needs to obtain the details of the patient's symptoms. A problem arises when a veteran has developed both PTSD and psychotic disorder or when a TBI patient with PTSD also has post-trauma psychotic symptoms due to damage to brain tissue.

Intrusive Thoughts

Intrusive thoughts, like other experiences of reliving, have some adaptive and survival value (Matsakis, 2007). They are a way of discharging the extensive energy generated by the body during combat and of releasing traumatic memories. Intrusive thoughts may also be a way of mentally reviewing the past in hope of figuring out how to avoid future dangers (i.e. repeating the trauma of war for the purpose of ego mastery). Reliving symptoms can also be a way of commemorating the war. Because many aspects of a soldier's war experiences are not known to others, symptoms serve to scream out that "it did happen" (Matsakis, 1994).

DISSOCIATION, AVOIDANCE, AND EMOTIONAL NUMBING

According to the *Diagnostic and Statistical Manual of Mental Disorders* (4th ed.) (DSM-IV), dissociation is, "a disruption in the usually integrated function of consciousness, memory, identity, or perception of the environment" (DSM-IV, 2000, p. 239). Generally, dissociation includes (a) dissociative amnesia (not remembering part or all of an event), (b) derealization, (c) fugue state (an altered state of consciousness in which one is not fully aware or alert to reality), and (d) depersonalization and dissociative identity disorder ([DID] the presence of two or more distinct identities or personalities).

In dissociative amnesia, a trauma victim may dissociate and isolate traumatic memories. Dissociated traumatic memories are split off, fragmented, and compartmentalized so the information does not become integrated with the rest of a person's memory, nor is it fully connected to the present awareness. Although the memory is walled off, this wall is highly permeable. It is analogous to a dam that has a leak; once in a while, the consciousness and awareness intrude and cause pain, flashbacks and hyperarousal (Schiraldi, 2009).

Flannery (1992) explains that people are more prone to dissociate if they are excessively fatigued, tired, drunk, sleepy, anxious, or deeply depressed. Dissociation can also disrupt interpersonal and occupational functioning and may be related to a number of dysfunctional behaviors such as aggression, shoplifting, eating disorders, and parasuicidal behaviors such as self-mutilation (Wagner & Linehan, 1998). Schapiro, Glynn, Foy, and Yavorsky, (2002) conducted research that provides preliminary empirical evidence for the connection between participation in war zone atrocity and trait dissociation. These authors believe that the tendency to dissociate, which can be considered an extreme form of avoidance behavior is more common among those soldiers whose war zone experiences were outside the limits of acceptable behavior, or "beyond the pale." They explain that soldiers who participated in more extreme acts of war-zone violence have had to employ dissociation as a mechanism to cope with memories that are so distressful they have never been integrated into their consciousness.

Derealization

Derealization may be a part of dissociation. In this case, a person looks at the event as if it is not really happening. The person may think that he or she is in a dream or far away or that the memory or event is happening in a foggy or dreamlike situation.

Fugue

Fugue may be considered a form of amnesia. In this process, an individual suddenly travels to another city with no recollection of how he or she got there. Some may even start a new life, develop a new identity, and then forget their own identity and life pattern.

AVOIDANCE AND EMOTIONAL NUMBING IN PTSD

In the diagnostic evaluation of PTSD, emotional numbing is currently classified in the avoidance symptom cluster, although some researchers question this wisdom. Recent research indicates that avoidance and numbing may be better explained as separate elements that differ in their clinical correlates and in their prognostic significance and response to treatment. These findings are also consistent with ideas that numbing arises from a biological mechanism associated with a response called "conditioned analgesia" (Asmundson, Stapleton & Taylor, 2004), which dampens arousal states. Numbing could also be considered a sensory dissociation and a survival device during combat (Schiraldi, 2009).

On the contrary, avoidance appears to be more of an intentional and conscious strategy for controlling distressing emotions (Asmundson & Taylor, 2008). The brain is believed to secrete a biochemical numbing material that touches all receptors of feeling in the brain, including both pain and joy receptors. As a result, these veterans may develop restricted range of affect, which is also referred to as psychic numbing or emotional anesthesia (Schiraldi, 2009).

Although in the short term, avoidance or denial alleviates anxiety and pain, it may also prevent the victim from developing the corrective information necessary for learning how to differentiate between a dangerous situation and a safe situation. Some clinicians believe avoidance may exacerbate or perpetuate the symptoms of PTSD, rather than promote adaptive behavior (Asmundson & Taylor, 2008).

INCREASED AUTONOMIC AROUSAL

Hyperarousal and Hypervigilance

High levels of hyperarousal are commonly associated with PTSD and often lead to self-medication. Those with hypervigilance symptoms feel vulnerable and frightened and frequently overreact to any stimulation. They anticipate a disaster and are unable to feel calm or relaxed in their own body and are very much guarded. Many veterans keep weapons with them or sleep with weapons in their beds or nearby. Although hypervigilance was a necessary survival skill during combat, in civilian life it causes problems both in interpersonal relationships and in the quality of life of the veterans (Schiraldi, 2009).

Exaggerated Startle Response

Combat veterans complain that when they hear a car backfiring or a door slam hard, they jump to the ground and "duck for cover." For veterans who have PTSD, these sounds may seem equal in intensity to the sounds of bombs exploding. Several research papers have found that startle reaction is one of the most frequent self-reported symptoms of PTSD (Pynoos et al., 1993). Startle reaction is also among the symptoms that best differentiate between individuals with PTSD and those without (Meltzer-Brody, Churchill & Davidson, 1999). The presence of startle reaction may therefore be a sort of barometer for PTSD. For example, there are some patients who will jump at the sudden sound of a slamming door. When this happens during an interview, it may be an indication of genuine symptoms of PTSD and may rule out the possibility of malingering. Not everyone who demonstrates startle reaction is suffering from PTSD, however; too much caffeine or sleep deprivation may also cause this symptom.

PTSD victims have sensitized nervous systems and may overreact to certain stimulation in a very frightening way (Schiraldi, 2009). Many spouses of veterans with PTSD indicate a reluctance to wake their spouse up by touching his or her face or shoulder, because their partner may instantly react by jumping up, getting into combat mode, and possibly even striking them. Families of veterans with PTSD are often aware that they cannot approach the veteran suddenly from behind. Instead they must take care to verbally inform him or her that they are approaching before getting physically close. As another precaution, family members may try to forewarn the veteran if they are about to create a loud noise, such as if they are using a hammer or other loud tool.

Anniversary Dates as Triggering Phenomena

As mentioned throughout this chapter, triggers can be of a sensory nature or be related to internal or external phenomenon. Triggering phenomenon can be connected with the various symptoms of PTSD. One of the common triggers that remind war veterans of the war experience are anniversary dates, such as the date they entered combat or were wounded, the date of the death of a comrade, or the date of a friendly fire incident or a particularly dangerous mission (Matsakis, 2007).

Veterans Administration (VA) nurse Kathleen Neason observed that Gulf War veterans may have "anniversary reactions" that cause them to become physically ill on specific dates relating to their service. A study of this phenomenon in Gulf War veterans found that 38 person experienced the most severe PTSD symptoms during the month that their wartime experience was most severe. The soldiers may not be consciously aware of a link between the dates when their symptoms of illness flare and the date of a past trauma. By reviewing the wartime records of a soldier, one could establish a link between reoccurring symptoms of illness and significant trauma-related dates (Neason, 2006).

CONCLUSION

PTSD may be considered one of the potential responses to the abnormal situation of war. Exposure to atrocity and friendly fire and witnessing the death of a civilian in collateral damage are among the most devastating elements that contribute to the development of PTSD. Symptoms of PTSD are demonstrated on an individual and unique basis. Some veterans use alcohol or drugs for self-medication and consider it a solution. Eventually this "solution" becomes a problem, however, to the point that alcohol and drug abuse may be considered one of the clinical characteristics of PTSD.

Although the clinical community is trying to adopt a protocol in regard to the criteria needed for diagnosis of PTSD, this may not always work. There is no recipe book or any cliché to diagnose PTSD. Recent observations indicate that although many veterans experience various symptoms of PTSD, one or two symptoms may be missing in order to qualify them with an official PTSD diagnosis, as defined by the DSM.

Every veteran with PTSD presents symptoms in his or her own way related to his or her individual psychology and biology. As Leo Tolstoy said, "All happy families resemble one another, each unhappy family is unhappy in its own way."

REFERENCES

Asmundson, G.J.G., Stapleton, J.A., and Taylor, S. (2004). Avoidance and numbing are distinct PTSD symptom clusters. *Journal of Traumatic Stress, 17,* 467–475.

Asmundson, G.J.G., and Taylor, S. (2008). Avoidance. In G. Reyes, J.D. Elhai, & J.D. Ford (Eds.), *The Encyclopedia of Psychological Trauma* (pp. 70–71). Hoboken, NJ: Wiley.

Blank, A.S. (1985). The unconscious flashback to the war in Vietnam veterans: Clinical mystery, legal defense and community problem. In S.M. Sonnenberg, A.S. Blank & J.A. Talbott (Eds.), *The Trauma of War: Stress and Recovery in Vietnam Veterans* (p. 297). Washington, DC: American Psychiatric Press.

Diagnostic and Statistical Manual of Mental Disorders. (4th ed.) (DSM-IV-TR.) (2000). Washington, DC: American Psychiatric Association.

Flannery, R.B. (1992). *Post-Traumatic Stress Disorder: The Victim's Guide to Healing and Recovering.* New York: Crossroads.

Housley, J. and Beutler, L.E. (2007). *Treating victims of mass disaster and terrorism.* Cambridge, MA: Hogrefe & Huber

Kobayashi, H., Boarts, J.M., and Delahanty, D.L. (2007). Polysomnographically measured sleep abnormalities in PTSD: A meta-analytic review. *Psychophysiology, 44,* 660–669.

Matsakis, A. (1994). *I can't get over it: A handbook for trauma survivors.* Oakland, CA: New Harbinger Publications.

Matsakis, A. (2007). *Back from the front: Combat trauma, love, and the family.* Baltimore, MD: Sidran Institute Press.

Meltzer-Brody, S., Churchill, E., and Davidson, J.R.T. (1999). Derivation of the SPAN, a brief diagnostic screening test for post-traumatic stress disorder. *Psychiatry Research, 88,* 63–70.

Neason, K. (2006, October 1). PTSD: Help patients break free [Online]. *www.RNWeb.com, 69*(10). Retrieved Oct. 29, 2011, from www.modernmedicine.com.

Nisenoff, C.D. (2008, July). Psychotherapeutic and adjunctive pharmacologic approaches to treating posttraumatic stress disorder. *Psychiatry, 5*(7), 42–51.

Peterson, K.C., Prout, M.F., and Schwarz, R.A. (1991). *PTSD: A Clinical Guide.* New York: Plenum.

Pynoos, R.S., Goenjiam, A., Tashjian, M., Karakashian, M., Manjikian, R., Maniu-kian, G., et al. (1993). Post-traumatic stress reaction in children after the 1988 Armenian earthquake. *British Journal of Psychiatry, 163,* 239–247.

Schapiro, J.A., Glynn, S.M., Foy, D.W., and Yavorsky, C. (2002). Participation in war-zone atrocities and trait dissociation among Vietnam veterans with combat-related posttraumatic stress disorder. *Journal of Trauma & Dissociation, 3*(2), 107–115.

Schiraldi, G.R. (2009). *The Post-Traumatic Stress Disorder Sourcebook.* New York: Mc-Graw-Hill.

Schreuder, B.J.N., Kleijn, W.C., and Rooijmans, H.G.M. (2000). Nocturnal re-experiencing more than forty years after war trauma. *Journal of Traumatic Stress, 13*(3), 453–462.

Scott, M.J., and Stradling, S.G. (1992). *Counseling for post-traumatic stress disorder.* London: Sage.

Vivian, R. (2010, March 5). War was always hell. *Psychiatric News, 45*(5), 18.

Wagner, A.W., and Linehan, M.M. (1998). Dissociative behavior. In V.M. Follette, J.I. Ruzek, and F.R. Abueg (Eds.), *Cognitive-Behavioral Therapies for Trauma* (pp. 191–225). New York: Guilford Press.

Wittman, L., Schredl, M., and Kramer, M. (2007). Dreaming in posttraumatic stress disorder: A critical review of phenomenology, psychophysiology and treatment. *Psychotherapy and Psychosomatics, 76*(1), 25–39.

Ziarowsky, P.A., and Broida, D.C. (1984, July). Therapeutic implications of nightmares of Vietnam combat veterans. *The V.A. Practitioner, 1*(7), 63, 67–68.

Chapter 4

SPIRITUAL DISTRESS AS A COMPONENT OF PTSD: THE NEED FOR SPIRITUAL HEALING

MARY PAQUETTE

INTRODUCTION

The return from battle is a slow ascent from hell.

James Hillman (2004, p. 33)

Service members fighting in any war are subject to extreme and some-times cold-blooded circumstances that test the limits of their psychological well-being. The reality of war leaves many of our military men and women physically, psychologically, and spiritually wounded. Immediate and long-term care helps to preserve the dignity and mental health of the war wounded.

Killing another human being is a requirement for survival when enemies are at war. Service members are prepared for this by way of rigorous and exhaustive military training, usually referred to as boot camp, where they learn to use their weapons to kill for protection, safety, and combat success (Grossman, 2009).

The specific and well-developed training takes normal young people and turns them into individuals who can dehumanize enemies sufficiently enough to kill them. Then, they are expected to believe they are good soldiers for doing so. The more adept service members are at killing, the more likely they are to be recognized as heroes and be awarded with military honors.

In a sense, the war continues within the service member even after returning home. The military is excellent at training and conditioning soldiers for war. Young lives are changed forever. What the military does not do well, however, is to reverse the process and turn the "trained killer" back into a well-adjusted civilian (McNair, 2002). During combat, service members find themselves dehumanizing and killing other human beings, often not only the enemy combatants but also innocent civilians (collateral damage). All this is done while acting as the good soldier: following orders, protecting comrades, and defending country. The inability to forget these experiences and what they did in the name of war and patriotism creates a private hell that a number of veterans endure for the rest of their lives. To the outside world, they are heroes, but to themselves they are not. They wake at night screaming with terror and guilt for having crossed a moral line that cannot be uncrossed. What makes a good soldier does not make a good citizen, and many service members need guidance to transition back to civilian life (Grossman, 2009).

RECOVERING FROM WAR

Who we are when we leave [the USA] is not who we
are . . . . when and if we are lucky enough to physically return.
You are completely changed by it [war].

Marine Corporal Sean Huze
(Mysko, 2006)

The expectations put upon returning service members are immense. They must maintain the military mindset and yet go back to hearth and home without worry or regret. They must also place their combat experience into a different perspective, with no instruction on how to do so. Ultimately, war veterans are asked to either exalt or ignore their actions in battle, which is usually not possible for them to do on their own. To many veterans, the brutality of war often seems impossible to integrate into their identity (Tick, 2005). Research has proved that the human nervous system is damaged by such traumatic and stressful experiences (van der Kolk, 2004). This is the beginning of PTSD, when a veteran's world view is shattered. There is an inner struggle to justify the actions that brought him glory but are so terrible that he cannot express them to those closest to him. A rage builds; negative ideation begins; and impulsive, destructive behavior replaces the reasonable, well-trained conduct of the person who shipped off to war (Paulson & Krippner, 2007). The acknowledgement of guilt, sorrow, and regret for killing people as a part of war is probably the safest thing veteran service members may do on their path to recovering their humanity. Those who recognize that war requires one to circumvent one's conscience may be able to more easily reintegrate into society. Learning to incorporate this life skill may be the beginning of true healing of the heart, soul, and body for those traumatized by war.

DOCUMENTARY FILMS: SOLDIERS' DISTRESS ABOUT KILLING

The average and healthy individual still has such an inner resistance that he will not take life if it is possible to turn away from that responsibility. At the vital point he becomes a conscientious objector.

Marshall (1947, 1978, p. 54)

Two recent documentaries discussed here capture the voices of returning veterans and still-enlisted service members about the difficulty of living with moral and spiritual distress.

The Ground Truth: After the Killing Ends

Soldiers who are speaking out in this film (Mysko, 2006) are vocal in their belief that their guilt fuels the fire to take action and make a difference for others who are still in the military and cannot safely speak. Twenty veterans were interviewed about the aftermath of war on their personal lives. All of the soldiers interviewed suffered psychological trauma, and many experienced physical injuries. Watching this documentary can be a disturbing experience that requires the viewer to reconsider the impact war has on soldiers. The war mind needs to be better understood by medical and psychological professionals in order to help the veteran resolve the guilt he or she may harbor.

It is heartbreaking to hear the veterans' confessions of guilt and the deep desire to compensate for actions that possibly were necessary during war but are difficult to accept after returning home. The veterans' public confessions in the documentary are no doubt powerful in releasing their guilt and helping them move on with their lives. They know that they were trained and conditioned to kill and that it was their jobs as a soldiers in a difficult and dangerous war. These veterans wanted to compensate for their wartime actions by living honorably in their civilian lives, with a renewed sense of their moral beliefs. Now home, they work hard to follow their conscience and to forget that their jobs once included "killing the enemy." Some are learning that speaking publicly about their combat experiences and postwar problems helps them to return to a normal life. They find some measure of redemption by helping others who face the same demons.

Soldiers of Conscience

Some soldiers decide to become conscientious objectors (COs) while they are still in the service. From 2001 to 2009, the military received about fifty CO requests each year and approved only half of them (Halloran, 2009). Active service members who claim CO status must prove that their change in belief occurred during military service; otherwise, they may face denial of their request or even a court-martial. *Soldiers of Conscience* (2007) recent documentary on this subject, made with the official permission of the U.S. Army, portrays the moral dilemma many service members face when they claim CO status while on active duty. Largely, these one-time combatants come to reject the requirement to kill. The film's stated mission is "to spark conversation and encourage healing around the taboo topic of killing in war" (*Soldiers of Conscience*, 2007).

Filmmakers Catherine Ryan and Gary Weimberg initially believed that only CO suffered moral pain from having to kill another human being. What they discovered, however, during their interviews with eight CO and a number of willing warriors, was that every soldier has a conscience and that soldiers must deal with the burden of culpability for killing during combat. Taking another's life is not easy for anyone, even when trained and conditioned to do so, as all service members are today. The issue of "justified killing" is appropriately analyzed in the film with compassion and intelligence, ultimately reaching the conclusion that both the COs and the willing warriors agree on one thing: killing has consequences, and there is more than one way to cope with them.

In the documentary, Major Pete Kilner, a West Point professor who admits to never killing anyone himself, addresses the morality and justification of killing during war. He also recognizes the damage it does to the psyches of service members:

> Now, we recruit people to serve their country and to kill. We train them how to kill . . . . but, we never explain to them why it's okay so that, when they do what they've been trained so well to do, they can be at peace with their consciences for the rest of their lives." (*Soldiers of Conscience*, 2007)

Major Kilner argues that war is usually the lesser of many evils. This film demonstrates that, although capable of great violence and malevolence, humans also have an amazing ability to rise above it all and follow their con-science and renounce killing. Watching the film is an eye-opener to the immense courage required to stand up for your moral beliefs and take a stand against killing even when such actions are met with dire consequences. Sergeant Camilo Mejia is one such individual. Mejia appears in both documentaries, *The Ground Truth and Soldiers of Conscience.* He gained notoriety as the CO who was imprisoned for deciding to go AWOL rather than go back to Iraq. His short time in battle–five months–was enough to convince him that his principles would not allow him to return. Soon after his case gained public attention in 2004, Mejia became the face of the antiwar movement. He took on the military establishment, was court-martialed, and served nine months of a one-year sentence. *Soldiers of Conscience* (2007) tells the story of how Mejia requested a discharge as a CO, which led to his imprisonment. Mejia's is one of several stories chronicled, each of which demonstrates immense courage and commitment to living one's values at any cost.

SPIRITUALITY AND SPIRITUAL DISTRESS

There are many definitions of spirituality, but perhaps the most all-encom-passing was developed by Barbara Dossey (2008). She calls spirituality a uni-fying force of the person, the essence of being that permeates all of life and is manifested in one's being, knowing, and doing. This force supplies the interconnectedness with self, others, nature, and a higher power. Notice that there is no mention of belief systems or religious faiths. Spirituality is about innate spirit regardless of demographic identifiers (e.g. national origin, reli-gious beliefs, race, etc.). The concept of spirit is unifying because it eliminates all the differences that exist among people of the world, including deeply held religious beliefs. There is a growing interest in holistic care and address-ing spirituality in a broad sense that does not separate spiritual treatment from psychotherapy, which may need to be implemented simultaneously (Tick, 2005).

Definition of Spiritual Distress

Smucker (2008), Clarke (2009), and O'Brien (2006) authors in the field of nursing, have contributed to the understanding of spiritual distress, which is defined by the North American Nursing Diagnosis Association (NANDA) as a disturbance in a person's belief system that causes "a disruption in the life principle that pervades a person's entire being and that integrates and tran-scends one's biological and psychological nature" (Smucker, 2008, p. 81). Many characteristics are suggested by NANDA, including:

• Guilt regarding behavior and its consequences
• Loss of connection and a feeling of emptiness and alienation
• Hopelessness and despair and terrible pain
• Anxiety resulting in a loss of peace, trust, and hope for the future
• A disturbance in one's perception of or relationship to a higher power
  (as he or she perceives it)

The 1980 inclusion of PTSD in the DSM-III produced specific language to describe the immediate and long-term effects of physiological and psychological traumatic experiences on the individual (American Psychiatric Association, 1980). The DSM's description of PTSD covers a wide variety of traumatic events but is not specific to war-induced PTSD, which is complicated by guilt that many soldiers feel for the compulsory killing of other human beings (McNair, 2002). Although trauma has an impact on every dimension of an individual, including the spiritual, the DSM characteristics do not provide language to diagnose spiritual distress. The manual addresses survivor guilt but not the anguish for having violated one's deepest values. Soul suffering and spiritual alienation are not captured by the physical and psychological symptoms of reexperiencing the trauma, arousal, and avoidance reactions. There is a need to expand the focus of PTSD treatment by developing new language and specific concepts to treat the deeper impact of combat experience on the entire person, including the spirit (Paulson & Krippner, 2007; Tick, 2005).

Spiritual Distress: A Case History

Dr. Ebrahim Amanat (2003) relates many veterans' stories in his book, *The Miracle of Love: A Spiritual Approach To PTSD*, which describes the powerful problems related to spiritual distress. In a particularly poignant case, Joe, an eighteen-year-old soldier, joined the Army because he felt small and insignificant next to his WW II–hero father. He viewed the military as a place where he could compensate for all his failings and do something important that would redeem him in his father's eyes and improve his self-image. While driving a military truck in Vietnam his platoon was ambushed and most of his friends were killed. Joe noticed a small group of "Vietcong regulars" and heard them shooting one of the men who was still alive. The Vietcong kicked the other bodies and laughed as they walked away, unaware that Joe was a witness to their behavior. Joe, feeling fearful, angry and humiliated, lost control and, by his own description, became a "killing machine" and killed all eight men, who were caught off guard. Joe reloaded and walked to a nearby village where he killed numerous men, women, and children. "There I wanted to remove any remaining signs of life. A shade of blood had blinded my eyes" (p. 86).

After the killing rampage, Joe retreated to the field and sobbed for hours until he was rescued. "By then I felt bewildered, confused, horrified. I shook so badly people had pity on me" (Amanat, 2003, p. 87). What was particularly confusing to Joe was that he feared being court-martialed for the atrocity he had committed. Instead, they decorated him with a medal and called him a hero. Joe later heard a news clip that reported eighteen Americans were killed in an ambush and forty-five Vietcong died that day. After returning home, Joe endured terrible nightmares and a constant feeling of emptiness. He identified himself as a monster and was unable to connect with his wife or children in any meaningful way. "Perversity, it seems, has bitten my heart. I am repulsive. I am disgusting" (p. 85). Surrounded by his suicide notes, he held a gun in his hand and cried of a "crushing guilt killing my soul every minute of the day" (p. 84).

THE LOSS OF SELF

People who have endured extreme trauma can suffer a profound break in the framework of the self, disrupting the unifying force of innate spirit, leading to the same alienation and self-hatred experienced by Joe (Wilson, Drozdek & Turkovic, 2006). Combat situations damage the soldier's belief in his invulnerability. Joe experienced being helpless in the face of danger. As a reaction to his feelings of fear, helplessness, rage, and humiliation, Joe committed an atrocity, killing innocent civilians. When his intense emotions subsided, Joe felt only horror and confusion at what he had done. He recalls, "I felt that my soul died that day" (Amanat, 2003, p. 87). It is an apt description of Joe's broken sense of self.

Long before PTSD was identified, Erik Erikson, who formulated the Eight Stages of Man developmental theory, referred to veterans he treated as having war neurosis that he describes as an identity disturbance (Tick, 2005). The experience of war can leave a young soldier doubting not only the meaning of life but also his own purpose and direction. Bessel van der Kolk speaks about the impact of trauma on a human being. "One cannot overestimate the degree to which trauma warps character. The most corrosive impact of horrific emotional trauma is to be found in the spiritual fabric of persons. The condition of PTSD is spiritual at its deepest level" (2009, p. 2).

Frank Snepp (2009), an investigative news producer and former CIA interrogator, admits to being plagued by his past when he states, "I am still haunted by what I did as a CIA interrogator during the Vietnam War" (p.

A21). He describes in detail the psychological manipulation and torment of a prisoner, which he believed was morally acceptable. In the end, Snepp concluded that "controlled brutality is a slippery slope, and once you pass through the moral membrane that should contain our worst impulses, it becomes so very easy to rationalize another step, and yet another, in the wrong direction" (p. A21). Loss of self seems to be connected to losing a boundary that keeps us from our most animalistic impulses.

Tick (2005) suggests that the war veteran experiences a loss of identity so profound that the individual needs to "embrace the experience of inner death and seek a new identity and a spiritual rebirth" (p. 108). Veterans know who they are before going to war, but after combat many of them no longer have a feeling of sameness, coherency, or continuity. The most perplexing and vital question that haunts them is "Who am I now?" Tick postulates that PTSD in veterans is a soul disorder and the root cause is moral pain that harms the soul. The loss of self is equivalent to the loss of the essence of being that is one's spiritual connection to life (Dossey, 2008). It manifests as confusion, emptiness, and a sense of deadness, isolation, and alienation. Joe captures the torment of this condition when he says, "Why should I go on? I have no name, no fortune, and no future" (Amanat, 2003, p. 85). The loss of self can result in suicidal ideation, substance abuse, and criminal behavior.

THE SEARCH FOR SELF

> *Some men never come home from war. Others become*
> *more fully human and wiser.*
>
> J.P. Wilson et al. (1988, p. 338)

The loss of self can trigger a search for meaning and purpose of one's life, which is known as an existential crisis (Fontana & Rosenheck, 2004). Amanat (2003) helps the reader see PTSD not as an illness but as an opportunity for growth. If a person attempts to make sense of his or her actions and experiences and tries to identify the meaning of his or her life, this search will trigger spiritual questioning. The search for meaning, however, is complicated by actions that are incongruent with one's moral values. Committing atrocities during battle is not deemed justifiable and looking for existential meaning for this behavior would naturally lead to acknowledging existential guilt (Wilson et al., 2006). The attempt to take responsibility for one's actions, no matter the circumstances, can produce feelings of self-hatred or, with guidance, may stimulate personal growth and ultimately, transformation.

For example, Lt. William Calley, dishonored by the 1969 My Lai massacre, acted against his moral values and lost his ability to cope after suffering heavy losses of fellow soldiers (Hendin & Haas, 2004). Calley experienced guilt when he realized that his actions were not morally justifiable. A confluence of factors left him vulnerable to raw emotionality and impulsive behavior. Guilt for one's actions, lack of action, or actions that fail is common with combat soldiers, who are often making rapid, life-changing decisions with very little information (Kubany, 1994). In 2009, Calley spoke for the first time in forty years, making a public apology during a speech at the Kiwanis Club of Greater Columbus. "There is not a day that goes by that I do not feel remorse for what happened that day in My Lai. I feel remorse for the Vietnamese who were killed, for their families, for the American soldiers involved and their families. I am very sorry" (Associated Press, p. A14). Calley had difficulty speaking to the group but addressed every question, visibly demonstrating his extreme remorse for his actions.

The search for self often begins with the painful process of taking responsibility for one's dark side. Daryl Paulson, one of the authors of *Haunted by Combat* (Paulson & Krippner, 2007), tells how he had to experience tremendous guilt, not only that he killed people but also how much he enjoyed doing so. Acknowledging the truth of one's behavior is essential to the healing process and reclaiming the loss of self. Accepting the unacceptable behaviors allows individuals to integrate the shadow aspect of their humanness and move toward a whole and balanced sense of self, which includes both the good and the bad. This process requires veterans to create new beliefs and myths that are positive frameworks for dealing with their experiences (Tick, 2005). The goal is to move beyond the trauma to higher levels of personality integration. The renewed self, situated in a new belief system, finds meaning in the traumatic events–meaning that can be embraced and used for personal growth (Paulson & Krippner, 2007).

POSTTRAUMATIC COMBAT GUILT

*To study psychological trauma is to come face to face both
with human vulnerability in the natural world and with the
capacity for evil in human nature.*

Judith Herman (1997, p. 7)

In 1994, Kubany developed a cognitive model of guilt typology in combat-related PTSD. This useful framework provides vocabulary that addresses the combat guilt that occurs, even when the soldier believes that the killing of another human being is necessary and justified. He defines combat guilt as "the veterans' intellectual, after-the-fact evaluations of their conduct during periods of trauma" (pp. 4–5). Kubany (1994) has identified eight different types of combat guilt: survivor, death, bystander, catch-22, betrayal/abandonment, moral/spiritual, hindsight bias, and demonic. In each instance, the veteran uses a faulty reasoning process whereby he concludes that he made a bad decision or used poor judgment. For purposes of this discussion only two identified types of guilt will be addressed: moral/spiritual and demonic.

Moral Guilt

Moral guilt is concerned with the principles of right and wrong behavior and the goodness or badness of human character and conduct. Spiritual conflict affects the human spirit or soul and is characterized by the loss of connection with the self (Kubany, 1994). This type of guilt occurs when a soldier violates normal human values such as "thou shall not kill." Studies show that killing another human being is the most damaging traumatic event of war (Grossman, 2009; McNair, 2002). Although not all soldiers suffer moral guilt from killing, those who do are more vulnerable to complicating their guilt with the other identified types of guilt. As with complicated grief, complicated guilt is more painful, longer lasting, and more difficult to resolve (Kubany, 1994).

The soldiers who became CO while enlisted gradually became aware of having a moral conflict that was not experienced earlier in their careers. Once this conflict was understood, it became impossible for the soldiers to continue to violate their values. Some soldiers may be able to justify killing the enemy but have difficulty with moral and spiritual guilt when exposed to or participating in atrocities of war. Lt. Col. Calley is a prime example of a soldier who participated in an atrocity and is still experiencing moral/spiritual guilt forty years later (Associated Press, 2009).

"The Beast Within"

Demonic guilt results from participation in despicable acts without regard to human spirituality (Amanat, 2003). It is guilt for having committed atrocities that are excessively brutal even for war. Examples of atrocities are the massacre at My Lai, as well as the village in Vietnam that Joe massacred, both of which occurred after participants suffered heavy losses of fellow soldiers. Rage and humiliation can provoke an attitude of retribution and feeling justified in implementing payback action, even horrendous actions such as the killing of innocent men, women, and children. Immediately following the rampage of killing, Joe experienced confusion and felt horrified that he lost his soul that day (Amanat, 2003). This demonic act ruptured Joe's connection to humanity and thus to himself, leaving him with the belief that he is a monstrous beast and his entire character is defective without possibility of redemption.

One Vietnam veteran explained the *beast within* this way: "As a soldier you lose your sense of safety, you lose your trust in your leaders, and worst you lose faith in yourself. You fear yourself because you know what you are capable of doing–horrible things that you did not know you could do. In combat, you feel not only helpless in the face of danger, but you know that the danger is also within because you have violated your morals and values. It is frightening to know how far we can go under circumstances of fury and rage; what we are willing to do to survive. Holding on to the guilt, never letting yourself off the hook is proof that you are not a monster; it is a testament to your character that you continue to feel guilty. Guilt makes me feel in control and it helps me not let loose the beast within, but does this at a very high cost to myself" (T.J. Baker, personal communication, March 13, 2009).

SPIRITUAL HEALING OF THE SOUL

Acknowledging that veterans need something *in addition* to traditional PTSD interventions opens the door to developing alternative approaches. Understanding the need to process the guilt and having rituals to help the veteran experience remorse, accept forgiveness, and forgive himself is crucial to the healing of the soul (Tick, 2005). The returning troops need to know there is a place where they can unburden their souls and receive forgiveness by "confessing" their transgressions (Paquette, 2008). The concept has been used by certain religions for centuries, and the modern therapeutic process often imitates the ritual, with a few adjustments.

Self-forgiveness occurs when the soldier finds a place within herself or himself to truly forgive the atrocities of war, accepting his/her behavior as human. Grieving the loss of life is necessary in recovering one's own humanity. The past cannot be changed or reversed; it can only be accepted. Self-forgiveness may become the goal, and accepting the unacceptable is the process. Mental health professionals can help facilitate the process of forgiveness by providing compassion, patience, and a readiness to listen to the "unacceptable." Veterans who gain a sense of forgiveness will find it easier to begin the process of healing and growth. There is a greater chance that the soldier will return to civilian life with a renewed sense of purpose and a reconnection to the goodness in others and himself.

CONCLUSION

Historically, the *Diagnostic Statistical Manual* (DSM-IV-TR), (American Psychiatric Association, 2000) has not recognized spiritual distress as a symptom of PTSD, and it is unlikely to do so in its next iteration, the DSM-V, due in 2013. Nevertheless, treatment approaches must eventually include methodologies that address how to relieve psychological and spiritual distress in returning service members. With the continuation of the Iraq War, more returning service people will have experiences with combat and killing. More research and greater understanding of PTSD and its symptoms will lead to better treatment. Meanwhile, military leaders who have become expert at creating and perpetuating the war mind will need to find ways to dismantle it. For the individual veteran, the beginning of recovery from PTSD and spiritual distress may come from, first, fully understanding that killing is a primary condition of war and, second, that the decision to suspend one's morality during battle does not mean one is condemned to an eternity of guilt, shame, and instability.

REFERENCES

Amanat, E. (2003). *The miracle of love: A spiritual approach to PTSD*. Huntington Beach, CA: Narangestan publisher.

American Psychiatric Association. (1980). *Diagnostic and statistical manual of mental disorders*. (DSM-III). Washington, DC: American Psychiatric Association.

American Psychiatric Association. (2000). *Diagnostic and statistical manual of mental disorders* (DSM-IV-TR). Washington, DC: American Psychiatric Association.

Associated Press (2009, August 22). Officer expresses remorse for My Lai. *The Los Angeles Times*, p. A14.

Clarke, J. (2009). A critical view of how nursing has defined spirituality. *Journal of Clinical Nursing, 18*(12), 1666–1673.

Dossey, B. (2008). *Holistic nursing: A handbook for practice* (5th ed.). Sudbury, MA: Jones and Bartlett.

Fontana, A., and Rosenheck, R. (2004). Trauma, change in strength of religious faith, and mental health service use among veterans treated for PTSD. *Journal of Nervous and Mental Disease, 192*(9), 579–584.

Grossman, D. (2009). *On killing: The psychological cost of learning to kill in war*. New York: Back Bay Books.

Halloran, L. (2009, November 13). *Will Hasan case prompt new look at objector rules?* Retrieved May 10, 2010, from NPR.org: http://www.npr.org/templates/story/story.php?storyId=120354216

Hendin, H., and Haas, A.P. (2004). Wounds of war: The aftermath of combat in Vietnam. In D. Knafo (Ed.), *Living with terror, working with trauma: A clinician's handbook*, 155–170. Lanham, MD: Jason Aronson.

Herman, J.L. (1997). *Trauma and recovery: The aftermath of violence - from domestic abuse to political terror.* New York: Basic Books.

Hillman, J. (2004). *A terrible love of war.* New York: Penguin Press.

Kubany, E.D. (1994). A cognitive model of guilt typology in combat-related PTSD. *Journal of Traumatic Stress, 7*(1), 3–19.

Marshall, S.L.A. (1947, 1978). *Men against fire.* Gloucester, Mass: Peter Smith.

McNair, R. (2002). *Perpetration-induced traumatic stress: The psychological consequences of killing.* Westpoint, CT: Praeger.

Mysko, A., Linderum, C., LaMagna, D., Lundberg, D.T., and Kayyem, F. (Producers), and Foulkrod, P. (Director). (2006). *The Ground Truth: After the Killing Ends* [Documentary]. USA: Universal Studios.

O'Brien, M.E. (2006). *Spirituality in nursing care: Standing on holy ground* (3rd ed.). Sudbury, MA: Jones and Bartlett.

Paquette, M. (2008). The aftermath of war: Spiritual distress. *Perspectives in Psychiatric Care, 44*(3), 143–145.

Paulson, D.S., and Krippner, S. (2007). *Haunted by Combat.* Westport, CT: Praeger Security International.

Smucker, C. (2008). A phenomenological description of the experience of spiritual distress. *International Journal of Nursing Terminologies and Classifications. 2*(7), 81–91.

Snepp, F. (2009, April 27). Tortured by the past. *Los Angeles Times,* p. A21.

Soldiers of Conscience. (2007). *Backgrounder: Soldiers at War in Soldiers of Conscience* Retrieved on April 10, 2010 from http://www.pbs.org/pov/soldiersofconscience/special_background.php

Tick, E. (2005). *War in the soul: Healing our nation's veterans from PTSD.* Wheaton, IL: Quest Books.

van der Kolk (2004). Psychobiology of posttraumatic stress disorder. In J. Panksepp, (Ed.), *Textbook of biological psychiatry.* Hoboken, NJ: John Wiley & Sons, Inc.

van der Kolk, B. (2009). A Biblical Response to Posttraumatic Stress Disorder. *Annual National Sponsored Chaplaincy Development Conference 2009.* North American Mission Board, Southern Baptist Convention. p. 2.

Wilson, J.P., Drozdek, B., and S. Turkovic (2006). *Posttraumatic shame and guilt. Trauma Violence, Abuse, 2,* 122–141.

Wilson, J.P., Harel, Z., & Kahana, B. (Eds.). *Human adaptation to extreme stress: From the Holocaust to Vietnam.* New York: Plenum Press.

Chapter 5

PROZAC ARMY: MEDICATED MILITARY IN COMBAT, A CONTROVERSIAL SUBJECT

Jamshid A. Marvasti

INTRODUCTION

Thompson (2008) reported in *TIME* magazine that, for the first time in history, "a sizable and growing number of U.S. combat troops are taking daily doses of antidepressants to calm nerves strained by repeated and lengthy tours in Iraq and Afghanistan." Apparently, the antidepressant drugs are provided to enable the military to preserve frontline soldiers and help the troops to "keep their cool" (Thompson, 2008). Lawrence Korb, Pentagon personnel chief under the Reagan administration said, "This is what happens when you try to fight a long war with an army that wasn't designed for a long war" (Thompson, 2008). Clayton and Nash (2007) stated that there is no pharmaceutical panacea for the spectrum of psychological, biological, spiritual, and existential injuries that war can cause. No magic pill can erase the image of a comrade's shattered body or decrease the guilt from having traded duty with your best friend on the day that he was injured or killed. Pharmacology has no ability to restore soldiers' trust in their mastery of their world or reestablish their lost innocence. Neither can it revive their shattered faith in a higher power or create wholeness in those who left pieces of themselves on the battlefield. They desperately wish to retrieve their lost parts for the purpose of becoming whole (Clayton & Nash, 2007).

COMBAT VETERANS ON MEDICATION

For many young soldiers deployed to these war zones, use of medication may constitute a serious problem. The U.S. Food and Drug Administration (FDA) urged drug companies to expand the warning labels on their antidepressant drugs due to the increased risks of suicide in children, adolescents, and young adults between the ages of eighteen and twenty-four years old. Drug companies complied by adding this warning in their updated label. The FDA also mandated suicide warnings on mood stabilizer medications (e.g. divalproex sodium [Depakote®], pregabalin [Lyrica®], carbamazepine [Tegretol®], lamotrigine [Lamictal®].) Thompson (2008) reported that nearly 40 percent of Army suicide victims in 2006 and 2007 had taken psychotropic drugs, such as the antidepressants fluoxetine hydrochloride (HCI) (Prozac®) and sertraline HCI (Zoloft®). According to a June 2010 Defense Department report, the number of active-duty troops on psychiatric medication was about 20 percent. This number represents a wide range of drugs, from antidepressants and antipsychotics to hypnotics, drugs that Army leaders and doctors fear could impair a soldier's judgment. Another military report made in July 2010 indicated that prescription medications were involved in one third of all active-duty suicides (Fox News, 2011).

A U.S. Central Command policy allows troops being deployed to Iraq and Afghanistan to bring with them a six-month supply of psychotropic drugs. Sending patients into combat on these medications amounts to "medical malpractice" says Dr. Peter Breggin, a New York psychiatrist and expert on the side effects of psychiatric drugs (Fox News, 2011). He adds that "the drugs simply shouldn't be given to soldiers." Breggin lists some of the side effects as anxiety, violent behavior, and impulsivity, "the latter being particularly dangerous in a war zone." For example, the antipsychotic medication quetiapine fumarate (Seroquel®) was approved by the Army in a low dose as a sleep aid. This happens to be the same drug that two Marines back from Iraq were prescribed before they died in their sleep (Fox, 2011). Dr. Breggin, who has testified before the House Committee on Veterans' Affairs about the risk of using antidepressants in the military, suggested that troops who are on these medications have two choices: they can either deploy without them or stay home (Fox, 2011). Dr. Joseph Glenmullen of Harvard Medical School commented on the military's distribution of drugs, saying "there is no question they're using them to prop people up in difficult circumstances." He also warned that "The high percentage of U.S. soldiers attempting suicide after taking SSRIs [selective serotonin reuptake inhibitors] should raise serious concerns" (Thompson, 2008).

CREATING A PRECEDENT FOR COMBAT MEDICATION

In 1994, Army psychiatrist E. Cameron Ritchie suggested that Army combat units administer SSRI antidepressant drugs. She felt that it would be preferable to treat "moderate and manageable" symptoms of depression with medication than to medically evacuate soldiers. Some Navy psychiatrists disagreed, arguing that the "real safety" of these medications in combat has not been proven (Thompson, 2008). One frequent side effect of SSRIs is excessive sweating/perspiring. In high-temperature areas, such as parts of Iraq, this may result in dehydration and electrolyte imbalances in the heat of combat. Case reports and anecdotal examples indicate that homicide and suicide have been committed by those who either were on these medications or going through withdrawal from them. The scientific basis of these reports, however, is not yet confirmed.

In civilian settings, SSRI antidepressant medication is considered to be only one aspect of treatment for PTSD. Counseling and psychotherapy need to be integrated with medication, and treatment should not be solely delegated to SSRIs. Under the best conditions, these medications only partially alleviate the symptoms, and it should be noted that 50 to 60 percent of patients do not respond to them at all.

Due to the documented side effect of suicide ideation in young people, frequent evaluation in the first few months of pharmacotherapy is a strongly required component. This is not possible in combat situations because of geographical isolation and the inability of the Pentagon to employ an adequate number of mental health counselors. For example, in 2007 when the troops in Iraq increased by 30,000, the number of mental health care workers remained the same. Dr. Kathy Platoni, a clinical psychologist and Army colonel who spent nearly twelve months in Iraq with the Army, stated that complications revolve around staffing for the mental health care system. She indicated that there is an estimated 40 percent vacancy in the active component among Army and Navy psychologists. She warned that such shortages result in long treatment delays, which are likely to continue (Platoni, 2007). In this sense, medical evacuation is the answer and may substantially decrease warrior suffering, unlike the use of SSRIs alone.

The motto of the Army Medical Corps is to "conserve the fighting strength," and there are those clinicians whose goal may be to keep military personnel from medical evacuation. However, critics of this policy believe this practice to be a violation of the Hippocratic oath and that the first loyalty of a physician should be to the patient and not to the mission.

HISTORY OF USING DRUGS IN MILITARY CONFLICT

During the Vietnam War, amphetamines were supplied to U.S. service-men at night to keep them awake, hypervigilant, and hyperalert. The following morning, however, they would need to use alcohol to counteract the effects of the stimulant medication and be able to sleep. It is now well-known that U.S. pilots, while flying in Afghanistan, were given amphetamines. This was disclosed by one of the pilot's lawyers after he mistakenly bombed Canadian soldiers. When he was brought to trial, his lawyer blamed the amphetamines for causing the fatal error (White, 2004).

PREVALENCE AND EPIDEMIOLOGY

According to a *Military Times* report (March 2010), prescription orders for psychiatric or pain medications for troops have increased since 2001. The report indicates that one in six service members is on some form of psychiatric medication. A Pentagon survey carried out in 2008 revealed that about 15 percent of soldiers said they had abused prescription drugs in the past month.

Data contained in the Army fifth MHAT report found that in an anonymous survey of U.S. troops taken during the fall of 2007, about 12 percent of combat troops serving in Iraq and 17 percent of those in Afghanistan reported taking prescription antidepressant drugs, sleeping pills, or both. Escalating violence and isolated missions in Afghanistan were described as some of the factors driving the soldiers there to rely on drugs to a greater extent than soldiers concurrently serving in Iraq. This increase in drug use indicates that America's forces in Iraq and Afghanistan are enduring a heavy price in the form of mental and psychological stress (Thompson, 2008 June 5).

WHAT MEDICATIONS ARE PRESCRIBED?

Many professionals are concerned about the amount of psychoactive medications that are being given to active duty troops. For example, according to the Military Health Plan, the rate of psychoactive drug prescriptions is up 85 percent in troops ages eighteen to thirty-four since 2003. Tricare, which provides medical benefits for service members and their families, reports that since 2001 more than 73,000 prescriptions for sertraline have been dispensed, more than 38,000 for fluoxetine, almost 18,000 for paroxetine HCl

(Paxil®), and a little more than 12,000 for duloxetine HCl (Cymbalta®). These data come from a 2009 report that includes family prescriptions. All of these drugs, which are SSRI antidepressants, carry a suicide warning label for young people (Rosenberg, 2010).

In addition to an increase in the use of SSRIs, the use of anticonvulsant medications such as topiramate (Topamax®) and gabapentin (Neurontin®) has risen 56 percent since 2005, as reported by Navy Times (Tilghman & McGarry, 2010). The FDA warned recently that these drugs may also cause suicidal thinking in patients. Statistics show that 4994 troops at Fort Bragg are currently on antidepressants; another 664 are on antipsychotic medications; and many soldiers are taking more than one type of prescription drug. There is additional speculation that troops may be prescribed the antismoking medication varenicline (Chantix®), which has been linked to violence and self-harm (Rosenberg, 2010).

Using SSRIs on PTSD patients is a controversial issue. Although much of the original research indicated that SSRIs have some effect on some of the symptoms of PTSD, the Institute of Medicine (IOM) (2008) report revealed the contrary. The IOM looked at fourteen SSRI studies on civilians and veterans that met its rigorous inclusion criteria. Half were judged to provide only modest information due to methodological limitations. Of the seven studies deemed to be most informative, four were positive and three were negative. Of more concern, however, is the fact that of the three negative studies, two were on veterans (Friedman, Marmer, Baker, Sikes & Farfel, 2007; Zohar et al., 2002). The IOM report concluded that the evidence was inadequate in terms of deciding the efficacy of SSRIs in treatment of PTSD. One criticism was that most of these studies had been sponsored by the pharmaceutical industry.

OFFICIALS' CONCERN ABOUT "MEDICATED ARMY"

Veterans Administration Secretary James Peake was forced to defend the military's use of medication before the House Committee on Veterans' Affairs in 2008, saying "even in drug trials the FDA has warned that widely prescribed medications such as asthma drugs (Singulair and Advair) are linked to suicide in young people." In hearings, Senator Jim Webb, a Democrat from Virginia, called the fact that one of every six troops is now on psychoactive drugs "pretty astounding and also very troubling." A *Marine Times* article reported that retired Col. Bart Billings, a former Army psychologist, testified before Congress, saying "I feel flat-out that psychiatrists are directly responsible for deaths in our military, for some of these suicides" (Rosenberg, 2010).

The U.S. Army Surgeon General expressed concern about "overmedication" of soldiers returning from combat. A *New York Times* article, citing interviews with soldiers and health-care workers, described the "warrior transition unit" at Fort Carson, Colorado, and similar posts as "warehouses of despair where damaged men and women are kept out of site, fed a diet of prescription pills, and treated harshly by noncommissioned officers" (Dao & Frosch, 2010). About 26 percent of the soldiers at the transition center in Fort Carson were on prescribed narcotics, as reported by Cameron Gimmie Keenan of the military hospital at Fort Carson (Agnece France-Presse, 2010).

Case History 1

Sergeant Christopher LeJeune, in an interview with *TIME* Magazine (Thompson, 2008), explained the impact of difficult situations that he and his comrades experienced in Iraq. "When you search someone's house, you have it built up in your mind that these guys are terrorists, but when you go in, there's little bitty tiny shoes and toys on the floor–things like that started affecting me a lot more than I thought they would." After having worked as a Scout in Baghdad for seven months, LeJeune began to become despondent. He had been protecting Iraqi police stations that were coming under heavy attack from rocket-propelled grenades. LeJeune explained, "We'd been doing some heavy missions, and things were starting to bother me." Thompson (2008) described the missions as extremely dangerous settings where soldiers were "acting as bait to lure insurgents into the open so the Army could target them." LeJeune was diagnosed with depression, and a military physician in Iraq gave him the antidepressant Zoloft as well as the antianxiety drug clonazepam and sent him back to combat.

Upon his return in 2004, LeJeune continued to take clonazepam and other medications, as 1 of 300,000 American veterans suffering from depression or PTSD. "PTSD isn't fixed by taking pills," he said, "it's just numbed." Ultimately he stopped taking the drugs.

Case History 2

In 2009, Specialist Michael Crawford looked forward to going to Fort Carson's warrior transition battalion to help him deal with his constant suicidal thoughts. Working as an Army sniper in Iraq, he had suffered two concussions from roadside bombs and watched several platoon mates burn to death. He had returned from his tour of duty emotionally broken. At Fort Carson he became 1 of 465 soldiers in the unit. For him, the program did not work. He was prescribed numerous medications for anxiety, depression, nightmares, and headaches that left him feeling listless and disoriented. He had one session a week with a nurse-manager to deal with his issues. He became increasingly unable to report for duty appropriately and was disciplined for not following his treatment plan. In August, he attempted suicide with alcohol and painkillers. He was begging to get out of the program (Dao & Frosch, 2010).

There are 7200 soldiers in thirty-two "warrior transition units" throughout the Army. These units were established as sheltering way stations where injured soldiers could recuperate before being returned to duty or processed for discharge. Because of their psychic as well as somatic wounds, however, soldiers in these units are very susceptible to depression and addiction. They complain that drugs are prescribed too easily by the medical staff and that the amount of psychotropic drugs and narcotics make exercise, waking, and attending class very difficult. Noncommissioned officers frequently discipline soldiers in all military ranks for failure to complete these tasks, often over objections by medical staff. This discipline exacerbates their depression and hopelessness. This practice has been supported by the unit commanders (Dao & Frosch, 2010).

EFFECTIVENESS OF PHARMACOTHERAPY: OPPOSING RESEARCH FINDINGS

SSRI antidepressants are the only medications approved by the FDA for treatment of PTSD; however, they are not a panacea. Research shows that, at best, these medications only decrease the symptoms of PTSD; they do not eliminate the disorder. Treatment resistance levels with SSRIs stands at around 50 percent in clinical trials of PTSD treatment (Asnis, Kohn, Henderson & Brown 2004).

An IOM (2007) committee reviewed thirty-seven randomized controlled trials (RCTs) of psychotropic drugs. Their conclusions indicated inadequate evidence for the efficacy of several medications used to control symptoms of PTSD. These were (a) alpha-adrenergic blockers (e.g. prazosin HCl), (b) benzodiazepines (e.g. alprazolam), (c) anticonvulsives (e.g. topiramate), and (d) monoamine oxidase inhibitors (MAOIs) (e.g. phenelzine sulfate). The committee also reviewed fourteen RCTs for SSRI antidepressants (e.g. sertraline/HCl, fluoxetine/HCl, paroxetine/HCl, and citalopram hydrobromide) and concluded that, here too, evidence of effectiveness is inadequate. In this case, seven studies documented a significant effect, but the seven other trials did not (IOM, 2007).

Riggs (2009) reviewed the results from several published studies indicating the effectiveness of sertraline HCl in decreasing PTSD symptoms (Brady et al., 2000; Davidson et al., 2001; Zohar et al., 2002). Paradoxically, in their clinical guidelines, the National Institute for Health and Clinical Excellence (NICE) did not find a significant effect or superiority of sertraline over a placebo (National Collaborating Centre, 2005). The reason for the discrepancy may have been that the NICE study included two unpublished research findings in their review (Bisson, 2007).

Research on the use of benzodiazepines for treatment of trauma survivors revealed one of two things: either there was no beneficial effect (Mellman, Clark & Peacock, 2003) or, as Gelpin, Bonne, Peri, Brandes, and Shalev (1996) reported, treatment with a benzodiazepine may have created a higher likelihood of subsequent PTSD. The negative aspects to all of these studies are limited sample size and also the lack of large-scale replications.

PREVENTION OF PTSD WITH DRUGS

In regard to prevention, there are theories that if the adrenergic response to a traumatic event is being blocked by medication, we might prevent its long-term encoding as a fear response (Pitman et al., 2002). Giving propranolol, a beta-adrenergic blocker, to trauma survivors who had an initial elevated heart rate within hours of a traumatic event failed to decrease the intensity of PTSD symptoms three months later. Another study done by Stein and colleagues (2007) indicated that neither propranolol nor the anticonvulsive medication gabapentin could decrease the symptoms of PTSD when administered within forty-eight hours of a traumatic injury. Schelling and associates (2004), however, used cortisol on patients with traumatic injury resulting in a lower level of PTSD symptoms at follow-up evaluation. This research was done on patients after cardiac surgery and may not be an appropriate comparison with veterans with months of exposure to combat trauma.

Shalev (2009) explains that, currently, there is no good evidence that medication intervention can prevent the development of PTSD, because the number of studies and also the quality of the studies are very limited. SSRIs are frequently used and recommended for treatment of chronic PTSD, but their impact on the treatment of acute stress disorder (ASD) is virtually unexplored. A study of escitalopram oxalate (Lexapro®) for acute PTSD treatment pointed to no positive effect of this drug over a placebo (Shalev, 2009).

Although many anecdotal case histories and clinicians' reports describe having been somewhat successful in decreasing or preventing the development of PTSD after the trauma, so far, pharmacological prevention of PTSD has not been substantiated.

DIFFERENCES IN PTSD: CIVILIAN AND COMBAT VETERAN

Friedman and colleagues (2007) indicated that combat-related PTSD may be more refractory to therapy than is PTSD related to other kinds of traumatic incidents. Combat trauma patients have high levels of severity and intensity and also much higher levels of comorbidity, including medical problems. Wilk and Hoge (2011) explained that most of the research on PTSD treatment has been based largely on patients who had a single traumatic event such as rape, car accident, or even a household emergency. These isolated incidents cannot be compared with veterans who have experienced multiple traumatic events over a significant period of time (Wilk & Hoge, 2011).

IS THERE AN ALTERNATIVE? RITUALS, RETREAT, THERAPEUTIC REVISITING, AND SHARING THE WAR BURDEN

Dr. Edward Tick, who facilitates a series of healing retreats for veterans, discussed our need for modern rituals as a way to heal our psychologically wounded warriors. He described PTSD as, in part, the tortured conscience of good people who did their best under conditions that would dehumanize anyone (Tick, 2008).

In Native American and other ancient and traditional cultures, returning warriors are put through significant rituals of purification before they can rejoin their families or reenter society. This implies an understanding that these warriors, if left unpurified, could in fact be dangerous. Dr. Tick believes that war is inherently a moral enterprise, and veterans in search of healing are on a profound moral journey.

He suggested that ultimately leaders, not ordinary troops, are held responsible for the result of battle and for the deaths that occurred (Tick, 2008).Without this transference of responsibility the veteran carries war's secret grief and guilt for us all.

CONCLUSION

When considering military use of medication, there is a need to differentiate between two populations. One uses medication to increase their capacity for fighting (e.g. increased energy, decreased tiredness, hypervigilance, mental sharpness or clarity, and hyperattentiveness). The other group uses medication to become "normal" and minimize the mental anguish that always comes with war. So, one group wants to achieve a higher than normal state, like pilots who take amphetamines during bombing missions, and the other group wishes to alleviate despair.

Civilians who experience PTSD as a result of some form of natural disaster may have a very different response from those who develop PTSD as combat veterans. For example, PTSD may manifest itself differently in victims of an earthquake or tsunami than in a combat veteran. The civilian may not have a rage-revenge and homicidal tendency or a desire to repeat the trauma by placing themselves in a dangerous situation (similar to a war zone) by reckless behaviors such as walking in a high crime neighborhood at midnight. Suicide and homicide may not be as frequent in civilians nor will self-blame and guilt be likely to be as prevalent. A victim of PTSD as the result of a flood or fire may not be inclined to hold his hands around the neck of his wife at midnight because he believes that she is an enemy combatant. Because of these differences, medications that have been effective for treatment of PTSD in civilians may not be helpful in treating combat PTSD.

One of the reasons for the rise in PTSD, suicides, and depression in veterans is due to the fact that when they reach the level of "breakdown" in combat they are not evacuated, given rest, or relieved from duty. Instead, they are given multiple drugs and sometimes forced to stay in combat, which may result in added trauma. It is well-known that the cumulative effect of trauma may be postponed with medication but is not nullified and is likely to affect the victim eventually.

The best treatment for war trauma and PTSD in combat veterans is prevention. If PTSD, depression, and suicide are the result of multiple deployments, exhaustion, witnessing civilian casualties, and exposure to atrocities, then "collateral damage" should be avoided at any cost. Invasion may need to be postponed until an adequate supply of healthy warriors is available, and evacuation of those veterans who are suffering should have priority, even if that means retreating and abandoning the mission.

REFERENCES

Agence France Press. (2010, April 27). *US military concerned about 'over-medication' of troops, The Raw Story*. Retrieved on November 3, 2011. http://www.rawstory.com/rs/2010/04/27military-concerned-overmedication-troops/

Asnis, G.M., Kohn, S.R., Henderson, M., and Brown, N.L. (2004). SSRIs versus non-SSRIs in post traumatic stress disorder: An update with recommendations. *Drugs, 64*(4), 383–404.

Bisson, J. I. (2007). Pharmacological treatment of post-traumatic stress disorder. *Advances in Psychiatric Treatment, 13*, 119–126.

Brady K., Pearlstein T., Asnis G.M., Baker, M.D., & Rothbaum, B. (2000). Efficacy and safety of sertraline treatment of posttraumatic stress disorder: a randomized controlled trial. *Journal of the America Medical Association, 283*, 1837–1844.

Clayton, N.M., and Nash, W.P. (2007). Medication management of combat and operational stress injuries in active duty service members. In C.R. Figley and W.P. Nash (Eds.), *Combat Stress Injury: Theory, Research, and Management* (pp. 219–245). New York: Routledge.

Davidson, J., Pearlstein, T., Londborg, P., Brady, K.T., Rothbaum, B., & Bell, J. (2001). Efficacy of sertraline in preventing relapse of posttraumatic stress disorder: Results of a 28-week double-blind, placebo-controlled study. *American Journal of Psychiatry, 158*(12), 1974–1981. doi:10.1176/appi.ajp.158.12.1974 PubMed

Dao, J., and Frosch, D. (2010, April 24, p. A1). Feeling warehoused in army trauma care units. *New York Times.*

Fox News. (2011, January 19). Concerns raised about combat troops using psychotropic drugs. *Fox News Politics.* Retrieved January 22, 2011, from http://www.foxnews.com/politics/2011/01/19/concerns-raised-combat-troops-using-psychotropic-drugs/

Friedman, M.J., Marmar, C.R., Baker, D.G., Sikes, C.R., and Farfel, G.M. (2007). Randomized, double-blind comparison of sertraline and placebo for posttraumatic stress disorder in a Department of Veterans Affairs setting. *Journal of Clinical Psychiatry, 68*(5), 711–20.

Gelpin, E., Bonne, O., Peri, T., Brandes, D., and Shalev, A.Y. (1996). Treatment of recent trauma survivors with benzodiazepines: A prospective study. *Journal of Clinical Psychiatry, 57*, 390–394.

Institute of Medicine (IOM). (2008). *Treatment of posttraumatic stress disorder: An assessment of the evidence.* Washington, DC: National Academies Press Committee on Treatment of Posttraumatic Stress Disorder.

Institute of Medicine (IOM) and National Research Council. (2007). *PTSD and Military Compensation.* Washington DC: National Academies Press.

Mellman, T., Clark, R., and Peacock, W. (2003). Prescribing patterns for patients with posttraumatic stress disorder. *Psychiatric Services, 54*, 1618–1621.

Military Times. (2010 March 17). Medicating the military: Use of psychiatric drugs has spiked; concerns surface about suicide, other dangers [Report]. Retrieved on May 10, 2011 from http://militarytimes.com/news/2010/03/military_psychiatric_drugs_0317 10w/

National Collaborating Centre for Mental Health, National Institute for Health and Clinical Excellence. (2005). *Post-traumatic stress disorder: The management of PTSD in adults and children in primary and secondary care.* London: Gaskell and the British Psychological Society.

Pitman, R., Sanders, K., Zusman, R., Healy, A., Cheema, F., Lasko, N., et al. (2002). Pilot study of secondary prevention of posttraumatic stress disorder with propranolol. *Biological Psychiatry, 51*(2), 189–192.

Platoni, K. (2007, April). Healing on the home front. *Clinical Psychiatry News, (35)*12.

Riggs, D.S. (2009). Treatment of anxiety disorders. In S.M. Freeman, B.A. Moore, and A. Freeman (Eds.). *Living and Surviving in Harms Way* (pp. 211–237). New York: Routledge.

Rosenberg, M. (2010, October 15). Are soldiers suicides caused by prescription drugs? *OpEdNews*. Retrieved on June 24, 2011 from http://www.opednews.com/articles/Are-Soldiers-Suicides-Caus-by-Martha-Rosenberg-101015-973.html

Schelling, G., Kilger, E., Roozendaal, B., de Quervain, D. J., Briegel, J., Dagge, A., Rothenhausler, H.B., Krauseneck, T., Nollert, G. & Kapfhammer, H.P. (2004). Stress doses of hydrocortisone, traumatic memories, and symptoms of posttraumatic stress disorder in patients after cardiac surgery: A randomized study. *Biological Psychiatry, 55,* 627–633.

Shalev, A.Y. (2009). Posttraumatic stress disorder and stress-related disorders. *Psychiatric Clinics of North America, 32,* 687–704.

Stein, M.B., Kerridge, C., Dimsdale, J.E., & Hoyt, D.B. (2007). Pharmacotherapy to prevent PTSD: Results from a randomized controlled proof-of-concept trial in physically injured patients. *Journal of Traumatic Stress, 20*(6), 923–932.

Thompson, M. (2008, June 5). America's Medicated Army. *Time*. Retrieved November 11, 2009 from http://www.time.com/time/printout/0,8816,1811858,00.html

Tick, E. (2008). Heal the warrior, heal the country. *Yes Magazine*. Retrieved February 8, 2011 from http://www.yesmagazine.org/issues/a-just-foreign-policy/heal-the-warrior-heal-the-country

Tilghman, A., & McGarry, B. (2010, March). Medicating the military: Use of psychiatric drugs has spiked; concerns surface about suicide, other dangers. *MilitaryTimes*. Retrieved on Nov 15, 2011 from http://www.armytimes.com/news/2010/03/military_psychiatric_drugs_031710w/

White, J. (2004 July 7). Air force pilot who bombed Canadians is fined $5,672. *Washington Post.*

Wilk, J.E., and Hoge, C.W. (2011). Military and veteran populations. In D.M. Benedek and G.H. Wynn (Eds.), *Clinical Manual for Management of PTSD* (pp. 349–369). Washington, DC: American Psychiatric Publishing, Inc.

Zohar, J., Amital, D., Miodownik, C., Kolter, M., Bleich, A., & Lane, R. (2002). Double-blind placebo-controlled pilot study of sertraline in military veterans with posttraumatic stress disorder. *Journal of Clinical Psychopharmacology, 22,* 190–195.

Chapter 6

PHARMACOTHERAPY FOR PTSD: ANTIDEPRESSANT MEDICATIONS

JAMSHID A. MARVASTI

SSRI ANTIDEPRESSANTS

SSRI medications are currently being used to decrease or control some of the symptoms of PTSD. In 1998 sertraline was the first medication approved by the FDA for this purpose, followed shortly by paroxetine. Although other SSRIs do not have approval from the FDA for PTSD treatment, there are a number of clinical reports indicating that they are just as effective.

When sertraline and paroxetine were compared with a placebo treatment, they decreased some of the symptoms associated with PTSD (Marshall, Beebe & Oldham, 2001). The clinical significance of these improvements was limited, however. The data for sertraline are more ambiguous than those of paroxetine (Bisson, 2007).

The Department of Veterans' Affairs and the Department of Defense (VA-DoD, 2004) considers SSRIs to have "significant benefit in therapy for PTSD." However, a number of clinical experiences bring into question just how significant this benefit is.

Ipser, Seedat, and Stein (2006) found evidence to support the use of SSRIs as first-line agents in the treatment of PTSD. SSRIs are thought to change the noradrenergic and serotonergic systems of the brain, which are involved in activating states of arousal. The effectiveness of these medications may also be related to the potency of serotonin over norepinephrine reuptake blockade (Crockett & Davidson, 2002).

Research suggests that PTSD symptoms, such as impulse control problem, sleep disorder, and repetitive response to intrusive recollections and traumatic memories, are considered to be disorders of 5-hydroxytryptophan (5-HTP), which may also explain the efficacy of SSRIs because 5-HTP is a precursor to serotonin. Animal studies have revealed that serotonin type 2 (5-HT2) receptor pathways are mediators of conditioned avoidance, resilience to stress, and the process of learned helplessness (Krystal, 1990). Essentially, SSRIs inhibit the reuptake of serotonin in the synapse, which causes a down-regulation of receptors, such as 5-HT2, while influencing other neurotransmitters, such as dopamine and norepinephrine.

EFFICACY OF SSRIs

It is documented that moderate or significant improvement is seen in approximately 60 percent of PTSD patients who are treated with SSRI antidepressants (Marshall et al., 2001). Remission rates, when the individual no longer meets the criteria for the diagnosis, are approximately 25 percent (Davidson, 2004). Response rates have been lower for Vietnam-era combat veterans with chronic, severe PTSD. There is some speculation that the limited response to SSRI treatment among civilians may be due to the opportunity for "secondary gain" through disability compensation (Schoenfeld, Marmar & Neylan, 2004).

In 2004, The VA-DoD guidelines recommended that SSRIs be tried for a period of at least twelve weeks before changing them or deeming them ineffective. While waiting for the therapeutic benefits to start, some patients may feel even worse for a period of time due to the initial adverse effects of SSRIs, which are common during the process of receptor down-regulation (VA-DoD, 2004).

MECHANISM OF SSRIs

SSRIs increase the brain-derived neurotrophic factor (BDNF), which is reduced in individuals exposed to extreme stress and may be associated with the atrophy of the hippocampus seen in some cases of PTSD. Serotonin may increase the availability of BDNF by initiating a signal transduction cascade that leads to its release. This action could also be increased by medications that elevate serotonin, such as SSRIs (Stahl & Grady, 2010). In addition to inhibiting the serotonin reuptake, SSRIs have other pharmacological properties, such as norepinephrine and dopamine reuptake inhibition. Each SSRI has a different set of secondary properties, that may contribute to its therapeutic or side effects profiles (Stahl & Grady, 2010).

REDUCTION OF SYMPTOMS OF PTSD BY SSRIs

In some studies, SSRIs have been shown decrease all three of the main symptom clusters of PTSD: reexperiencing, hyperarousal, and emotional numbness and avoidance. Some clinicians have called SSRIs the "shock absorbers" of the mind, because they have been documented to cause a reduction in anger even before depression or other PTSD symptoms are diminished (Hierholzer, 2010). Veterans with PTSD who take SSRIs report that their "fuse" seems longer. This change has been observed within a few days of starting treatment and in patients who have received a lower dose than usually prescribed for depression.

Sometimes it is the friends and family of the veteran who first notice that anger has decreased. Often this effect is confirmed if the patient discontinues the medication. The veteran's loved ones may suspect that he or she has become noncompliant with medication when they see an abrupt increase in the patient's anger. A former Vietnam War medic explained that when he stopped his sertraline he perceived that people around him were suddenly "lots more angry and difficult." Later on he realized that it was his appraisal of others that had suddenly changed. In this sense, one may conclude that SSRIs may induce emotional dampening and reduction of anger (Hierholzer, 2010). It is also possible that these changes may be due to the initial alleviation of depression, beginning with a change in the level of anger and rage.

Sertraline

Sertraline has weak dopamine reuptake properties and is approved for treatment of PTSD, panic disorder, social anxiety disorder, obsessive-compulsive disorder (OCD), major depression, and premenstrual dysphoric disorder (Stahl & Grady, 2010).

In several studies, sertraline has demonstrated efficacy in the short-term and long-term treatment of PTSD, regardless of the nature of the trauma or the age of the traumatic occurrence. One study (Stein, van der Kolk, Austin, Fayyad & Clary, 2006) compared the effects of sertraline among adult patients with different index traumas and found this medication to be significantly more effective than the placebo was, regardless of whether patients had experienced interpersonal trauma or childhood abuse. Rothbaum and colleagues (2006) conducted a study to compare the benefit of augmenting sertraline with prolonged exposure (PE) therapy to sertraline alone. Patients who received sertraline alone reported a significant reduction in PTSD symptoms after ten weeks but no further reduction after an additional five weeks. Those who received a combination of sertraline and PE, however, did report a further reduction in symptoms after five additional weeks (Rothbaum et al., 2006).

Dosage. The recommended dosage of sertraline is between 50 and 200 mg per day for adults.

Drug interactions. Because it is tightly bound to plasma proteins, one should be cautious when using this medication in combination with those drugs that have similar characteristics, such as warfarin sodium (Coumadin®). A prothrombin time should always be used to monitor blood clotting when sertraline and warfarin are used together. When sertraline is combined with other SSRIs or migraine medications, such as triptans, there may be a concern regarding the development of serotonin syndrome. The administration of sertraline with MAOIs is contraindicated, because it may significantly increase the risk of serotonin syndrome. Sertraline may increase toxicity of diazepam, tolbutamide, and warfarin. This increase may be due to the capacity of sertraline to inhibit the cytochrome P-450 enzymes or displacement from plasma protein binding (Gore & Lucas, 2010).

Precaution. Sertraline is listed as category C for pregnancy. Fetal risk was revealed in animals but has not yet been established in human beings. It is generally accepted that if the benefit outweighs the risk, sertraline may be used during pregnancy. Other precautions should be used with patients who have preexisting seizure disorder, recent myocardial infarction, hepatic or renal impairment, or an unstable heart problem (Gore & Lucas, 2010). In young people, increased risk of suicide is associated to SSRIs medication.

Paroxetine

Paroxetine is a potent inhibitor of presynaptic serotonin (5-HT) reuptake. It is also a norepinephrine reuptake inhibitor, especially in higher doses, which leads some professionals to think that it should be included in the new class of dual serotonin and norepinephrine reuptake inhibitors (SNRIs). Paroxetine was originally approved for depression; since it came onto the market, however, it has been used for the treatment of panic disorder, OCD, PTSD, social anxiety disorder, and generalized anxiety disorder (GAD). It is also effective in treating postmenopausal hot flashes (Ehmke & Nemeroff, 2009).

Marshall and colleagues (2001) conducted a large randomized placebo-control trial on patients with chronic PTSD, with significant improvements found in paroxetine-treated patients who were given dosages of 20 mg and 40 mg a day. Paroxetine was effective in treating the three main cluster groups of reexperiencing, hyperarousal and avoidance and numbing, in comparison with the placebo. In their research, Tucker and associates (2001) indicated that paroxetine was superior to the placebo. They revealed that in an open label trial, this medication not only caused improvements in subjective symptoms but also normalized elevated heart rate and blood pressure reactivity in PTSD patients with comorbid depression. Bremne, Vermetten, and Charney (2003) reported that the year-long treatment of PTSD patients with 10 to 50 mg a day of paroxetine was associated with improvement in verbal declarative memory and increases in hypocampal volume.

Pharmacokinetics. Paroxetine has an anticholinergic effect, which contributes to its anxiolytic efficacy. Paroxetine is a norepinephrine reuptake inhibitor, a nitric oxide synthesis inhibitor and a potent Cyp-450-2d6 inhibitor. Paroxetine may have a rapid decline in the plasma level and contribute to withdrawal symptoms upon sudden discontinuation (Gore & Lucas, 2010). Paroxetine is well-absorbed from the gastrointestinal tract, and its absorption is not influenced by the presence or absence of food in the stomach (Kaye, Haddock & Langley, 1989).

Dosage. The recommended dose of paroxetine is 20 to 50 mg. Adults generally start with 20 mg per day, which may be increased in 10-milligram intervals every week.

Drug interactions. Medical literature recommends that individuals taking paroxetine should avoid alcohol, tryptophan, and thioridazine. Paroxetine may cause hyperreflexia, weakness, and lack of coordination when it is mixed with sumatriptan. Caution should be used when mixing with drugs that are metabolized by Cyp-450-2d6. In addition, caution should be used when mixed with lithium, digoxin, diuretics, phenobarbital, warfarin, phenytoin, guanidine, and monotheophylline.

SSRI DISCONTINUATION SYNDROME

Withdrawal syndrome is possible with abrupt discontinuation of SSRI medications, with the exception of fluoxetine because of its long half-life. This syndrome has several characteristics, including flulike symptoms, such as headache, lightheadedness, chills, and body aches. Neurological symptoms such as paresthesias, an "electric shock-like" sensation, may also occur. These symptoms disappear without specific treatment over one to two weeks after discontinuation. There are reports that some patients do experience more protracted discontinuation syndrome, especially those who were treated with paroxetine. One strategy is to decrease the medication gradually. Another is to substitute the SSRI for a brief course of fluoxetine, for example, 10 mg for one to two weeks, then discontinue the fluoxetine (Schatzberg, Blier & Delgado, 2006).

Because withdrawal symptoms are often misdiagnosed as a return of depression or anxiety, a mnemonic device has been employed to improve detection of SSRI withdrawal symptoms. Clinicians are advised to watch for symptoms of HANGMAN, where the H stands for headache, the A for anxiety, the N for nausea, the G for gait instability, the M for malaise, the A for asthenia (fatigue), and the N for numbness (paresthesias) (Marvasti & Cunningham, 2008).

Specific Side Effects of SSRI Antidepressives

Gastrointestinal problems. These may include nausea, vomiting, and diarrhea and are generally dose dependent and tend to decrease in severity over the first few weeks of treatment. In some patients, however, diarrhea may persist. SSRIs may predispose people to bleeding disorders by blocking the uptake of serotonin into platelets.

Activation/insomnia. These medications sometimes exacerbate restlessness and may precipitate aggression and sleep disorder. Akathisia (restless leg syndrome) is another side effect of SSRIs and at any time may contribute to the development of suicidal behavior (Lineberry, Ramaswamy, Bostwick & Rundell, 2006). Akathisia is sometimes treated using a beta-blocker or benzodiazepines. In regard to insomnia as sign of SSRI activation, some patients responded well to melatonin and others to trazodone or sedative hypnotic medication (Caley, 1997).

Sexual side effects. Erectile or ejaculatory dysfunction, loss of libido, and anorgasmia may be complications of antidepressant medication. In a veteran population, any sexual disorder needs to be evaluated in detail and on a case-by-case basis. Many of these veterans have PTSD, which by itself may cause sexual disorder. Some may have underlying medical problems that cause sexual disorder. Still others have drug or alcohol addiction or are using medication for pain or hypertension, which may have side effects of sexual disorder. At times, a disturbance in marital relationship may be the primary cause of sexual problem.

Since genital anesthesia is a side effect of SSRIs, these medications have also been used to reduce obsession with sexuality in the treatment of sexual offenders and uncontrollable paraphilias. Citalopram may be contraindicated for these populations, because it has been associated with spontaneous orgasms, yawning, and clitoral priapism.

A recent Cochrane Data Base review reveals that some trials suggest that the addition of sildenafil or bupropion may reduce antidepressant-induced erectile dysfunction in men (Rudkin, Taylor & Hawton, 2004). A sexual side effect of paroxetine is a dose-dependent element and does not appear to decrease with prolonged administration of this medication. Recommendations for decreasing the impact of SSRI medication on sexual functioning include:

1. Decreasing the dosage
2. Changing to a different antidepressant with lesser side-effect liability
3. Adding an agent. These agents are sildenafil, yohimbine, buspirone, cyproheptadine, amantadine, methylphenidate, bupropion and tadalafil. These medications may be helpful in reversing arousal difficulty, erectile dysfunction, or orgasmic problem (Balon & Segraves, 2008; Rosen, Lane & Menza, 1999; Segraves, 2007). However, some controlled studies indicate that the efficacy of these agents is lacking, with one exception. Apparently, ephedrine, which has been previously shown to enhance genital blood flow in women, was used in nineteen women who had sexual dysfunction as a side effect of an SSRI. Ephedrine significantly improved self-reported scores of desire and orgasm intensity, compared with baseline scores. It should be noted, however, that these measures were also similarly enhanced by a placebo (Meston, 2004).

Neurological side effects. SSRIs may precipitate migraine and tension headaches. These effects tend to be temporary and in most cases will gradually decrease within the first few weeks of treatment and may disappear altogether. There are some reports that with continued treatment, SSRIs may actually help to prevent or even treat migraine headaches (Doughty & Lyle, 1995). SSRIs may also cause extrapyramidal side effects, including akathisia, parkinsonism, dystonia, and tardive dyskinesia (Gerber & Lynd, 1998). The incidence of such side effects is generally low; however, with older patients, especially those with Parkinson's disease this incidence may be higher.

Serotonin syndrome. In rare cases, an SSRI may contribute to the development of serotonin syndrome, which is due to an excess of central nervous system serotonergic activity. The signs and symptoms of this syndrome are abdominal pain, flushing, sweating, diarrhea, hyperthermia, lethargy, change in mental status, rhabdomyolysis, tremor, myoclonus, renal failure, cardiovascular shock, and possibly death (Boyer & Shannon, 2005). Serotonin syndrome has been reported when SSRIs are coadministered with medication such as tramadol HCl (Ultram®), high-dose triptans (migraine medications), or the antibiotic linezolid (Zyvox®), which also has some ability to inhibit MAO.

Amotivational syndrome. Lack of motivation (amotivational syndrome) and apathy have been reported as potential side effects of SSRIs. These side effects may surface after several months of treatment and are frequently misdiagnosed as recurrence of initial depression. Because amotivational syndrome is often dose oriented, increasing the dose may exacerbate these symptoms. According to Popper (1998), apathy and amotivational syndrome may also be misdiagnosed as marijuana-induced amotivational syndrome if the patient was also known to be using cannabis for self-medication.

Nocturnal Bruxism. Grinding of the teeth is another potential side effect of SSRIs. The headaches associated with bruxism need to be differentiated from migraine or nonmigraine headaches, because these conditions can also be exacerbated by SSRIs. Some individuals will be unaware of grinding their teeth during sleep and may present with complaints of a morning headache.

OTHER ANTIDEPRESSANT MEDICATIONS

SNRIs: Venlafaxine

Davidson and colleagues (2006) conducted a six-month, double-blind, placebo-controlled trial among 329 adult outpatients with a primary diagnosis of PTSD to determine the efficacy of venlafaxine (Effexor®) extended release (ER), an SNRI. Researchers concluded that when compared with the placebo group, the treatment group improved significantly on cluster symptoms, such as reexperiencing, avoidance, and numbing, but not hyperarousal. Also, the remission rate among the venlafaxine ER group was higher than with the placebo, and the medication was well-tolerated over the course of the study (Davidson et al., 2006). The VA-DOD (2004) guidelines consider venlafaxine to have "some benefit" for treatment of PTSD (Malberg & Schechter, 2005).

Side Effects of SNRIs

The side effects of SNRIs are similar to those of SSRIs; however, SNRIs are more likely to cause side effects that reflect noradrenergic activity, including increased pulse rate, dilated pupils, excessive sweating, constipation, dry mouth, and hypertension.

Mirtazapine

Mechanism of Action

Mirtazapine (Remeron®) is structurally unrelated to any other psychotropic medication. It enhances noradrenergic and serotonergic transmission and has no significant affinity for dopamine receptors, low affinity for muscarinic cholinergic receptors, and high affinity for histamine-1 (De Boer, 1996).

By blocking alpha-2 receptors, mirtazapine increases both serotonin and norepinephrine. However, because 5-HT receptors are also blocked by these medications, the net stimulation falls on 5-HT1A receptors. This results in the release of dopamine, the element that may help with depression and anxiety. In turn it may contribute to anxiolytic, antidepressant, and sleep-restoring properties. Histamine-1 receptor antagonism may help insomnia and anxiety but may also cause sedation and contribute to weight gain (Stahl & Grady, 2010).

Mirtazapine has a different mechanism of action in comparison with SSRIs, and there are some expectations that if combat-related PTSD does not respond to SSRIs, or SSRIs increase the PTSD hyperactivity and hyperarousal, then mirtazapine may be a better choice of treatment. It absorbs well from the gastrointestinal tract, and the presence of food in the stomach does not interfere with the absorption of this medication.

Effectiveness

Mirtazapine has been approved for the treatment of major depression. In one trial, those who had developed side effects of sexual problems when taking an SSRI medication were put on mirtazapine after discontinuation of the SSRI. Fifty-four percent of these patients described improvements in sexual functioning (Fava, Dunner & Greist, 2001); however, it was not as effective in reversing the SSRI-associated sexual side effects in those patients who were taking fluoxetine (Michelson, Kociban & Tamura, 2002). It was found to be effective in those patients with depression who also had symptoms of anxiety, and reduced their anxiety as early as the first week of treatment (Goodnick, Puig & DeVane, 1999).

In an eight-week open label study of six patients who had severe and chronic PTSD, this medication resulted in reductions on a scale of PTSD severity (Connor, Davidson, Weisler & Ahearn, 1999). Another six-week double-blind comparison study compared mirtazapine with sertraline in Korean veterans who were suffering from PTSD. Mirtazapine was statistically significantly superior to sertraline on several measures and its efficacy was maintained to twenty-four weeks (Chung, Min, Kim, Kim, & Jun, 2004).

Due to its sedating properties, mirtazapine has been used for treatment of patients with primary sleep disorders. In a double-blind cross-over study of seven patients with obstructive sleep apnea, this medication produced significantly greater reduction in apnea-hypopnea index scores in comparison with a placebo. The dosage was 4.5 mg to 50 mg a day (Carley, Olopade & Ruigt, 2007).

It is possible that, due to its anxiolytic and sedative effect, mirtazapine may be useful for treatment of PTSD. It may also be helpful for those with comorbidity of obstructive sleep apnea (Maher, Rego & Asnis, 2006). In a small study on treatment of combat related PTSD, mirtazapine was found to be effective in decreasing the symptoms of PTSD (Kim, Pae, Chae, Jun & Bahk, 2005). Additionally, Lewis found it helpful in decreasing the nightmares and associated insomnia in a population of refugee patients with PTSD (Lewis, 2002). The VA-DoD (2004) guidelines also consider mirtazapine to have "some benefit" for treatment of PTSD (Malberg & Schechter, 2005).

Side effects. The most commonly reported side effects of mirtazapine are somnolence, increased appetite, weight gain, and dry mouth (Fava et al. 2001). Most of these side effects generally decreased over time; however, there are reports that weight gain associated with this medication is greater than with other antidepressants. Mirtazapine may increase cholesterol levels in some patients (Davis & Wilde, 1996). The risk of weight gain is believed to decrease if the dosage is lower than 30 mg per day (Barkin, Schwer & Barkin, 2000). The noradrenergic effect of this medication is dose dependent and may increase at dosages of more than 50 mg per day (Kent, 2000).

Tricyclic Antidepressants

There are relatively few controlled studies (Davidson, Kudler & Smith, 1990; Kosten, Frank, Dan, McDougle & Gille, 1991) investigating the effectiveness of TCAs in reducing symptoms associated with PTSD. TCAs were among the first antidepressant medications used to treat comorbid symptoms of anxiety. The use of other anxiolytics, such as benzodiazepines, however, became more commonplace due to their ability to immediately diffuse symptoms of panic and acute anxiety. Symptoms such as tension, apprehension, and worry are more responsive to antidepressants; somatic symptoms associated with anxiety disorders are responding better to benzodiazepines.

TCA medications, including amitriptyline (Elavil®) and imipramine (Tofranil®) were used in the treatment of PTSD for their sedative and hypnotic effects. There are not enough studies, however, to show their effectiveness, and side effects are a concern. An overdose of these medications can also be lethal (Bisson, 2007; Lerer, Bleich & Kotler, 1987).

Side effects. The cardiac and anticholinergic effects associated with these medications limit their use. Other side effects associated with TCAs include orthostatic hypotension, sedation, weight gain, and cardiotoxicity.

Monoamine Oxidase Inhibitors

Although MAOIs were initially used to promote abreaction among Vietnam veterans with combat-related PTSD, a few small controlled trials found that these medications were also effective in reducing symptoms associated with comorbid disorders such as depression and anxiety (Hogben & Cornfield, 1981; Kosten et al., 1991; Shestatzsky, Greenberg & Lerer, 1988). There has been a lack of large placebo-controlled trials investigating the efficacy of MAOIs with PTSD because the dietetic restrictions and risk of hypertensive crises associated with this class of medications has decreased interest in their use as first-line agents. According to Davidson and colleagues (2006), MAOIs may be useful as an adjunctive therapy among patients who have a minimal response to SSRIs after four to six weeks of treatment.

Phenelzine

In one trial, phenelzine (Nardil®) showed significantly reduced intrusion and re-experiencing symptoms of PTSD but had no effect on avoidance symptoms. Usually this medication is reserved for those who did not respond to SSRI or TCA medication.

The recommended adult dosage for phenelzine is 15 mg three times per day. Co-administration with foods containing tyramine can cause hypertension crisis. Concurrent use with tryptophan should be approached with caution because it may result in serotonin syndrome. Phenelzine may enhance the effect of meperidine, and concomitant prescription of these two drugs should be avoided. This medication is contraindicated for those who have alcohol problems, congestive heart failure, and pheochromocytoma. Additionally, it may decrease the seizure threshold, a concern when treating patients who have epilepsy (Gore & Lucas, 2010).

The VA-DoD (2004) guidelines explained that older antidepressant medications such as TCAs and MAOIs have "some benefit" in treatment of PTSD. Research shows that both of these medications may reduce insomnia and symptoms of re-experiencing. MAOIs outperformed TCAs when the two were compared; however, neither was effective in decreasing emotional numbing and avoidance of PTSD (Coope, Carty & Creamer, 2005). The pregnancy risk for phenelzine is category C.

Augmentation

For those who cannot tolerate SSRI medications or show no improvement, second-line augmentation medications have been used, such as TCAs or MAOIs (Ruzek, Curran & Friedman, 2004). Augmentation may also be considered for those who have partial response to SSRIs. Augmentation with an adrenergic-inhibiting agent may help those who have excessive arousal, hyperactivity, or dissociation. Those who demonstrate emotional lability, impulsivity, or aggression may benefit from augmentation with an anticonvulsant agent (Ruzek et al., 2004).

COMBAT CONSIDERATIONS

Clayton and Nash (2007) explained that each military service has its own regulation concerning deployment of personnel who are taking SSRI antidepressants. They report that many military personnel who are taking SSRIs are able to carry out their duty; however, service members who engage in special high-risk duty (e.g. aviation and handling of nuclear weapons) are restricted from taking SSRIs while performing their jobs (Clayton & Nash, 2007). This discrepancy is somewhat disturbing, because one veteran on medication may be restricted from aviation but may be allowed to drive a bus full of personnel on narrow roads in dangerous areas of Afghanistan. Reportedly, SSRI medications are not toxic to any organs and apparently do not interfere with cognitive or motor functioning (Wadsworth, Moss, Simpson & Smith, 2005). Clinicians have identified multiple cases of abnormal blood electrolytes, however. In addition, pharmacological literature documents multiple side effects such as agitation, blurred vision, pounding heartbeat, muscle tenderness/weakness, trembling, nausea/vomiting, dizziness, akathisia, and excessive sweating (*The Complete Pill Guide*, 2003). These side effects are not compatible with combat duty regardless of the level of risk of a specific mission.

SNRIs (e.g. venlafaxine) have a warning of hypertension. This risk appears to be greater when doses are more than 150 mg per day (Thase, Tran & Wiltse, 2005).

Due to significant side effects of TCAs, including life-threatening toxicity at high doses as well as danger of overdose, these medications are considered less than optimal for active duty veterans.

REFERENCES

Balon, R., and Segraves, R.T. (2008). Survey of treatment practices for sexual dysfunction(s) associated with antidepressants. *Journal of Sex and Martial Therapy*, 34, 353–365 [G].

Barkin, R.L., Schwer, W., Barkin, S.J. (2000). Recognition and management of depression in primary care: A focus on the elderly. A pharmacotherapeutic overview of the selection process among the traditional and new antidepressants. *American Journal of Therapeutics, 7,* 205–226.

Bisson, J.I. (2007). Pharmacological treatment of post-traumatic stress disorder. *Advances in Psychiatric Treatment, 13,* 119–126.

Boyer, E.W., and Shannon, M. (2005). The serotonin syndrome. *New England Journal of Medicine, 352,* 1112–1120.

Bremner, J.D., Vermetten, E., and Charney, D.S. (2003). Long-term treatment with paroxetine increases verbal declarative memory and hippocampal volume in posttraumatic stress disorder. *Biological Psychiatry,* 54, 693–702.

Caley, C.F. (1997). Extrapyramidal reactions and the selective serotonin-reuptake inhibitors. *Annals of Pharmacotherapy, 31,* 1481–1489 [F].

Carley, D.W., Olopade, C., and Ruigt, G.S. (2007). Efficacy of mirtazapine in obstructive sleep apnea syndrome. *Sleep, 30,* 35–41.

Chung, M.Y., Min, K.H., Kim, S.S., Kim, W.C., and Jun, E.M. (2004). Efficacy and tolerability of mirtazapine and sertraline in Korean veterans with posttraumatic stress disorder: a randomized open label trial. *Human Psychopharmacology, 19,* 489–494.

Clayton, N.M., and Nash, W.P. (2007). Medication management of combat and operational stress injuries in active duty service members. In C.R. Figley and W.P. Nash (Eds.), *Combat Stress Injury: Theory, Research, and Management* (pp. 219–245). New York: Routledge.

Connor, K.M., Davidson, J.R.T., Weisler, R.H., and Ahearn, E. (1999). A pilot study of mirtazapine in post-traumatic stress disorder. *International Clinical Psychopharmacology, 14,* 29–31.

Cooper, J., Carty, J., and Creamer, M. (2005). Pharmacotherapy for posttraumatic stress disorder: Empirical review and clinical recommendations. *Australian and New Zealand Journal of Psychiatry, 39,* 674–682.

Crockett, B.A., and Davidson, J.R. (2002). Pharmacotherapy for posttraumatic stress disorder. In D.J. Stein and E. Hollander (Eds.), *Textbook of Anxiety Disorder,* pp. 387–402. Washington DC: American Psychiatric Publishing.

Davidson, J.R.T. (2004). Remission in post-traumatic stress disorder (PTSD): Effects of sertraline as assessed by the Davidson trauma scale, clinical global impressions and the clinician-administered PTSD scale. *International Journal of Psychopharmacology, 19,* 85–87.

Davidson, J., Kudler, H., and Smith, R. (1990) Treatment of post-traumatic stress disorder with amitriptyline and placebo. *Archives of General Psychiatry, 47,* 259–266.

Davidson, J.R., Rothbaum, B.O., & Tucker, P., Asnis, G., Benatia, I., & Musgnung, J. (2006). Venlafaxine extended release in posttraumatic stress disorder: A 6-month randomized controlled trial. *Journal of Clinical Psychopharmacology, 26*(3), 259-267.

Davis, R., and Wilde, M.I. (1996). Mirtazapine: A review of its pharmacology and therapeutic potential in the management of major depression. *CNS Drugs, 5,* 389–402 [F].

De Boer, T. (1996). The pharmacologic profile of mirtazapine. *Journal of Clinical Psychiatry, 57*(suppl 4), 19–25.

Department of Veterans Affairs & Department of Defense (VA-DoD). (2004). *VA/DoD Clinical Practice Guideline for the Management of Post Traumatic Stress.* Washington, DC: Office of Quality and Performance. Available at http://www.oqp.med.va.gov/cpg/PTSD/PTSD_Base/htm

Doughty, M.J., and Lyle, W.M. (1995). Medications used to prevent migraine headaches and their potential ocular adverse effects. *Optom Vis Sci , 72*, 879–891 [F].

Ehmke, C.J. and Nemeroff, C.B. (2009). Paroxetine. In A.F. Schatzberg and C.B. Nemeroff (Eds.), *Textbook of Psychopharmacology* (pp. 321–352). Washington, DC: American Psychiatric Publishing, Inc.

Fava, M., Dunner, D.L., and Greist, J.H. (2001). Efficacy and safety of mirtazapine in major depressive disorder patients after SSRI treatment failure: An open-label trial. *Journal of Clinical Psychiatry, 62*, 413–420.

Gerber, P.E., and Lynd, L.D. (1998). Selective serotonin-reuptake inhibitor-induced movement disorders. *Annals of Pharmacotherapy, 32*, 692–698

Goodnick, P.J., Puig, A., and DeVane, C.L. (1999). Mirtazapine in major depression with comorbid generalized anxiety disorder. *Journal of Clinical Psychiatry, 60*, 446–448.

Gore, A., and Lucas, J.Z. (2010, July 1). Posttraumatic stress disorder. *eMedicine Psychiatry.* Retrieved on Nov. 15, 2011 from https://emedicine.medscape.com/article/288154-overview.

Hierholzer, R. (2010, May). Do Antidepressants alter emotional processing in PTSD? *The American Journal of Psychiatry.* Retrieved May 7, 2010, from http://ajp.psychiatryonline.org/cgi/content/short/167/5/599?rss=1

Hogben, G.L., and Cornfield, R.B. (1981). Treatment of traumatic war neurosis with phenelzine. *Archives of General Psychiatry, 38*(4), 440–445.

Ipser, J., Seedat, S., and Stein, D.J. (2006, October). Pharmacotherapy for post-traumatic stress disorder—a systematic review and meta-analysis. *South Africa Medical Journal, 96*(10), 1088–1096.

Kaye, C.M., Haddock, R.E., and Langley, P.F. (1989). A review of the metabolism and pharmacokinetics of paroxetine in man. *Acta Psychiatrica/ Scandinavica Supplementum, 350*, 60–75.

Kent, J. M. (2000). SNaRIs, NaSSAs, and NaRIs: New agents for the treatment of depression. *Lancet, 355*, 911–918.

Kim, W., Pae, C.U., Chae, J.H., Jun, T.Y., and Bahk, W.M. (2005). The effectiveness of mirtazapine in the treatment of post-traumatic stress disorder: A 24-week continuation therapy. *Psychiatry and Clinical Neurosciences, 59*(6), 743–747.

Kosten, T.R., Frank, J.B., Dan, E., McDougle, C.J., and Gille, E.L. Jr. (1991). Pharmacotherapy for posttraumatic stress disorder using phenelzine or imipramine. *Journal of Nervous and Mental Disease, 179*(6), 366-370.

Krystal, H. (1990) Animal models for posttraumatic stress disorder. In Giller, E.L. (Ed.), *Biological Assessment and Treatment of Posttraumatic Stress Disorder* (pp. 3–26). Washington, DC: American Psychiatric Press.

Lerer, B., Bleich, A., and Kotler, M. (1987). Posttraumatic stress disorder in Israeli combat veterans. Effect of phenelzine treatment. *Archives of General Psychiatry, 44*(11), 976–981.

Lewis, J.D. (2002). Mirtazapine for PTSD nightmares. *American Journal of Psychiatry, 159*, 1948–1949.

Lineberry, T.W., Ramaswamy, S., Bostwick, J.M., and Rundell, J.R. (2006, May). Traumatized troops: How to treat combat-related PTSD. *Current Psychiatry, 5*(5), 39–40, 45–48, 51–53.

Maher, M.J., Rego, S.A., and Asnis, G.M. (2006). Sleep disturbances in patients with posttraumatic stress disorder: Epidemiology, impact and approaches to management. *CNS Drugs, 20*(7), 567–590.

Malberg, J.E., and Schechter, L.E. (2005). Increasing hippocampal neurogenesis: A novel mechanism for antidepressant drugs. *Current Pharmaceutical Design, 11*, 145–155.

Marshall, R.D., Beebe, K.L., and Oldham, M. (2001). Efficacy and safety of paroxetine treatment for chronic PTSD: A fixed-dose, placebo-controlled study. *American Journal of Psychiatry, 158*(12), 1982–1988.

Marvasti, J.A. and Cunningham, K.M. (2008). Trauma of terrorism: Pharmacotherapy in acute trauma and PTSD. In J.A. Marvasti (Ed.), *Psycho-Political Aspects of Suicide Warriors, Terrorism and Martyrdom* (pp. 241–268). Springfield, IL: Charles C Thomas Publisher.

Meston, C.M. (2004). A randomized, placebo-controlled, crossover study of ephedrine for SSRI-induced female sexual dysfunction. *Journal of Sex Marital Therapy, 30*, 57–68.

Michelson, D., Kociban, K., and Tamura, R. (2002). Mirtazapine, yohimbine or olanzapine augmentation therapy for serotonin reuptake-associated female sexual dysfunction: A randomized, placebo controlled trial. *Journal of Psychiatric Research, 36*, 147–152.

Popper, C.W. (1998). Management of SSRI-induced apathy in a child with OCD. *Masters in Psychiatry* (pp. 4–11). Greenwich, CT: Cliggott Connection.

Rosen, R.C., Lane, R.M., and Menza, M. (1999). Effects of SSRI's on sexual function: A critical review. *Journal of Clinical Psychiatry, 19*, 67–85.

Rothbaum, B.O., Cahill, S.P., Foa, E.B., Davidson, J.R., Compton, J., Connor, K.M., Astin, M.C., and Hahn, C.G. (2006). Augmentation of sertraline with prolonged exposure in the treatment of posttraumatic stress disorder. *Journal of Traumatic Stress, 19*(5), 625–638.

Rudkin, L., Taylor, M.J., and Hawton, K. (2004). Strategies for managing sexual dysfunction induced by antidepressant medication. *Cochrane Database Systematic Reviews, 4*:CD003382.

Ruzek, J.I., Curran, E., and Friedman, M.J. (2004). Treatment of the returning Iraq war veteran. *Iraq War Clinician Guide.* White River Station, VT: Department of Veterans Affairs, National Center for PTSD.

Schatzberg, A.F., Blier, P., and Delgado, P.L. (2006). Antidepressant discontinuation syndrome: Consensus panel recommendations for clinical management and additional research. *Journal of Clinical Psychiatry, 67* (suppl 4):27–30 [G].

Schoenfeld, F.B., Marmar, C.R., and Neylan, T.C. (2004). Current concepts in pharmacotherapy for posttraumatic stress disorder. *Psychiatric Services, 55*, 519–531.

Segraves, R.T. (2007). Sexual dysfunction associated with antidepressant therapy. *Urology Clinics of North America, 34*, 575–579, vii [F].

Shestatzsky, M., Greenburg, D., and Lerer, B. (1988). A controlled trial of phenelzine in posttraumatic stress disorder. *Psychiatric Research, 24*, 149–155.

Stahl, S.M., and Grady, M.M. (2010). *Stahl's Illustrated: Anxiety, Stress, and PTSD*. New York: Cambridge University Press.

Stein, D.J., van der Kolk, B.A., Austin, C., Fayyad, R., and Clary, C. (2006). Efficacy of sertraline in posttraumatic stress disorder secondary to interpersonal trauma or childhood abuse. *Annals of Clinical Psychiatry, 18*(4), 243–249.

Thase, M.E., Tran, P.V., and Wiltse, C. (2005). Cardiovascular profile of duloxetine, a dual reuptake inhibitor of serotonin and norepinephrine. *Journal of Clinical Psychopharmacol, 25*, 132–140 [E].

The Complete Pill Guide. (2003). Fluoxetine. New York: Barnes & Noble Publishing, Inc. pp. 452–456.

Tucker, P., Zaninelli, R., Yehuda, R., Ruggiero, L., Dillingham, K., and Pitts, C.D. (2001). Paroxetine in the treatment of chronic posttraumatic stress disorder: Results of a placebo-controlled, flexible-dosage trial. *Journal of Clinical of Psychiatry, 62*, 860–868.

Wadsworth, E.J.K., Moss, S.C., Simpson, S.A., & Smith, A.P. (2005). SSRIs and cognitive performance in a working sample. *Human Psychopharmacology: Clinical and Experimental, 20*, 561–572.

Chapter 7

PHARMACOTHERAPY FOR PTSD: MOOD STABILIZERS AND ANTIADRENERGICS

Jamshid A. Marvasti

INTRODUCTION

A number of anticonvulsant drugs (mood stabilizers) have been used for management of PTSD symptoms. These include carbamazepine, valproic acid, lamotrigine, topiramate, oxcarbazepine, phenytoin, and gabapentin. These medications may be useful for mood stabilizing and to control moderating rage and aggressive impulsive behavior. They are also thought to have an antikindling effect. The kindling effect refers to the theory that seizures can be triggered by small repeated events. Seizures are thought to be caused by excessive firing in the neural pathways mediated by glutamate, the brain's primary excitatory neurotransmitter (Loscher, 1998). The kindling phenomenon happens when the repetitive stimulation of a neuron results in a gradual lowering of seizure threshold, thereby requiring less and less stimulation to trigger seizure activity (Friedman, 2001). Due to prolonged and excessive stress, a high level of cortisol will also be present in the body and will cause a similar sensitization and vulnerability to excitotoxicity. The kindling mechanism is believed to contribute to symptoms of physiological hyperactivity, spontaneous intrusive memories, and flashbacks, all of which are present in PTSD (Schoenfeld, Marmar & Neylan, 2004).

ANTISEIZURE MEDICATIONS AND MOOD STABILIZERS IN PTSD

At the present time, these anticonvulsant medications are not approved or officially marketed for use in treatment of PTSD; in reviewing the literature, however, there are some indications that topiramate and lamotrigine may be considered for those patients whose symptoms are refractory and do not respond to first-line agents (Tucker et al., 2007). Schoenfeld and colleagues (2004) reported that anticonvulsant medications may have the potential to prevent the development of PTSD if the victim receives it within the first days after the traumatic event. Despite these assertions, the VA-DoD guideline classified anticonvulsant medications as having "unknown benefits" in PTSD treatment (Department of Veterans Affairs & Department of Defense [VA-DoD], 2004).

MOOD STABILIZERS

Valproate

Valproate is an antiseizure medication and mood stabilizer indicated in the treatment of bipolar disorder. It may be helpful for control of irritability, aggression, and impulsive behavior in PTSD (Forster, Schoenfeld, Marmar & Lang, 1995). Valproate is known to increase the function of the brain's inhibitory neurotransmitter gamma-aminobutyric acid (GABA) and may decrease hyperarousal symptoms in PTSD (VA-DoD, 2004).

Research investigating the effectiveness of valproate in PTSD has been conducted primarily among combat veterans because they are more likely to report symptoms of impulsivity, irritability, and severe reexperiencing of combat-related trauma (Fesler,1991; Petty, Davis & Nugent, 2002). Fesler (1991) conducted a study to determine the effectiveness of adjunctive valproate among sixteen Vietnam combat veterans with moderate to severe hyperarousal and reexperiencing symptoms. Half of the patients reported a significant reduction in the core symptoms of PTSD, and nine participants also reported significant improvement in the duration and quality of their sleep. Eleven out of the fourteen reported a significant reduction in hyperarousal symptoms, and none of the participants reported any serious or long-term side effects (Fesler, 1991).

Side effects. Dizziness, drowsiness, hair loss and thinning, nausea, tremor, weight gain, hyperammonemia, thrombocytopenia, vomiting, hepatotoxicity, and pancreatitis are side effects. Adding zinc on daily basis may inhibit hair loss.

A 2008 FDA meta-analysis found that patients taking anticonvulsant drugs had about twice the risk for suicidal behavior or ideation compared with those patients receiving a placebo. The FDA required new labeling to include warnings for suicide.

Topiramate

Topiramate has shown efficacy in treatment of civilian PTSD (Berlant, 2004). It is thought to increase GABA activity and may decrease nightmares in individuals with PTSD (VA-DoD, 2004). In a double-blind, randomized, controlled study with veterans of the Iran/Iraq war, topiramate (up to 500 mg daily) was a more effective treatment when compared with a placebo group. The study revealed that those who were treated with topiramate reported a significant decrease in intrusive nightmares and memories and a decrease in flashbacks, insomnia, irritability, anger, and startle reaction compared with those receiving a placebo (Akuchekian & Amanat, 2004). Furthermore, Johnson and colleagues (2007) reported in their research that topiramate was beneficial in decreasing harmful alcohol use. This may be an additional benefit for combat veterans with PTSD who frequently develop comorbidity of substance abuse. This medication can also alleviate physical pain associated with comorbidity of PTSD, especially migraine headaches.

Side effects. Weight gain, metabolic acidosis and kidney stones, tinnitus, hearing loss, and sedation are side effects. Suicide warning is another side effect.

Lamotrigine

Lamotrigine inhibits the production and release of glutamate from presynaptic neurons and attenuates the entry of calcium at the *N*-methyl-*d*-aspartate (NMDA) receptor (Brenner & Stevens, 2006). This medication was found effective in decreasing the avoidance and numbing symptoms of PTSD, and also had an impact on the control of intrusive memories (VA-DoD, 2004).

Side effects. Dizziness, ataxia, diplopia, fatigue, insomnia, vomiting, somnolence, suicide warning, and rare instances of Stevens-Johnson syndrome are side effects.

Carbamazepine

Carbamazepine is used to treat seizures, nerve pain, and bipolar disorder and is thought to have an antikindling effect. Currently, there is little clinical information available about the use of carbamazepine as a treatment for PTSD; at least one study, however, showed that it may reduce the reexperiencing of symptoms, irritability, impulsivity, and violent behavior in PTSD patients (Cooper, Carty & Creamer, 2005).

Side effects. Dizziness, vomiting, ataxia, asthenia, amnesia, pancytopenia, diarrhea, and suicide risk are side effects.

Lithium

Lithium is used as a mood stabilizer in bipolar disorder and has been indicated as an agent that may decrease anger, irritability, and hyperarousal in PTSD patients (Schoenfeld et al., 2004). As with antidepressant medications, long-term use of lithium indicates an increase in hippocampal neurogenesis (Malberg & Schechter, 2005).

Side effects. Tremor, vomiting, diarrhea, drowsiness, muscular weakness, and polyuria are side effects.

COMBAT CONSIDERATIONS

Use of mood-stabilizing medications during combat duty may not be appropriate. Some medications require regular monitoring of blood levels because therapeutic levels and toxic levels are very close to each other. Any drug that has a narrow therapeutic window (e.g. lithium) should be avoided as treatment for military personnel who are directly or indirectly involved in combat. If a service member is on lithium prior to deployment, it should be discontinued or the personnel should not be assigned to a combat mission. Lithium is a salt and therefore competes with sodium in kidney transactions. When sodium decreases (due to perspiration, diarrhea, vomiting, or starvation) the level of lithium will increase and may reach a level of toxicity. The level of lithium in the blood may also fluctuate due to an individual's activity, climate, and nutrition. Given the drastically varied climate in Afghan- istan, a soldier may be in combat in hot weather one day and on R&R in cool weather the next. If the soldier is on lithium, hot weather may cause him or her to perspire, depleting the body of salt, and resulting in an elevated lithium level. Cooler weather and less physical activity may cause the level of lithium to be lower. These inconsistencies can be dangerous to the health of the soldier and should be avoided. Side effects of lithium, such as tremors and bradykinesia (slowness of reaction, movement), may be a barrier for performance in combat.

If an antiseizure/mood stabilizer needs to be prescribed to combat personnel, oxcarbazepine (Trileptal®) or gabapentin may be preferred, because they do not require frequent measuring of blood levels. Valproic acid, carbamazepine, and phenytoin (Dilantin®) require frequent monitoring of blood levels. The *Physician's Desk Reference* lists some of the side effects for these medications as ataxia, amnesia, dizziness, diplopia, asthenia, and hearing loss, all of which may place a veteran at risk during combat. All anticonvulsant medications carry a warning from the FDA concerning an increase in risk of suicide.

ADRENERGIC MODULATOR MEDICATIONS

Antiadrenergic Medications

Antiadrenergic medications (alpha- or beta-blockers) have been used for the treatment of hypertension. They are also used in psychiatry to decrease anxiety, particularly performance anxiety, social anxiety, and panic attacks. In addition, they can decrease unwanted side effects of some medications, such as tremors and restlessness (Kelly, 1985).

Rationale for Using Antiadrenergic Medications

Autonomic dysregulation is theorized to be the primary event seen in patients with PTSD. Elevated levels of plasma norepinephrine at rest and significant increase of this element when exposed to trauma-related stimuli have been documented (Yehuda et al., 1998). Patients who have sustained periods of higher norepinephrine levels may be at increased risk of PTSD through a process that overconsolidates memories of the traumatic event (Pitman, 1989). In this sense, medication that decreases the effects of norepinephrine may also decrease the symptoms of PTSD by modulating central and peripheral adrenergic activity. Adrenergic blockers, such as beta-blockers, may decrease anxiety and arousal in PTSD patients. Medications that reduce the release of brain norepinephrine such as clonidine (Catapres®) and guanfacine (Tenex®) may do the same job.

Research indicates that an individual whose level of adrenergic activity (sympathetic nervous system activity) remains elevated following a traumatic event is at higher risk of eventually developing PTSD, compared with someone whose adrenergic activity returns to baseline. Those with chronic traumatic stress disorder continue to have persistently higher levels of norepinephrine and epinephrine. These are thought to contribute to symptoms of hyperarousal and interfere with memory processing of trauma. Memory processing is vital in integrating and healing from traumatic memories

(Southwick et al., 1999). On this basis, any medication that inhibits the effect of sympathetic nerves, (i.e. the effect of norepinephrine in the brain) may be helpful in decreasing the symptoms of traumatic stress (VA-DOD, 2004).

BETA-BLOCKERS: PROPRANOLOL

Propranolol (Inderal®) has an effect on both beta-1 and beta-2 receptors but neither of the alpha receptors. It easily penetrates the blood–brain barrier and is effective both centrally and peripherally. As indicated in research, propranolol may decrease exaggerated startle reaction, explosiveness, nightmares, and intrusive reexperiencing in some patients with PTSD.

Charney (2002) found that the use of beta-blockers among individuals with PTSD reduced the consolidation of their fear memories and augmented psychotherapy. One study found that propranolol significantly impaired the memory of an emotionally arousing story but did not affect the memory of an emotionally neutral story (Cahill as cited in Kilgore, 2005). These findings support the long-standing assumption that memories associated with emotionally charged experiences become overconsolidated as a result of the activation of the beta-adrenergic stress hormone systems, particularly in the amygdala.

Propranolol has been used to treat symptoms of anxiety, especially in cases of public speaking, performance anxiety, fear of flying, and other phobias. It is the only known beta-blocker that can cross the blood–brain barrier. Clinical researchers have hypothesized that blocking beta-adrenergic receptors might tone down consolidation of emotional memories.

There has been research in the administration of propranolol immediately after severe trauma with the hope that it may reduce the likelihood of development of PTSD (Vaiva et al., 2003). Pitman and Delahanty (2005) report the use of propranolol with emergency room trauma patients within six hours of their exposure to the traumatic event. This was done with the hope that it would prevent the development of PTSD or at least decrease the somatic reaction to the traumatic event. At least one study, however, showed no significant effect in preventing the subsequent development of PTSD (Stein, 2006).

In small open trials, propranolol was effective in decreasing hypervigilence, startle reaction, angry outbursts, and intrusive recollections (Schoenfeld et al., 2004). Its benefit in decreasing sleep disorders, nightmares, and avoidance/emotional numbing has been mixed, however. In fact, sleep disturbance and vivid dreams have been seen in nonpsychiatric literature as a common side effect of beta-blocker medications (Stoschitzky et al., 1999).

Dosage. The dosage is 40 to 80 mg per day in a divided dose. It may be increased up to 120 to160 mg for optimal effect.

Side effects and warnings. Propranolol may decrease effects if coadministered with aluminum salt, barbiturates, penicillin, cholestyramine, nonsteroidal antiinflammatory drugs, and rifampin. It may increase the toxicity of calcium channel blockers, cimetidine, and loop diuretics when coadministered. Beta-blockers may also increase the toxicity of haloperidol, benzodiazepines, hydralazine, and phenothiazines.

Beta-adrenergic blockers may decrease the warning signs of hypoglycemia and hyperthyroidism in diabetics or those with thyroid problems. Abrupt withdrawal may exacerbate hyperthyroidism, including thyroid storm. Drugs should be withdrawn slowly and monitored closely (Gore & Lucas, 2010).

Clinical use of propranolol:

1. Patients with certain disorders should be excluded. These disorders include bronchial asthma, chronic obstructive pulmonary disease, congestive heart failure, hyperthyroidism, insulin-dependent diabetes mellitus, persistent angina, and significant peripheral vascular disease.
2. For patients with clinical concerns of hypotension or bradycardia, an initial single test dose of 20 mg should be administered. Dosage may then be increased by 20 mg/d every three days.
3. For patients without cardiovascular or cardiopulmonary disorder, propranolol may be initiated on a schedule of 20 mg three times per day. Dosage may then be increased by 60 mg/d every three days.
4. Do not increase medication if the pulse rate is reduced to lower than 50 beats/min or systolic blood pressure is less than 90 mm Hg.
5. Do not administer propranolol if symptoms of severe dizziness, ataxia, or wheezing occur. If these symptoms persist, medication should be reduced or discontinued.
6. Dosage may be increased to 12 mg/kg of patient's body weight, or until aggressive behavior has diminished. No more than 800 mg is usually necessary to control aggressive behavior.
7. Some patients may respond rapidly to propranolol. In other cases, use of propranolol should be maintained on the highest dose for at least 8 weeks before concluding that the patient is not responding to the medication.
8. Use concurrent medications with caution. Blood levels of all antipsychotic and anticonvulsive medications should be monitored.

(Silver, Hales & Yudofsky, 2002)

ALPHA-ADRENERGICS: PRAZOSIN

Prazosin, an alpha–1 antiadrenergic agent, is a highly lipid-soluble element that can cross the blood–brain barrier and is known to decrease norepinephrine hyperactivity. Raskind and coworkers (2003) reviewed the literature and found that overstimulation of the alpha-1 receptor may be involved in disrupted sleep, nightmares, and increased release of anxiety-producing hormones such as corticotropin releasing factor (CRF).

Norepinephrine hyperactivity may be a central mechanism in nightmares and other sleep disorders. Placebo-controlled, double-blind studies on combat veterans revealed that prazosin reduced nightmares, physiological arousal, intrusive memories, emotional numbing, and avoidance behavior (Raskind et al., 2003, 2007).

Dosage. The precise dosing regimen for prazosin has not yet been established, however, clinicians have used it in doses of 2 mg at bedtime, with titration to 10 to 15 mg at night (Geppert, 2009).

Side effects. Side effects are orthostatic hypotension, light headedness, dizziness, and falls (Geppert, 2009 Oct 2).

ALPHA–2 ADRENERGIC AGONISTS: CLONIDINE AND GUANFACINE

Clonidine and guanfacine are centrally acting medications that activate the presynaptic alpha-2 receptors. The effectiveness of these medications may be due to the tendency for presynaptic alpha-2 receptors to become down-regulated under chronic stress. This assists the brain's own mechanism of "turning off" the sympathetic outflow of norepinephrine (Friedman, Davidson & Mellman, 2000; Raskind et al., 2007). PTSD psychopathology is thought to be connected to dysregulation in noradrenergic mechanisms, with particular respect to hyperarousal and memory function (Raskind et al., 2000). On the basis of this theory, the alpha-2 adrenergic agonist clonidine has been used for management of PTSD because it may decrease the central nervous system's noradrenergic activity. Clonidine was used among severely traumatized Cambodian refugees with some benefit (Kinzie & Leung, 1989). In other studies, it was shown to decrease symptoms of hyperarousal and improve sleep disorder (Boehnlein & Kinzie, 2007).

Khoshnu (2006) referred to a study from the Yale University PTSD Unit that provided evidence to support the use of clonidine if used within three days of the traumatic event, for the duration of seven to nine days. However, a large placebo-controlled trial of guanfacine for treatment of PTSD in veterans did not show any effectiveness (Neylan et al., 2006).

Side effects of clonidine. The most common side effects are dry mouth, sedation, constipation, headache, fatigue, and dizziness. Less common side effects include anorexia, nausea, weight gain, hallucinations, anxiety, depression, nightmares, leg cramps, heart failure, and reduced sex drive.

Side effects of guanfacine. The side effects are fatigue, sedation, dizziness, headache, dry mouth, nausea, dyspepsia, hypotension, atrioventricular block, bradycardia, impotence, anorexia, constipation, irritability and asthma.

COMBAT CONSIDERATION

These medications decrease blood pressure and may cause dizziness and falls. Propranolol decreases the cardiac contractions and velocity of conduction. The result may be poor physical performance and early fatigue if the patient tries to exercise in the hours immediately following the administration of this medication. The alpha-2 agonists can also cause exercise fatigue because they increase alpha-2 activation, which causes bradycardia. Taking these drugs may decrease the power and endurance of service members in active duty. Propranolol causes mild bronchoconstriction and bronchospasms in patients who have asthma or reactive airway disease (Clayton & Nash, 2007).

REFERENCES

Akuchekian, S., and Amanat, S. (2004). The comparison of topiramate and placebo in the treatment of posttraumatic stress disorder: A randomized, double-blind study. *Journal of Research in Medical Sciences, 9*(5), 240–244.

Berlant, J.L. (2004). Prospective open-label study of add-on and monotherapy topiramate in civilians with chronic nonhallucinatory posttraumatic stress disorder. *BMC Psychiatry, 4*(1), 24.

Boehnlein, J., and Kinzie, J. (2007). Pharmacologic reduction of CNS noradrenergic activity in PTSD: the case for clonidine and prazosin. *Journal of Psychiatric Practice, 13*(2), 72–78.

Brenner, G.M., and Stevens, C.W. (2006). *Pharmacology* (2nd ed.). Philadelphia: Saunders Elsevier.

Charney, D.S. (2002). Update on treatment of anxiety disorders. *The Journal of Clinical Psychiatry CNS Discourses, 2*(1), 1–4.

Clayton, N.M. and Nash, W.P. (2007). Medication management of combat and operational stress injuries in active duty service members. In C.R. Figley and W.P.

Nash (Eds.), *Combat Stress Injury: Theory, Research, and Management* (pp. 219–245). New York: Routledge.

Cooper, J., Carty, J., and Creamer, M. (2005). Pharmacotherapy for posttraumatic stress disorder: Empirical review and clinical recommendations. *Australian and New Zealand Journal of Psychiatry, 39,* 674–682.

Department of Veterans Affairs and Department of Defense (VA-DoD). (2004). *Clinical Practice Guidelines for the Management of Post Traumatic Stress.* Washington, (DC): Veteran Health Administration, DoD.

Fesler, F. A. (1991). Valproate in combat-related posttraumatic stress disorder. *Journal of Clinical Psychiatry, 52*(9), 361–364.

Forster, P.L., Schoenfeld, F.B., and Marmar, C.R., and Lang, A.J. (1995). Lithium for irritability in post-traumatic stress disorder. *Journal of Traumatic Stress, 8*(1),143–149.

Friedman, M.J. (2001). Allostatic versus empirical perspectives on pharmacotherapy for PTSD. In J.P. Wilson, M.J. Friedman, and J.D. Lindy (Eds.), *Treating Psychological Trauma & PTSD,* 94–124. New York: Guilford Press.

Friedman, M.J., Davidson, J.R.T. & Mellman, T.A. (2000) Pharmacotherapy. In E.B. Foa, T.M. Keane, and M.J. Freidman (Eds.), *Effective Treatments for PTSD: Practice Guidelines from the International Society for Traumatic Stress Studies.* (pp. 84–105). New York: Guilford Press.

Geppert, C.M.A. (2009, October 2). From war to home: Psychiatric emergencies of returning veterans. *Psychiatric Times, 26*(10), 1–5.

Gore, A., and Lucas, J.Z. (2010, July 1). Posttraumatic stress disorder. *Medicine Psychiatry.* Retrieved on Nov. 15, 2011 from: http://emedicine.medscape.com/article/288154-overview.

Johnson, B.A., Rosenthal, N., Capece, J.A., Wiegand, F., Mao, L., and Beyers, K. (2007).Topiramate for treating alcohol dependence: A randomized controlled trial. *JAMA, 298*(14), 1641–1651.

Kelly, D. (1985). Pharmacology of stress: Beta-blockers in anxiety. *Stress Medicine, 1,* 143–152.

Khoshnu, E. (2006). Clonidine for treatment of PTSD. *Clinical Psychiatry News,* 34(10), p. 22.

Kilgore, C. (2005). Propranolol, other drugs eyed to block PTSD: Idea is that blocking B-adrenergic receptors might tone down consolidation of emotional memories. *Clinical Psychiatry News, 33,* 67. Retrieved March 10, 2011. www.clinicalpsychiatry.com/article/PIIS0270664405703015/fulltext

Kinzie, J.D., and Leung, P. (1989). Clonidine in Cambodian patients with posttraumatic stress disorder. *Journal of Nervous Mental Disease, 177,* 546–550.

Loscher, W. (1998). Pharmacology of glutamate receptor antagonists in the kindling model of epilepsy. *Progress in Neurobiology, 54,* 721–741.

Malberg, J.E., and Schechter, L.E. (2005). Increasing hippocampal neurogenesis: A novel mechanism for antidepressant drugs. *Current Pharmaceutical Design, 11,* 145–155.

Neylan, T.C., Lenoci, M., Samuelson, K.W., Metzler, T.J., Henn-Haase, C., Hierholzer, R.W., Lindley, S.E., Otte, C., Schoenfeld, F.B., Yesavage, J.A., &

Marmar, C.R. (2006). No improvement of posttraumatic stress disorder symptoms with guanfacine treatment. *American Journal of Psychiatry, 163*(12), 2186–2188.

Petty, F., Davis, L., and Nugent, A.L. (2002). Valproate therapy for chronic combat induced posttraumatic stress disorder. *Journal of Clinical Psychopharmacology, 22*(1), 100–101.

Pitman, R.K. (1989). Post-traumatic stress disorder, hormones, and memory [Review]. *Biological Psychiatry, 26*, 221–223.

Pitman, R.K., and Delhanty, D.L. (2005). Reevaluating the association between emergency department heart rate and the development of posttraumatic stress disorder: A public health approach. *Biological Psychiatry, 10*(2), 99–106.

Raskind, M.A., Dobie, D.J., Kanter, E.D., Petrie, E.C., Thompson, C.E., Peskind, E.R. & et al. (2000). The alpha1-adrenergic antagonist prazosin ameliorates combat trauma nightmares in veterans with posttraumatic stress disorder: a report of 4 cases. *Journal of Clinical Psychiatry, 61*(2), 129-133.

Raskind, M.A., Peskind, E.R., Kanter, E.D., Petrie, E.C., Radant, A., Thompson, C.E., et al. (2003). Reduction of nightmares and other PTSD symptoms in combat veterans by prazosin: A placebo controlled study. *American Journal of Psychiatry, 160*, 371–373. Available from: http://ajp.psychiatryonline.org/cgi/content/ full/160/2/371. Accessed April 23, 2009.

Raskind, M.A., Peskind, E.R., Hoff, D.J., Hart, K.L., Warren, D., Shofer, J., O'Connell, J., Taylor, F., Gross, C., Rohde, K., and McFall, M.E. (2007). A parallel group placebo controlled study of prazosin for trauma nightmares and sleep disturbance in combat veterans with post-traumatic stress disorder. *Biological Psychiatry, 61*, 928–934.

Schoenfeld, F.B., Marmar, C.R., and Neylan, T.C. (2004). Current concepts in pharmacotherapy for posttraumatic stress disorder. *Psychiatric Services, 55*, 519–531. Available from: http://ps.psychiatryonline.org/cgi/content/full/55/5/519. Accessed April 11, 2011.

Silver, J.M., Hales, R.E., and Yudofsky, S.C. (2002). Neuropsychiatric aspects of traumatic brain injury. In S.C. Yudofsky and R.E. Hales (Eds.), *Neuropsychiatry and Clinical Neurosciences* (pp. 625–672). Washington, DC: American Psychiatric Publishing, Inc.

Southwick, S.M., Bremner, J.D., Rasmusson, A., Morgan, C.A., Amsten, A., and Charney, D.S. (1999). Role of norepinephrine in the pathophysiology and treatment of post-traumatic stress disorder. *Biological Psychiatry, 46*, 1192–1204.

Stein, M. (2006, November). *Pharmacoprevention of Adverse Psychiatric Sequelae of Physical Injury.* Presented at the 21st Annual Meeting of International Society for Traumatic Stress Studies, Toronto.

Stoschitzky, K., Sakotnik, A., Lercher, P., Zweiker, R., Maier, R., Liebmann, P., et al. (1999). Influence of beta-blockers on melatonin release. *European Journal of Clinical Pharmacology, 55*, 111–115.

Tucker, P., Trautman, R.P., Wyatt, D.B., Thompson, J., Capece, J.A., & Rosenthal, N.R. (2007). Efficacy and safety of topiramate monotherapy in civilian posttraumatic stress disorder: a randomized, double-blind, placebo-controlled study. *Journal of Clinical Psychiatry, 68*(2), 201–206.

Vaiva, G., Ducrocq, F., Jezequel, K., Benoit, A., Lestavel, P., Brunet, A., and Marmar, C.R. (2003). Immediate treatment with propranolol decreases posttraumatic stress disorder. *Biological Psychiatry, 54* (9), 947–949.

Yehuda, R., Siever, L.J., Teicher, M.H., Levengood, R.A., Gerber, D.K., Schmeidler, J., et al. (1998). Plasma norepinephrine and 3-methoxy-4-hydroxyphenylglycol concentrations and severity of depression in posttraumatic stress disorder and major depressive disorder. *Biological Psychiatry, 44,* 56–63.

Chapter 8

PHARMACOTHERAPY FOR PTSD: TRANQUILIZERS, HYPNOTICS AND NEUROLEPTIC MEDICATIONS

Jamshid A. Marvasti

INTRODUCTION

Benzodiazepines have been used to treat symptoms of anxiety for many years. Researchers suggest that these medications can also reduce acute somatic symptoms associated with anxiety. Although benzodiazepines are generally not indicated for long-term treatment of anxiety disorders or PTSD, they are perhaps the most effective therapy for the acute relief of anxiety and anxiety-driven somatic complaints. It is also known that benzodiazepines have no therapeutic effect on core PTSD symptoms (Clayton & Nash, 2007).

INEFFECTIVENESS OF BENZODIAZEPINES IN TREATMENT OF TRAUMA

Research on using benzodiazepines for treatment of trauma revealed either no beneficial effect (Mellman, Clark & Peacock, 2003) or an even higher likelihood of subsequent development of PTSD (Gelpin, Bonne, Peri, Brandes & Shalev, 1996). There are indications that benzodiazepines may interfere with a patient's ability to desensitize his or her fear response to triggers that may bring up traumatic memories (Schoenfeld, Marmar & Neylan, 2004). There is no research to indicate that benzodiazepines control PTSD symptoms. For example, studies on alprazolam (Xanax®) for treatment of PTSD symptoms did not reveal any significant benefit (Braun, Greenberg, Dasberg & Lerer, 1990). Another study was done using clonazepam that revealed that it did not have an impressive effect on sleep-related PTSD symptoms (Cates, Bishop, Davis, Lowe & Wooley, 2004).

Benzodiazepines are able to decrease arousal and anxiety and also to increase, or even create, sedation. Their effectiveness in the treatment of nightmares, however has not been conclusive, and they can worsen sleep apnea (Maher, Rego & Asnis, 2006). Although at times benzodiazepines may induce sleep rapidly, they can also cause the quality of sleep to worsen. This is due to their tendency to increase the time spent in stages 1 and 2 and to decrease the time spent in stages 3, 4, and REM (Brenner & Stevens, 2006). For this reason, benzodiazepines may interfere in a negative way with the process of healing from PTSD.

The VA-DoD guidelines (Department of Veterans Affairs and Department of Defense [VA-DoD], 2004) do not support the use of benzodiazepines and place them in the "no benefit/harm" category for treatment of PTSD but in the "unknown benefit" category for acute stress disorder.

Side Effects of Benzodiazepines

The common side effects of benzodiazepines include drowsiness, ataxia, behavioral problems, hyperactivity, hypersalivation, psychosis, and antero-grade amnesia or memory loss for the period of time that the medication is active in the brain. Blood dyscrasias and hepatic dysfunction are also possible idiosyncratic side effects associated with the use of clonazepam. This medication should not be discontinued rapidly because as doing so may result in withdrawal symptoms, rebound anxiety, insomnia, irritability, and headache (Brenner & Stevens, 2006).

COMBAT CONSIDERATIONS WITH BENZODIAZEPINES

Because of the side effects involved with use of these medications, they should be avoided by active duty military personnel. In addition to the previous side effects, benzodiazepines have a quality of developing dependency and addiction and impaired cognitive and motor function and may cause rebound anxiety, impaired judgment, and impaired planning capacity, as well as negative effects to sleep patterns (Clayton & Nash, 2007). Sometimes these medications, like alcohol, cause emotional and behavioral disinhibition.

Although, in general, benzodiazepines should be avoided in combat situations, there may be some benefit to their use during medical evacuation or in managing severe agitation. In any case, they should only be used for short periods due to dependency and addiction as well as side effects (Clayton & Nash, 2007).

NONBENZODIAZEPINE SEDATIVE/HYPNOTIC MEDICATION FOR INSOMNIA

Many military personnel in combat suffer from sleep deprivation. Those with PTSD have persistent nightmares, anxiety, irritability, and interrupted sleep. REM sleep deprivation, in particular, may cause disruption in hippocampal function and plasticity (McDermott et al., 2003). Sleep deprivation and disruption of sleep architecture have been shown to be connected with physical health problems (Friedman & Schnurr, 1995) and have been associated with an increase in motor, learning, and cognitive impairment (Durmer & Dinges, 2005).

NONBENZODIAZEPINE HYPNOTICS

Hypnotic drugs such as zaleplon (Sonata®), zolpidem (Ambien®), eszopiclone (Lunesta®) and zopiclone (Imovane; Canada only) are different from benzodiazepines from a structural point of view. Much like benzodiazepines, however, they cause sedation by potentiating the activity of GABA. These medications do not cause a significant increase in tolerance, nor do they cause withdrawal syndrome upon discontinuation. The half-lives of these medications are varied. Zaleplon has the shortest half-life, around one hour, and eszopiclone has the longest, which is five to seven hours.

OTHER SEDATIVE/HYPNOTIC MEDICATIONS: TRAZODONE

Trazodone HCl (Deseryl) is used as an antidepressant medication in high doses (400–500 mg/d), but can be used in low doses (50–100 mg) for sleep disorders. Trazodone is a potent antagonist at serotonin-2a receptors. It also blocks serotonin-2c receptors and serotonin transporters. Additionally, it blocks histamine-1 receptors (which are responsible for sedation), and alpha-1–adrenergic receptors, which may contribute to efficacy for treating nightmares. There are reports that trazodone may have eliminated nightmares in combat veterans; however, there is not enough research to support this finding (Geppert, 2009).

Side effects. Sedation is the most common side effect of trazodone. The cardiovascular side effects include orthostatic hypotension, especially among the elderly or those with preexisting heart disease. Trazodone has been associated with life-threatening ventricular arrhythmias in several case reports (Mendelson, 2005). It has additional side effects, such as nasal congestion, dry mouth, blurred vision, and constipation, which make some patients uncomfortable enough to request a change in medication. Sexual side effects, including erectile dysfunction in men and, in rare cases, priapism, may occur. Priapism may require surgery.

ALPHA-1 ANTAGONIST FOR NIGHTMARES: PRAZOSIN

Prazosin (Minipress®) is a non-sedating alpha-1 adrenoreceptor antagonist that crosses the blood–brain barrier and decreases the response of the brain to norepinephrine. Research reveals that prazosin does not cause "daytime hangover" and has the capacity to enable restorative sleep in some individuals without decreasing alertness, an important factor for soldiers who need to be alert in combat situations. Prazosin is approved for treatment of high blood pressure, not for treatment of PTSD or sleep disorder.

Trauma nightmares and sleep disorders in PTSD may be due to excessive brain response to released norepinephrine, which results in disrupted REM and other sleep stages (Taylor et al., 2008). Noradrenergic neurons originate in the locus coeruleus and are involved in the autonomic output of fear. They also innervate the amygdala and the prefrontal cortex, both of which are important to anxiety mechanisms. Alpha-adrenergic blockers may modulate the anxiogenic effect of noradrenergic hyperactivation. Alpha-adrenergic receptors may have a role in insomnia in patients with PTSD, because they are involved in sleep responses (Stahl & Grady, 2010).

Calohan and colleagues (2010) prescribed prazosin to thirteen soldiers who had distressing trauma nightmares and impaired military function in northern Iraq, and the results indicated improvement in sleep disorder. Prazosin has been shown to be helpful in treating nightmares in Vietnam combat veterans (Raskind et al., 2007); however, the precise dosing has not yet been established. Clinicians have used 2 mg at bedtime with titration up to 15 mg (Geppert, 2009).

Side effects. The most common side effects of prazosin are lightheadedness, dizziness, syncope, and hypotension. The pregnancy category is C.

DOXEPIN

Although doxepin HCl (Sinequan®) is one of the TCAs that inhibit serotonin and norepinephrin reuptake, it is also an antagonist at histamine-1, muscarine-1, and alpha-1–adrenergic receptors. New research reveals that at a very low dose (3–6 mg at night) it may be useful in the treatment of insomnia because of its binding potency to the histamine-1 receptor (Markov & Doghramji, 2010). Although doxepin has not been studied in PTSD, its hypnotic property could be desirable for states of hyperarousal, especially at night (Stahl & Grady, 2010).

Side effects. Side effects of doxepin include drowsiness, dizziness, dry mouth, loss of appetite, constipation, and nausea. It should not be used in patients with narrow-angle glaucoma. Doxepin has a pregnancy risk of category C.

WHEN MEDICATIONS CAUSE NIGHTMARES

Clinicians should be aware that some medications may also cause side effects such as nightmares and sleep disorders. A few of these that are associated with nightmares are as follows:

1. Beta-blockers such as atenolol (Tenormin®) and propranolol
2. SSRI antidepressants such as fluoxetine and sertraline
3. Antipsychotics such as risperidone (Risperdal®)
4. Dopamine agonists such as levodopa and amantadine (Symmetrel®)
5. Antihistamines such as chlorpheniramine
6. ACE inhibitors and ARB such as enalapril and losartan
7. Miscellaneous drugs such as digoxin, naproxen, verapamil, and fleroxacin

ANTIPSYCHOTIC MEDICATIONS: INDICATIONS FOR COMBAT TRAUMA

Antipsychotic medications, especially those that are atypical, have been used for their sedative properties, particularly with PTSD patients with severe symptoms or those who did not respond to other medications. They have also been used with patients who have comorbidities such as bipolar disorder, psychotic illness, or even borderline personality disorder. These medications are not the first-line treatment for PTSD intervention (Baldwin et al., 2005).

There have been reports of improvement in some cases in which antipsychotics were used as adjunctive treatment in combination with antidepressants (SSRIs), especially in those PTSD patients who had explosive, aggressive, or violent behavior (Schoenfeld et al., 2004). There are also reports that atypical antipsychotic medication may have augmented SSRI therapy for those with trauma-related hallucinations, violent behavior, or hypervigilance and paranoia (Friedman, 2001).

Hamner (cited by Sherman, 2006) recommends the use of atypical antipsychotic medications as a third- or fourth-line treatment for patients who have been refractory to adequate trials of other medications. Patients with persistent symptoms of hyperarousal, aggressiveness, or mood swings or those with pronounced dissociative symptoms may be considered candidates for atypical antipsychotic medication. Hamner argues that one-third to one-half the customary dosage for schizophrenia or acute bipolar disorder is usually effective when treating patients with PTSD. When patients clearly demonstrate symptoms of psychosis, however, he recommends the highest dose that can be tolerated by the patient (Sherman, 2006).

The VA-DoD guidelines (2004) classified typical antipsychotic medications as "no benefit/harm" for treatment of PTSD.

ATYPICAL ANTIPSYCHOTIC MEDICATION IN CONTROLLING PTSD SYMPTOMS/COMORBIDITY

A handful of atypical antipsychotic medications, olanzapine (Zyprexa®), risperidone, aripiprazole (Abilify™), and quetiapine have been used in treatment of PTSD and its comorbidities in combat veterans. The available evidence may point to the use of risperidone as a preferred drug for the management of PTSD (Hamner, Dietsch, Brodrick, Ulmer & Lorberbaum, 2003; Monelly, Ciraulo, Knapp & Keane, 2003; Pivac, Kozaric -Kovacic & Muck-Selel, 2004).

In a relatively small study, SSRI medications were augmented with olanzapine which appeared to be beneficial in treating SSRI-resistant, combat-related PTSD symptoms, especially sleep disorders (Stein, Klein & Matloff, 2002). In another study, monotherapy with antipsychotic medication indicated a reduction in psychotic and PTSD symptoms. There is no psychotic subtype of combat-related PTSD; however, PTSD with hallucinations and delusions that has resisted previous SSRI antidepressive therapy may benefit from the addition of an antipsychotic medication (Pivac & Kozaric-Kovacic, 2006).

Quetiapine

Quetiapine has alpha-1 blocking and antihistamine properties and has reportedly been used to improve quality of sleep and reduce nightmares in combat veterans with PTSD. It is prescribed in low doses as a hypnotic (Robert et al., 2005).

There is evidence supporting the use of adjunctive quetiapine among patients with combat- and noncombat-related PTSD. Ahearn, Mussey, Johnson, Krohrn, and Krahn (2006) evaluated the effectiveness of quetiapine among patients with PTSD who continued to experience PTSD symptoms even though they were taking an SSRI. Research participants had a mix of combat and noncombat-related PTSD and were on a stable dose of an SSRI for at least six weeks at the onset of the study. After eight weeks of receiving a moderate dose of quetiapine, research participants reported an overall improvement in PTSD symptoms (Ahearn et al., 2006).

Risperidone

Risperidone has a function of blocking alpha-2–adrenergic receptors, which may contribute to its efficacy in treatment of depression. It also blocks alpha-1–adrenergic receptors, which may contribute to orthostatic hypotension and sedation but could also potentially be used to treat sleep disturbance in PTSD (Stahl & Grady, 2010). In a randomized, double-blind, placebo-controlled trial, Hamner and associates (2003, January) found that risperidone was effective for treating comorbid psychotic symptoms among patients with PTSD.

Aripiprazole

Lambert (2006) conducted a study to determine the effects of aripiprazole in the management of PTSD in returning veterans. This medication was found to be well-tolerated and was effective in the management of sleep disorders, nightmares, and agitated behavior during sleep and was also helpful in decreasing hyperarousal. Because one research participant experienced a paradoxical excitation response to the medication, it was suggested that aripiprazole should be studied further.

Chlorpromazine

During the Vietnam War, chlorpromazine (Thorazine®) was widely used for treatment of highly agitated soldiers or those who were injured and were excessively agitated during evacuation. Chlorpromazine has a very powerful sedating effect, with no addictive or dependency quality; therefore, it was used freely for sedation and sleep disorder during combat in Vietnam (Clayton & Nash, 2007).

Side Effects of Atypical Antipsychotic Medications

The side effects associated with atypical antipsychotic medications include weight gain, sedation, metabolic syndrome, hyperlipidemia, hyperprolactinemia, obesity, increased blood sugar, tremor, muscle spasms, muscle rigidity, tardive dyskinesia, and rare complications such as agranulocytosis and neuroleptic malignant syndrome.

COMBAT CONSIDERATIONS

Practical considerations concerning the use of atypical antipsychotics in combat include side effects, such as weight gain, asthenia/tiredness, tremor, blurred vision, persistent grogginess (sedation after sleep has ended), and "hangover." These may be detrimental to military personnel, who need to be vigilant, alert, and in good physical shape (Clayton & Nash, 2007). Atypical antipsychotics are also associated with a possible increase in the risk of diabetes. Unlike lithium and SSRIs, antipsychotics have not been shown to increase the neurogenesis of cells in the hippocampus (Malberg & Schechter, 2005), which decreases its benefit in treating PTSD.

REFERENCES

Ahearn, E.P., Mussey, M., Johnson, C., Krohn, A., and Krahn, D. (2006). Quetiapine as an adjunctive treatment for post-traumatic stress disorder: An 8-week open-label study. *International Journal of Clinical Psychopharmacology, 21*(1), 29–33.

Baldwin, D.S., Anderson, I.M., Nutt, D.J., Bandelow, B., Bond, A., Davidson, J.R.T., et al. (2005). British Association for Psychopharmacology. Evidence-based guidelines for the pharmacological treatment of anxiety disorders: recommendations from the British Association for Psychopharmacology. *Journal of Psychopharmacology, 19*(6), 567–596.

Braun P., Greenberg, D., Dasberg, H., and Lerer, B. (1990). Core symptoms of post-traumatic stress disorder unimproved by alprazolam treatment. *Journal of Clinical Psychiatry, 51*, 236–238.

Brenner, G.M., and Stevens, C.W. (2006). *Pharmacology* (2nd ed.). Philadelphia: Saunders Elsevier.

Calohan, J., Peterson, K., Peskind, E.R., and Raskind, M.A. (2010). Prazosin treatment of trauma nightmares and sleep disturbance in soldiers deployed in Iraq. *Journal of Traumatic Stress, 23*(5), 645–648.

Cates, M.E., Bishop, M.H., Davis, L.L., Lowe, J.S., and Wooley, T.W. (2004). Clonazepam for treatment of sleep disturbances associated with combat-related posttraumatic stress disorder. *Annals of Pharmacotherapy, 38*, 1395–1399.

Clayton, N.M., and Nash, W. P. (2007). Medication management of combat and operational stress injuries in active duty service members. In C.R. Figley and W.P. Nash (Eds.), *Combat Stress Injury: Theory, Research, and Management* (pp. 219–245). New York: Routledge.

Department of Veterans Affairs and Department of Defense (VA-DoD). (2004). *VA/DoD Clinical Practice Guideline for the Management of Post Traumatic Stress.* Washington, DC: Office of Quality and Performance. Retrieved from http://www.oqp.med.va.gov/cpg/PTSD/PTSD_Base/htm

Durmer, J. S., and Dinges, D. F. (2005). Neurocognitive consequences of sleep deprivation. *Seminars in Neurology, 25*, 117–129.

Friedman, M.J. (2001). Allostatic versus empirical perspectives on pharmacotherapy for PTSD. In J.P. Wilson, M.J. Friedman, and J.D. Lindy (Eds.), *Treating Psychological Trauma & PTSD* (pp. 94–124). New York: Guilford Press.

Friedman, M.J., and Schnurr, P.P. (1995). The relationship between trauma, posttraumatic stress disorder, and physical health. In M.J. Friedman, D.S. Charney, and A.Y. Deutch (Eds.), *Neurobiological and clinical consequences of stress: From normal adaptation to posttraumatic stress disorder* (pp. 507–524). Philadelphia: Lippincott-Raven.

Gelpin, E., Bonne, O., Peri, T., Brandes, D., and Shalev, A.Y. (1996). Treatment of recent trauma survivors with benzodiazepines: A prospective study. *Journal of Clinical Psychiatry, 57*, 390–394.

Geppert, C.M.A. (2009, October 2). From war to home: Psychiatric emergencies of returning veterans. *Psychiatric Times, 26*(10), 1–5.

Hamner, M.B., Dietsch, S.E., Brodrick, P.S., Ulmer, H.G., and Lorberbaum, J.P. (2003). Quetiapine treatment in patients with posttraumatic stress disorder: An open trail of adjunctive therapy. *Journal of Psychopharmacology, 23*, 15–20.

Hamner, M.B., Faldowski, R.A., Ulmer, H.G., Frueh, B.C., Huber, M.G., and Arana, G.W. (2003, January). Adjunctive risperidone treatment in post-traumatic stress disorder: A preliminary controlled trial of effects on comorbid psychotic symptoms. *International Clinical Psychopharmacology, 18*(1), 1–8.

Lambert, M.T. (2006). Aripiprazole in the management of post-traumatic stress disorder symptoms in global war on terrorism veterans. *International Journal of Clinical Psychopharmacology, 21*(3), 185–187.

Maher, M.J., Rego, S.A., and Asnis, G.M. (2006). Sleep disturbances in patients with posttraumatic stress disorder: epidemiology, impact and approaches to management. *CNS Drugs, 20*(7), 567–590.

Malberg, J.E., and Schechter, L. E. (2005). Increasing hippocampal neurogenesis: A novel mechanism for antidepressant drugs. *Current Pharmaceutical Design, 11*, 145–155.

Markov, D., and Doghramji, K. (2010, October). Doxepin for Insomnia. *Current Psychiatry, 9*(10), 67–77.

McDermott, C.M., LaHosgte, G.J., Chen, C., Musto, A., Bazan, G.N., and Magee, J.C. (2003). Sleep deprivation causes behavioral, synaptic, and membrane excitability alterations in hippocampal neurons. *Journal of Neuroscience, 23*, 9687–9695.

Mellman, T., Clark, R., and Peacock, W. (2003). Prescribing patterns for patients with posttraumatic stress disorder. *Psychiatric Services, 54*, 1618–1621.

Mendelson, W.F. (2005). A review of the evidence for the efficacy and safety of trazodone in insomnia. *Journal of Psychiatry, 66*, 469–476.

Monelly, E.P., Ciraulo, D.A., Knapp, C., and Keane, T. (2003). Low-dose risperidone as adjunctive therapy for irritable aggression in posttraumatic stress disorder. *Journal of Clinical Psychopharmacology, 23*, 193–196.

Pivac, N., Kozaric-Kovacic, D., and Muck-Seler, D. (2004). Olanzapine versus fluphenazine in an open trial in patients with psychotic combat-related post-traumatic stress disorder. *Psychopharmacology 175*, 451–456.

Pivac, N., and Kozaric -Kovacic , D. (2006). Pharmacotherapy of treatment-resistant combat-related posttraumatic stress disorder with psychotic features. *Croatian Medical Journal, 47*(3), 440–451.

Raskind, M.A., Peskind, E.R., Hoff, D.J., Hart, K.L., Warren, D., Shofer, J., O'Connell, J., Taylor, F., Gross, C., Rohde, K., and McFall, M.E. (2007). A parallel group placebo controlled study of prazosin for trauma nightmares and sleep disturbance in combat veterans with post-traumatic stress disorder. *Biological Psychiatry, 61*, 928–934.

Robert, S., Hamner, M.B., Kose, S., Ulmer, H.G., Deitsch, S.E. and Lorberbaum, J.P. (2005). Quetiapine improves sleep disturbances in combat veterans with PTSD: sleep data from a prospective, open-label study. *Journal of Clinical Psychopharmacology, 25*(4), 387–388. doi:10.1097/01. jcp.0000169624.37819.60 PubMed.

Schoenfeld, F.B., Marmar, C.R., and Neylan, T.C. (2004). Current concepts in pharmacotherapy for posttraumatic stress disorder. *Psychiatric Services, 55*, 519–31.

Sherman, C. (2006). Antidepressants often just a first step in PTSD: Following initial SSRIs, adrenergic antagonists, anticonvulsants, atypical antipsychotics often used [Online]. *Clinical Psychiatry News, 34*, 25. Retrieved December 11, 2009. Available from: www.clinicalpsychiatrynews.com/article/PIIS02706644067133 15/fulltext

Stahl, S.M., and Grady, M.M. (2010). *Stahl's illustrated: Anxiety, stress, and PTSD.* New York: Cambridge University Press.

Stein, M.B., Kline, N.A. and Matloff, J.L. (2002). Adjunctive olanzapin for SSRI-resistant combat-related PTSD: A double-blind, placebo-controlled study. *American Journal of Psychiatry, 159*, 1777–1779.

Taylor, F.B., Martin, P., Thompson, C., Williams, J., Mellman, T.A., Gross, C., and et al. (2008). Prazosin effects on objective sleep measures and clinical symptoms in civilian trauma PTSD: A placebo-controlled study. *Biological Psychiatry, 63*, 629–632.

Chapter 9

PHARMACOTHERAPY FOR ALCOHOL PROBLEMS AS A COMORBIDITY OF PTSD

JAMSHID MARVASTI & KHAIRUL NUAL

MILITARY PERSONNEL AND ALCOHOL

For years people have used alcohol to alleviate or numb trauma and its comorbidities. Although the pleasure it brings may seem gratifying, the long-term or even immediate results of alcohol can cause one's life to crumble into pieces. A report issued by the U. S. Centers for Disease Control and Prevention estimated that medium and high intake of alcohol contributed to 75,754 deaths in the United States in 2001 (Centers for Disease Control, 2004). Alcohol serves as an integral part of society and a norm in Western culture and does appear to have some positive effects. Many statistics show that the risk of alcohol misuse is far greater than any potential benefit, however.

The effect of alcohol on brain chemistry is widespread. Studies show that soldiers with PTSD who use alcohol can be detrimentally affected, both mentally and physically. Literature indicates that those with substance abuse problems may show an increase in other dangerous behaviors such as self-harm and suicidal inclinations (Ruzek, Polusny & Abueg, 1998).

Studies suggest that alcohol contributes to the loss of focus among soldiers and may induce other negative effects during military wartime duties, including an adverse impact on unit effectiveness (Jacobson et al., 2008). The misuse of alcohol has also been linked with soldier misconduct and withdrawal from military service (Hoge et al., 2005). Misuse of alcohol by veterans with PTSD and TBI complicates treatment and recovery (Taft et al., 2007). One study focusing on veterans from the first Gulf War found that intense alcohol consumption led to increased mortality rates (Bell et al., 2001).

It has been shown that soldiers with preexisting alcohol or other substance abuse problems experience a higher and faster rise in stress level when deployed compared with nonalcoholic soldiers. Also, if in the war zone there is easy access to drugs or alcohol, negative behaviors may continue and accelerate. Alcohol users will also develop tolerance, which requires greater quantities be consumed in order to achieve an effect. Additionally, there are withdrawal symptoms associated with sudden discontinuation after a prolonged period of alcohol use. These can include anxiety, depression, insomnia, shakiness or tremors, sweating, nausea and vomiting, heart palpitations, and convulsions (Clayton & Nash, 2007).

Clinicians in Iraq report that not only is alcohol readily available, but also black market diazepam is inexpensive and easily accessible (Lande, Martin & Ruzek, 2004). In Afghanistan, opium poppies and marijuana remain the two largest cash crops, as reported by Sorenson (2004). Medical and military programs differ in their approaches when addressing alcohol and drug use disorders in military personnel. Alcohol or drug misuse is a medical disorder, it is often treated as an administrative issue in the U.S. military, however. Anyone failing to comply with orders (alcohol counseling and treatment) can be discharged from the military (Santiago et al., 2010). Military officials claim it is necessary to take such actions because noncompliance by a minute number of soldiers can greatly harm the whole unit.

DOES ALCOHOL HAVE BENEFITS?

Simon and Gorman (2004) explain that, in some studies, alcohol use (not abuse or dependency) has been shown to actually prevent the development of PTSD after a disaster, especially if the individual was drinking before the disaster occurred (McFarlane, 1998). Research was done on epidemiological cohorts of 127 victims of a ballroom fire seven to nine months after the disaster. It showed that alcohol consumption and intoxication each independently decreased the incidence of PTSD (Maes, Delmeire, Mylle & Altamura, 2001).

Explanations of this finding generally focus on memory- and arousal-related mechanisms. As with benzodiazepines, alcohol has an attenuating effect on stress-induced increases in norepinephrine turnover at the amygdala and the locus coeruleus (Shirao et al., 1988). In this sense it minimizes symptoms of pretraumatic anxiety and arousal. Alcohol may also inhibit the storage of memories and subsequent fear conditioning by inhibiting encoding consolidation or retrieval of previously conditioned or contextually related traumatic memories (Maes et al., 2001). In addition, some researchers think that alcohol inhibits NMDA-mediated synaptic channels at the amygdala, and in this direct way inhibits long-term potentiation (Faingold, N'Gouemo & Riaz, 1998).

Drinking alcohol after a disaster, however, is not advised by any clinician, and studies show that an increase in pathological alcohol use post disaster is not helpful. After a traumatic event, alcohol use may even inhibit the healthy and necessary recording of memories in the same manner as benzodiazepine use. Although a small amount of alcohol may decrease anxiety, it is not known how much can be used before it begins to inhibit the healthy recording of memories.

PTSD AND ALCOHOL CONNECTIONS

Many individuals with PTSD use alcohol or mind-altering drugs to cope with emotional arousal and decrease the disturbing impact of traumatic memories. However, researchers have reported that substance abuse by itself may trigger or exacerbate PTSD symptoms (Saladin, Brady, Dansky & Kilpatrick, 1995).

Both the postdeployment health reassessment and the two-item conjoint screen test conducted on military veterans affirmed that alcohol misuse was higher after deployment than it was before (Hoge et al., 2004). Studies indicate that, especially among male combat veterans and civilians exhibiting PTSD, alcohol abuse or dependence is the most common co-occurring disorder. Alcohol abuse appears to be a greater problem compared with depression, anxiety disorders, conduct disorders, and nonalcohol substance abuse (Kessler, Sonnega, Bromet, Hughes & Nelson, 1995). Seventy-five percent of combat veterans with lifetime PTSD were also facing the problem of alcohol abuse or dependence (Kulka et al., 1990).

The relationship between alcohol or drug use and PTSD symptoms is supported by the concept of self-medication. Psychiatric disorders self-medicated with alcohol are common among psychiatric patients (Bremner, Southwich, Darnell & Charney, 1996). However, there is another theory that each disorder arises independently, without any causal relationship between them. One disorder may worsen or improve the other, even if they are not caused by one another (Najavits, 2008).

The National Center for PTSD (Department of Veterans Affairs) reports that soldiers with PTSD who use alcohol risk putting themselves and their families in serious danger (Price, 2007). Researchers from King's College in London have stated that alcohol misuse is now a greater problem than PTSD itself (Jeremy, 2010). A recent study from the *Journal of Military Medicine* examined the rates of PTSD in 120 service men and women who returned from Iraq and Afghanistan. Within this sample, 6 percent of soldiers had PTSD, 27 percent showed dangerous alcohol use, and another 6 percent had problems with PTSD and alcohol use (Erbes, Westermeyers, Engdahl & Johnsen, 2007). They also found that 62 percent of the service members were receiving some kind of mental health care, such as individual, group, or family therapy or medication.

Studies showed three quarters of surviving soldiers who suffered abusive or violent trauma in war were reported to have drinking problems. Soldiers diagnosed with PTSD who consume alcoholic beverages are more prone to having anxiety and mood disorders, disruptive behaviors, and chronic physical illness (Kofoed, Friedman & Peck, 1993).

SUBSTANCE ABUSE, PTSD, AND TBI

In TBI, damage to the frontal and temporal lobes may cause a decrease in self-control and an increase in impulsivity. These structural changes associated with TBI may contribute to substance abuse. The relationship between PTSD and substance abuse may be indirect or direct or occur through the TBI mechanism. Corrigan and Cole (2008) indicated that one key feature of PTSD is hyperarousal, which may lead to substance abuse problems as a self-medication technique. Hyperarousal can lead to hypervigilance, which in turn may lead to avoidance of stimuli associated with a high level of distress. These factors can promote substance abuse through attempts to self-medicate anxiety, avoid traumatic memory, or increase emotional numbing and detachment from a painful environment.

ALCOHOL USE IN AMERICA

Epidemiological research reveals that individuals with PTSD are at increased risk of having an alcohol or substance use disorder (SUD). Current rates of PTSD are thought to be much higher (25 to 55%) in those with a SUD diagnosis than in the general population. In addition, 65 to 80 percent of individuals seeking PTSD treatment are shown to have a SUD (Ouimette & Brown, 2003).

PTSD and substance abuse are frequently described as comorbid. Within the U.S. population, men with PTSD have a 52 percent lifetime rate of AUD and a 35 percent rate of drug use disorder. Among women these rates are lowered to 28 percent and 27 percent respectively.

In the United States, it has been estimated that the prevalence of a lifetime SUD ranged from nearly 22 percent to 43 percent among those diagnosed with PTSD, in comparison with 8 to 25 percent for people without PTSD (Breslau, Davis, Peterson & Shultz, 1997). It has been found that rates of PTSD appear to be more prevalent (up to 43%) among those in inpatient substance abuse treatment programs (Dansky, Saladin, Brady, Kilpatrick & Resnick, 1995). Further testing shows that individuals with PTSD and SUD suffer from more severe PTSD symptoms than do those with PTSD alone (Saladin et al., 1995). It is also documented that 60 to 80 percent of Vietnam veterans who are in treatment have problems with alcohol (Evans & Sullivan, 1995).

ALCOHOL AND SLEEP DISORDER

Alcohol's effects are similar to those of benzodiazepines and may cause side effects such as loss of motor coordination, impaired cognitive processing, impaired judgment/planning, dizziness, drowsiness, disinhibition of emotion and behavior, and anterograde amnesia. Alcohol has negative effects on sleep, causing fragmentation of sleep patterns, shorter duration of sleep, reduction in stages 3 and 4, and disturbances in REM sleep (Landolt & Gillin, 2001). It is also documented that alcohol can continue its deteriorating effect on sleep patterns for months, or even years, after a chronic drinker has stopped drinking. Schmitz, Sepandj, Pickler, and Rudas (1996) indicated that alcohol inhibits the pineal gland's ability to secrete melatonin, which serves to initiate sleep. This inhibition of melatonin can remain during abstinence in chronic alcohol drinkers. It is documented that even moderate alcohol intake disrupts the hippocampal function and may lead to impairment in learning and memory (White et al., 2000). Many individuals with trauma drink alcohol to be able to sleep, but alcohol ultimately works against this goal. Military personnel should be made aware of this fact (Clayton & Nash, 2007).

TREATMENT DIFFICULTIES

SUD can mask the symptoms of PTSD, which can create a barrier for treatment. In most situations, PTSD generally precedes substance abuse and substance abuse is often a form of self-medication for PTSD. Some individuals report that PTSD symptoms may trigger substance abuse, which may in turn intensify the PTSD symptoms. Self-medication often does not adequately alleviate the symptoms of PTSD, and the substance itself becomes a problem.

The outcome of treatment is much worse when the dual diagnosis of PTSD and SUD is present. In addition, many patients who have a dual diagnosis with PTSD and drug abuse may have third, fourth, or fifth diagnoses, such as depression, anxiety, and antisocial behavior. Hence, the term dual diagnosis may be a misnomer and the term co-occurring diagnosis may be more accurate (Najavits, 2008).

It is recommended that therapists explain the nature of each disorder and the link between them to the patients, teaching them healthier coping skills and problem-solving behaviors and giving attention to all disorders, regardless of the exact nature of the treatment program. For the treatment of PTSD and AUD, it is ideal to treat both disorders integrally. Clinical researchers have developed integrated PTSD-AUD therapy, with or without exposure therapy elements. As the name implies, exposure therapy is a type of treatment involving exposure to the context or object responsible for the trauma in a safe therapeutic environment. In cases of PTSD, exposure therapy may be contraindicated if SUD is present due to a concern that exposure may increase the potential for alcohol or drug relapse (Ouimette & Read, 2008).

Another difficulty for individuals who are suffering from a dual diagnosis of PTSD and SUD arises when the professionals who are treating them are not equipped to treat both disorders simultaneously. PTSD patients who are suffering from alcohol problems are generally referred to an alcohol treatment program because clinicians often feel that the patient first needs to address the alcohol or SUD problem before treating PTSD. It is our strong recommendation, however, that both disorders be treated simultaneously. We feel that neglecting to do so has contributed to the high failure rate in treatment of dual diagnoses of PTSD and SUD or AUD.

Some clinicians explain that improvement in one disorder does not necessarily imply improvement in the other. Studies suggest that individuals with both AUD or SUD and PTSD consume more alcohol, relapse more quickly, have less social support, are more likely to be unemployed, and have treatment readmission rates that are higher than those for AUD or SUD patients without PTSD.

PHARMACOTHERAPY: ALCOHOL AS A COMORBIDITY OF PTSD

Three medications are currently approved by the FDA for treatment of alcohol dependence: (a) disulfiram (Antabuse®); (b) naltrexone HCl (ReVia®,

Depade®); oral or long-acting injectable; and (c) acamprosate (Campral®). In addition, the anti-seizure medication topiramate is also being used for the management of alcohol dependence.

Some studies indicate that antidepressive medications combined with naltrexone were effective in treating PTSD-AUD comorbidity. In one study, a total of sixty-nine patients from two VA sites were randomized and given doses of either 40 mg per day of paroxetine or 200 mg per day of the TCA desipramine HCl. The two groups later received either 50 mg per day of naltrexone or a matching placebo. The preliminary results suggested that both paroxetine and desipramine were evenly matched in safely decreasing symptoms of PTSD and alcohol consumption (Brauser, 2009).

Disulfiram

Disulfiram was approved in 1951 by the U.S. FDA and has been used clinically for the past fifty years for patients who suffer from alcoholism (Meyer, 1989). The effectiveness of disulfiram varies from person to person. If taken as directed, it can help a patient completely stop drinking by increasing the number of days the recipient abstains from drinking (Petrakis, Gonzalez, Rosenheck & Krystal, 2002).

Randomized, controlled trials of this medication have been few, and the results show a mixed efficacy (Peachy & Naranjo, 1984). The most comprehensive research in the treatment of alcoholism was conducted by the VA on male veterans with alcohol problems. In terms of total abstinence, length of abstinence before relapse, employment, or social stability, they found little difference between disulfiram and a placebo group (Fuller, et al., 1986). Despite this finding, it is thought that with supervised dosing, or with patients who are highly motivated, disulfiram can be an effective treatment in the prevention of relapse (Banys, 1988; Fuller, et al., 1986).

One study of disulfiram on patients who had dual disorders of alcohol and schizophrenia, bipolar disorder, anxiety, or personality disorders show- ed no worsening of their symptoms as a result of this medication (Kofoed et al., 1986). Another report suggested that there was miniscule evidence of interaction between disulfiram and medications commonly given to treat major psychiatric disorders, which included antidepressants, antimania agents, and antipsychotics (Larson, Olincy, Rummans & Morse, 1992).

As Goodwin (1992) explained, one of the main problems with disulfiram is that it is easy for the patient to discontinue the medication and start drinking; therefore, the relapse rate may be very high. On that basis, it is effective when used in clinical settings that focus on abstinence and have control over the patient's compliance in taking the medication. Sometimes it is helpful for the patient to have the medication dispensed from a treatment center or doctor's office on a daily basis or to have it administered by a partner or family member.

Mechanism of Action

Treatment with disulfiram is a type of aversive therapy. The normal breakdown of alcohol produces a by-product named acetaldehyde, which becomes highly toxic if mixed with disulfiram. This toxicity can produce a significant amount of aversive reactions, including severe headaches, nausea, vomiting, flushing, and anxiety. No treatment is needed for mild reactions; however, if the symptoms are serious (e.g. arrhythmia or respiratory depression), immediate treatment with supportive measures should be administered.

It is assumed that these negative reactions motivate the patients to stop drinking; however, one drawback is that they also provide a good reason to stop taking the medication (Chick, 1999; Chick et al., 1992; O'Farrell & Bayog, 1986). On that note, disulfiram may work more effectively on impulsive drinkers (Krampe, Stawicki & Wagner, 2006).

Dosage

The usual adult dose for alcohol dependence is 500 mg once per day. This dosage is continued for one to two weeks after the abstinence of ethanol, when it may be decreased to 250 mg per day and continued for six months to a year. The 500-mg dose is the maximum recommended by the manufacturer (Drugs.com, 2010e).

Side effects

The side effects of disulfiram include blurred vision, headache, heart palpitation, sweating, dry mouth, nausea, confusion, and weakness. Older clinical reports (prior to 1970) suggest that disulfiram may cause several psychiatric symptoms, including depression, anxiety, mania, psychosis, and delirium (Larson et al., 1992). In these cases, it is important to keep in mind that the standard dose was one to two grams, compared to current dose of 250 to 500 mg, and that that these symptoms were likely the result of the higher dose. It should also be noted that prior to 1970 the definitions of psychiatric symptoms were not standardized (Petrakis et al., 2002).

Naltrexone

Naltrexone was approved by the FDA in 1994 as a specific opiate receptor antagonist that can be used for rectifying alcoholic misuse. Its effectiveness is based on its ability to decrease the euphoric effects of alcohol. Alcohol is believed to stimulate the release of endogenous opioid beta-endorphin, and naltrexone may have a blocking impact on endogenous endorphin. Clinically, this medication appears to reduce the "high" feeling associated with alcohol. It may also reduce the likelihood of relapse in heavy drinkers (O'Brien et al., 1996; Pettinati et al., 2006).

Naltrexone reduces cravings and enhances the ability to maintain abstinence. Patients may prefer to take naltrexone over disulfiram because it does not create the same adverse reaction (Petrakis et al., 2002). Although naltrexone seems to have some advantages over disulfiram, reports also indicate that patient compliance may be an issue (Volpicelli et al., 1997). Several studies have been conducted to determine the impact of naltrexone on comorbidities such as psychosis and anxiety disorders, but no controlled studies have been evaluated to determine its effect on PTSD. One study found that it did not worsen symptoms of schizophrenia (Sernyak et al., 1998). Another study reported that naltrexone does not precipitate panic attacks, either alone or when given with sodium lactate (Liebowitz et al., 1984).

Long-acting injectable forms of naltrexone are available, and monthly injections of 380 mg may result in a stable therapeutic dose for twenty-eight to thirty days. Long-acting treatment may be more helpful, because it guarantees compliance with the medication (O'Malley et al., 2002). This medication may be more effective if the patient achieved at least seven days of abstinence prior to starting it.

Mechanism of Action

Naltrexone inhibits the regions of the brain that creates the pleasure one feels from consuming narcotics or alcohol. When these parts of the brain are blocked it eliminates the euphoria the person experiences, making it easier to stop drinking. Unlike disulfiram, naltrexone does not make the patient feel ill if he or she drinks alcohol while taking it (Robert, 2009).

Dosage

The usual adult dosage for alcohol dependence is administered in oral tablets of 50 mg once per day. It is also available in 380-mg doses that can be given once every month by intramuscular injection (Drugs.com, 2010f).

Side Effects

The most common side effect of naltrexone is nausea. Other side effects include headache, diarrhea, dizziness, nervousness, drowsiness, and anxiety. Some users may become depressed, get cramps, have rashes, and experience joint and muscle pain. One should avoid taking this medicine with disulfiram, because it may increase liver toxicity and liver damage (Raber, 2003).

Acamprosate

Acamprosate was approved in the United States based on three double-blind, placebo-controlled trials that were conducted in Europe. These studies showed that acamprosate was superior to the placebo with respect to the number of dropouts, relapse rate, and total days of abstinence from alcohol (O'Brien & Dackis, 2009). Acamprosate reduces excitatory glutamate neurotransmission and increases GABA neurotransmission, which may make it a possible "substitute" for alcohol during withdrawal. It may mitigate the adverse effects of withdrawal and increase the likelihood of abstinence (Stahl & Grady, 2010).

One U.S. trial of acamprosate was not very promising; however, a meta-analysis of all controlled trials indicates its usefulness (Bouza, Angeles, Munoz & Amate, 2004). One placebo-controlled group study involving more than 4500 patients indicated that detoxified patients who were given acamprosate were less likely to drop out of treatment and had much higher success rates of abstinence than did those who were not given the medication. Taking acamprosate may facilitate the patient's ability to remain in abstinence by minimizing withdrawal symptoms (Mason & Ownby, 2000). The FDA, however, suggests that acamprosate does not reduce withdrawal symptoms.

Some reports suggest that acamprosate works only when patients attend support groups or therapy and simultaneously abstain from alcohol (Mason, 2001). Although the FDA has stated that acamprosate may not be effective to those who are actively drinking while in treatment, reports from several studies have reaffirmed its benefits. Twenty-four randomized control trials were reviewed with 6915 alcohol-dependent patients, who also suffered from psychosocial problems. The results indicate that acamprosate prevented relapse in one of every nine patients who had stopped drinking. It also increased the number of days patients abstained from alcohol by an average of three days a month (Science Daily, 2010).

Mechanism of Action

Acamprosate is believed to reduce relapses among alcohol-dependent individuals (Rösner et al., 2010) by stabilizing brain chemistry that has been altered because of alcohol dependence. It works by antagonizing the action of glutamate, a neurotransmitter that is hyperactive in the postwithdrawal phase (Mason & Heyser, 2010). It also normalizes imbalances in other neurotransmissions that can remain long after acute alcohol withdrawal. If left untreated, this physiological dysregulation may prompt relapse (Littleton & Zieglgansberger, 2003).

Dosage

The usual adult dosage is 666 mg taken orally three times per day, in two 333-mg tablets (Drugs.com, 2010g).

Side Effects

Serious side effects are anomalous heartbeat, allergic reactions, low or high blood pressure, shortness of breath, self-destructive ideas, severe anxiety/depression, confusion, and decrease in urinating.

Less-concerning side effects include nausea, vomiting, stomach pain, loss of appetite, constipation, diarrhea, headache, dizziness, drowsiness, vision problems, problems with memory or thinking, weakness, cold or flulike symptoms, back pain, joint or muscle pain, dry mouth, decreased or distorted sense of taste, insomnia, impotence, loss of interest in sex, sweating, mild skin rash, or numbness or tingly sensation (Drugs.com, 2010a).

Topiramate

Topiramate is an anticonvulsant medication that is reported to have beneficial effects in alcohol treatment. Along with its use for binge eating and treating obesity, this drug has been investigated to help alcohol-dependent individuals (Johnson et al., 2003, 2007) and has also been specifically used on PTSD victims in clinical trials (Berlant & van Kammen, 2002).

Johnson and associates (2003, 2007) from the University of Virginia conducted a study on 371 alcohol-dependent patients by administering either topiramate or a placebo and having them go to a counselor every week for fourteen weeks. Both groups showed improvement, but in the topiramate patients, their percentage of heavy drinking days dropped from 81.9 percent to 43.8 percent. In the placebo group, heavy drinking days dropped from 82 percent to 51.8 percent. This study further showed that patients did not drink heavily for twenty-eight days and some abstained from alcohol completely for twenty-eight or more days (Drugs.com, 2010b). Johnson and associates, stated that a large number of alcoholics have hypertension, and in addition to reducing drinking significantly, topiramate decreases blood pressure. It can also decrease the risk of heart disease in alcohol-dependent people. Johnson stated that topiramate acts as many medications rather than just one (Med India, 2008).

Mechanism of Action

While the exact functioning and mechanism is unknown, topiramate is known to decrease alcohol cravings and alcohol withdrawal symptoms (Kenna et al., 2009).

Dosage: Average adult dosage usually begins with a 25-mg morning dose and increases gradually to a total of 300 mg given twice daily, in divided doses.

Side effects: The most common side effects of topiramate include constipation, diarrhea, headache, dry mouth, nausea, fatigue, trouble sleeping, and weight loss. More severe side effects are allergic reactions, blood in urine, irregular heartbeat, loss of consciousness, chest pains, speech problems, and suicidal thoughts (Drugs.com, 2010c). This drug may cause kidney stones, decreased sweating with increased body temperature, and glaucoma (French et al., 2004). Avoiding alcohol is recommended because it may increase certain side effects and also increase the risk of developing seizures (Drugs.com, 2010c).

CONCLUSION

Alcohol should be considered a drug that is used without a prescription. It is obvious that alcohol is used by those with a history of trauma as a way to self-medicate. Although the numbing effect may alleviate feelings of suffering, it does not cure the trauma. On the contrary, this temporary solution becomes a permanent problem for many veterans and victims of war trauma.

REFERENCES

Banys, P. (1988). The clinical use of disulfiram (Antabuse): A review. *Journal of Psychoactive Drugs, 20*(3), 243–261.

Bell, N.S., Amoroso, P.J., Wegman, D.H., & Senier, L. (2001). Proposed explanations for excess injury among veterans of the Persian Gulf War and a call for greater attention from policymakers and researchers. *Injury Prevention 7*, 4–9.

Berlant, J., and van Kammen, D.P. (2002, January). Open-label topiramate as primary or adjunctive therapy in chronic civilian posttraumatic stress disorder: A preliminary report. *The Journal of Clinical Psychiatry, 63*(1), 15–20.

Bouza, C., Angeles, M., Munoz, A., and Amate, J.M. (2004). Efficacy and safety of naltrexone and acamprosate in the treatment of alcohol dependence: A systematic review. *Addiction, 99*(7), 811–828.

Brauser, D. (2009, September 4). Naltrexone, disulfiram decrease alcohol dependence symptoms in veterans with PTSD. *Medscape Medical News.* Retrieved on 11/11/11 from http://www.medscale.com/viewarticle/708427.

Bremner, J.D., Southwick, S.M., Darnell A., and Charney, D.S. (1996). Chronic PTSD in Vietnam combat veterans: Course of illness and substance abuse. *American Journal of Psychiatry; 153*, 369–375.

Breslau, N., Davis, G.C., Peterson, E.L., and Schultz, L. (1997). Psychiatric sequelae of posttraumatic stress disorder in women. *Archives of General Psychiatry, 54*, 81–87

Centers for Disease Control and Prevention. (2004, September 24). Alcohol-attributable deaths and years of potential life lost: United States, 2001. *MWWR. Morbidity and Mortality Weekly Report, 53*(37); 866–870.

Chick, J. (1999). Safety issues concerning the use of disulfiram in treating alcohol dependence. *Drug Safety, 20*(5), 427–435.

Chick, J., Gouch, K., Falkowski, W., Kershaw, P., Hore, B.M., Ritson, B., et al. (1992). Disulfiram treatment of alcoholism. *British Journal of Psychiatry, 161*, 84–89.

Clayton, N.M., & Nash, W.P. (2007). Medication management of combat and operational stress injuries in active duty service members. In C.R. Figley and W.P. Nash (Eds.), *Combat stress injury: Theory, research, and management* (pp. 219–245). New York: Routledge.

Corrigan, J.D., and Cole, T.B. (2008). Substance use disorders and clinical management of traumatic brain injury and posttraumatic stress disorder. *JAMA, 300*, 720–721.

Dansky, B.S., Saladin, M.E., Brady, K., Kilpatrick, D.G., and Resnick, H.S. (1995). Prevalence of victimization and posttraumatic stress disorder among women with substance use disorders; comparison of telephone and in-person assessment samples. *International Journal of Addiction, 30*, 1079–1099.

Drugs.com (2010, a). Acamprosate information from drugs.com micromedex™ [Updated October, 1 2010], Cerner Multum™ [Updated October, 20 2010], Wolters Kluwer™ [Updated November, 4 2010]. Available from http://www.drugs.com/mtm/acamprosate.html

Drugs.com (2010, b). Epilepsy drug holds promise as treatment for alcoholism; c2000-10 Micromedex™ [Updated October, 1 2010], Cerner Multum™ [Updated October, 20 2010], Wolters Kluwer™ [Updated November, 4 2010]. Available from http://www.drugs.com/news/epilepsy-holds-promise-alcoholism-9605.html

Drugs.com (2010, c). Topiramate side effects; c2000-10 Micromedex™ [Updated October 1, 2010], Cerner Multum™ [Updated October, 20 2010], Wolters Kluwer™ [Updated November 4, 2010]. Available from http://www.drugs.com/sfx/topiramate-side effects.html

Drugs.com (2010, d). Topiramate information; c2000-10 Micromedex™ [Updated October 1, 2010], Cerner Multum™ [Updated October 20, 2010], Wolters Kluwer™ [Updated November 4, 2010]. Available from http://www.drugs.com/mtm/topiramate.html

Drugs.com (2010, e). Disulfiram dosage; c2000-10 [Updated October 20, 2010; cited: December 19, 2010]. Available from www.drugs.com/dosage/disulfiram.html

Drugs.com (2010, f). Naltrexone dosage information; c2010 [Updated October 20, 2010; cited: December 19, 2010]. Available from http://www.drugs.com/dosage/naltrexone.html

Drugs.com (2010, g). Acamprosate dosage; c2000-10 [Updated: October 20, 2010; cited: December 19, 2010]. Available from www.drugs.com/dosage/acamprosate.html

Erbes, C., Westermeyer, J., Engdahl, B., and Johnsen, E. (2007). Post-traumatic stress disorder and service utilization in a sample of service members from Iraq and Afghanistan. *Military Medicine, 172*, 359–363.

Evans, K., and Sullivan, J.M. (1995). *Treating addicted survivors of trauma.* New York: Guilford Press.

Faingold, C.L., N'Gouemo, P., and Riaz, A. (1998). Ethanol and neurotransmitter interactions-from molecular to integrative effects. *Progress in Neurobiology, 55*(5), 509–535.

French, J.A., Kanner, A.M., Bautista, J., Abou-Khalil, B., Browne, T., Harden, C.L., et al. (2004). Efficacy and tolerability of the new antiepileptic drugs I: Treatment of new onset epilepsy. Report of the Therapeutics and Technology Assessment Subcommittee and Quality Standards Subcommittee of the American Academy of Neurology and the American Epilepsy Society. *Neurology, 62*(8), 1252–1260.

Fuller, R.K., Branchey, L., Brightwell, D.R., Derman, R.M., Emrick, C.D., Iber, F.L., et al., (1986). Disulfiram treatment of alcoholism. A Veterans Administration cooperative study. *JAMA, 256*(11), 1449–1455.

Goodwin, D.W. (1992). Alcohol: Clinical aspects. In J. H., Lowinson, P., Ruiz, and R. B. Millman (Eds.) *Substance Abuse–A Comprehensive Textbook* (pp 144–151). Baltimore, MD: Williams & Wilkins.

Hoge, C.W., Castro C.A., Messer, S.C., McGurk, D., Cotting, D.I., & Koffman, R.L. (2004). Combat duty in Iraq and Afghanistan, mental health problems, and barriers to care. *New England Journal of Medicine, 351*, 13–22.

Hoge, C.W., Toboni, H.E., Messer, S.C., Bell, N., Amoroso, P. & Orman, D.T. (2005). The occupational burden of mental disorders in the US military: Psychiatric hospitalizations, involuntary separations, and disability. *American Journal of Psychiatry, 162*, 585–59.

Jacobson, I.G., Ryan, M.A., Hooper, T.I., Smith, T.C., Amoroso, P.J. Borko, E.J., et al. (2008). Alcohol use and alcohol-related problems before and after military combat deployment. *JAMA, 300*, 663–675.

Jeremy, L. (2010, May 13). Alcohol a problem for war veterans, study finds. *The Independent on Sunday.* Retrieved December 4, 2010, from http://www.independent.co.uk/life-style/health-and-families/health-news/alcohol-a-problem-for-war-veterans-study-finds-1972190.html

Johnson, B., Aitdaoud, N., Bowden, C., DiClemente, C.C., Roache, J.D., Lawrom, K., et al. (2003). Oral topiramate for treatment of alcohol dependence: A randomized controlled trial. *The Lancet, 361,* 1677–1685.

Johnson, B.A., Rosenthal, N., Capece, J.A., Wiegand, F., Mao, L., Beyers, K., et al. (2007). Topiramate for treating alcohol dependence: A randomized controlled trial. *JAMA, 298,* 1641–51.

Kenna, G.A., Lomastro, T.L., Schiesl, A., Leggio, L., & Swift, R.M. (2009, May). Review of topiramate: an antiepileptic for the treatment of alcohol dependence. *Current Drug Abuse Reviews, 2*(2), 135–42.

Kessler, R.C., Sonnega, A., Bromet, E., Hughes, M., and Nelson, C.B. (1995): Post traumatic stress disorder in the National Comorbidity Survey. *Archives of General Psychiatry, 52*; 1048–1060.

Kofoed, L., Friedman, M.J., and Peck, R. (1993, Summer). Alcoholism and drug abuse in patients with PTSD. *Psychiatric Quarterly, 64*(2), 151–171.

Kofoed, L., Kania, J., Walsh, T., and Atkinson, R.M. (1986). Outpatient treatment of patients with substance abuse and coexisting psychiatric disorders. *American Journal of Psychiatry, 143*(7), 867–872.

Krampe, H., Stawicki, S., and Wagner, T. (2006, January). Follow-up of 180 alcoholic patients for up to 7 years after outpatient treatment: Impact of alcohol deterrents on outcome. *Alcoholism, Clinical and Experimental Research, 30*(1), 86–95.

Kulka, R.A., Schlenger, W.E., Fairbank, J.A., Hough, R.L., Jordan, B.K., Marmar, C.R., and Wiess, D.S. (1990). *Trauma and the Vietnam War Generation: Report of Findings From the National Vietnam Veterans Readjustment Study.* New York, Brunner/Mazel.

Lande, R.G., Marin, B.A., and Ruzek, J.I. (2004). Substance abuse in the deployment environment. In *Iraq War Clinician Guide* (2nd ed., pp. 79–82). White River Station, VT: National Center for Post-Traumatic Stress Disorder, Department of Veterans Affairs.

Landolt, H.P., and Gillin, J.C. (2001). Sleep abnormalities during abstinence in alcohol-dependent patients: Aetiology and management. *CNS Drugs, 15,* 413–425.

Larson, E.W., Olincy, A., Rummans, T.A., and Morse, R.M. (1992). Disulfiram treatment of patients with both alcoholic dependence and other psychiatric disorders: A review. *Alcoholism: Clinical and Experimental Research, 16*(1), 125–130.

Liebowitz, M.R., Gorman, J.M., Fyer, A.J., Dillon, D.J., & Klein, D.F. (1984). Effects of naloxone on patients with panic attacks. *American Journal of Psychiatry, 141*(8), 995–997.

Littleton, J., and Zieglgansberger, W. (2003). Pharmacological mechanisms of naltrex-one and acamprosate in the prevention of relapse in alcohol dependence. *American Journal on Addiction, 12*(Suppl 1), S3-S11.

Maes, M., Delmeire, L., Mylle, J., and Altamura, C. (2001). Risk and preventive factors of post-traumatic stress disorder (PTSD): Alcohol consumption and intoxication prior to a traumatic event diminishes the relative risk to develop PTSD in response to that trauma. *Journal of Affective Disorders, 63,* 113–121.

Mason, B.J. (2001). Treatment of alcohol-dependent outpatients with acamprosate: A clinical review. *Journal of Clinical Psychiatry, 62* (Suppl 20), 42–48.

Mason, B.J., and Heyser, C.J. (2010, January). The neurobiology, clinical efficacy and safety of acamprosate in the treatment of alcohol dependence. *Expert Opinion on Drug Safety, 9*(1), 177–188.

Mason, B.J. and Ownby, R.L. (2000). Acamprosate for the treatment of alcohol dependence: A review of double-blind, placebo-controlled trials. *CNS Spectrums, 5*(2), 58–69.

McFarlane, A.C. (1998). Epidemiological evidence about the relationship between PTSD and alcohol abuse: the nature of the association. *Addictive Behaviors, 23*(6), 813–825.

Med India (2008, June 11). Topiramate may be useful in treating alcohol addiction. MeDIndia Retreived from http://www.medindia.net/news/Topiramate-may-Be-Useful-in-Treating-Alcohol-Addiction-37854-1.htm

Meyer, R.E. (1989). Prospects for a rational pharmacotherapy of alcoholism. *Journal of Clinical Psychiatry, 50*(11), 403–412.

O'Brien, C.P., Volpicell, L.A., and Volpicelli, J.R. (1996). Naltrexone in the treatment of alcoholism: A clinical review. *Alcohol, 13*(1), 35–39.

O'Brien, C.P., and Dackis, C.A. (2009). Treatment of substance-related disorders. In A.F. Schatzberg and C.B. Nemeroff (Eds.), *Textbook of Psychopharmacology* (pp. 1213–1229). Washington, DC: American Psychiatric Publishing, Inc.

O'Farrell, T.J., and Bayog, R.D. (1986). Antabuse contracts for married alcoholics and their spouses: A method to maintain Antabuse ingestion and decrease conflict about drinking. *Journal of Substance Abuse Treatment, 3*, 1–8.

O' Malley, S.S., Krishnan-Sarin, S., Farren, C., et al. (2002). Naltrexone decreases craving and alcohol self-administration in alcohol-dependent subjects and activates the hypothalamo-pituitary-adrenocortical axis. *Psychopharmacology* (Berl), *160*, 19–29.

Ouimette, P., and Brown, P.J. (2003). *Trauma and Substance Abuse: Consequences, and Treatment of Comorbid Disorders.* Washington, DC: American Psychological Association.

Ouimette, P., and Read, J.P. (2008). Alcohol use disorders. In G. Reyes, J.D. Elhai, and J.D. Ford (Eds.), *The Encyclopedia of Psychological Trauma* (pp. 20–22). Hoboken, NJ: Wiley.

Peachy, J.E., and Naranjo, C.A. (1984). The role of drugs in the treatment of alcoholism. *Drugs, 27*, 171–182.

Petrakis, I.L., Gonzalez, G., Rosenheck, R., and Krystal, H. (2002). Comorbidity of alcoholism and psychiatric disorders. *Alcohol Research and Health, 26*(2), 81–89.

Pettinati, H.M., O'Brien, C.P., Rabinowitz, A.R., et al. (2006). The status of naltrexone in the treatment of alcohol dependence: Specific effects on heavy drinking. *Journal of Clinical Psychopharmacology, 26*(6), 610–625.

Price, J.L., (2007, January 1) *Findings from the National Vietnam Veterans Readjustment Study.* Retrieved November 6, 2011 http://www.ptsd.va.gov/professional/pages/vietnam-vets-study.asp

Raber, J., (2003) Naltrexone, Gale Encyclopedia of Mental Disorders. Retrieved on Nov. 11, 2011 from http://www.encyclopedia.com/topic/Naltrexone.aspx

Robert, B. (2009). Information. from Familydoctor.org. c2000-10 American Academy of Family Physicians. Retrieved on Nov. 11, 2011 from: http://familydoctor.org/familydoctor/en/drugs-procedures-devices/prescription-medicines/naltrexone-for-alcoholism.html

Rösner, S., Hackl-Herrwerth, A., Leucht, S., Lehert, P., Vecchi, S., & Soyka, M. (2010). Acamprosate for alcohol dependence. *Cochrane Database of Systematic*

Reviews (9). Retrieved on Nov. 11, 2011 from: http://www2.cochran.org/reviews/en/ab004332.html

Ruzek, J.I., Polusny, M.A., and Abueg, F.R. (1998). Cognitive behavioral therapies for trauma. In V.M. Follette, J.I. Ruzek, and F.R. Abueg (Eds.), *Assessment and Treatment of Concurrent Posttraumatic Stress Disorder and Substance Abuse* (pp. 226–255). New York: Guilford.

Saladin, M.E., Brady, K.T., Dansky, B.S., and Kilpatrick, D.G. (1995). Understanding comorbidity between PTSD and substance use disorders: Two preliminary investigations. *Addictive Behaviors, 20*, 643–655.

Santiago, P.N., Wilk, J.E., Milliken, C.S., Castro, C.A., Engel, C.C., & Hoge, C.W. (2010) *Combat Veterans. Psychiatric Services, 61*(6): 575-581

Schmitz, M.M., Sepandj, A., Pichler, P.M., and Rudas, S. (1996). Disrupted melatonin-secretion during alcohol withdrawal. *Progress in Neuro-psychopharmacology and Biological Psychiatry, 20*, 983–995.

ScienceDaily (2010, September 17). Acamprosate prevents relapse to drinking in alcoholism, review finds. Retrieved on July 20, 2011 from http://www.science-daily.com/releases/2010/09/100907210819.htm.

Sernyak, M.J., Glazer, W.M., Heninger, G.R., Charney, D.S., Woods, S.W., Petrakis, I.L. et al. (1998). Naltrexone augmentation of neuroleptics in schizophrenia. *Journal of Clinical Psychopharmacology, 18*(3); 248- 251.

Shirao, I., Tsuda, A., Ida, Y., Tsujimaru, S., Satoh, H., Oguchi, M., et al. (1988). Effect of acute ethanol administration on noradrenaline metabolism in brain regions of stressed and nonstressed rats. *Pharmacology, Biochemistry, and Behavior, 30*(3), 769–773.

Simon, A., and Gorman, J. (2004). Psychopharmacological possibilities in the acute disaster setting. *Psychiatric Clinics of North America, 27*, 425–458.

Sorenson, G. (2004). Afghanistan veteran returns. *Vet Center Voice, 25*(2), 6–15.

Stahl, S.M., and Grady, M.M. (2010). *Stahl's illustrated: Anxiety, stress, and PTSD.* New York: Cambridge University Press.

Taft, C.T., Kaloupek, D.G., Schumm, J.A., Marshall, A.D., Panuzio, J. & Keane, T.M. (2007). Posttraumatic stress disorder symptoms, physiological reactivity alcohol problems, and aggression among military veterans. *Journal of Abnormal Psychology, 116*, 498–507.

Volpicelli, J.R., Rhines, K.C., Rhines, J.S., Volpicelli, L.A., Alterman, A.I., & O'Brien, C.P. (1997). Naltrexone and alcohol dependence. Role of subject compliance. *Archives of General Psychiatry, 54*(8), 737–742.

White, H.S., Brown, S.D., Woodhead, J.H., Skeen, G.A. & Wolf, H.H. (2000) Topiramate modulates GABA-evoked currents in murine cortical neurons by a nonbenzodiazepine mechanism. *Epilepsia, 41*(Suppl), S17–S20.

Chapter 10

FIGHTING FOR YOUR LIFE: CLINICAL ISSUES IN WAR TRAUMA BEREAVEMENT

Karen L. Carney and William J. Pilkington

You end up doing things that you never thought you would do. You do them to survive. You promise that you won't leave anyone behind. But then you do. You try not to think about it. You come home and get busy with your life. But there are times when it hits you. You wonder why you survived but some of your buddies didn't. It's hard.

Richard J. Darmofal
U.S. Air Force, Vietnam veteran

You're trained to look at the enemy as an object. They're not human. You detach yourself. Don't ever ask a vet if he killed anyone.

Anonymous Gulf War veteran

INTRODUCTION

The basic function of any system is survival. What makes bereavement from war trauma extraordinary is that it involves survival on many dimensions. The soldiers' instinct to protect themselves may be at odds with a moral compass that makes them wish to preserve the lives of comrades and civilians. Religious beliefs, philosophies of life, and cultural and personal values may be challenged. Dedication to the mission may put soldiers at odds with the instinct to preserve their own life and the lives of comrades, creating a battlefield on many fronts: the external threats to survival and the internal conflicts of the psyche. Bereaved veterans and their families may struggle with issues of greater meaning. Their perception of how and why their loved one suffered or were killed will affect the course of their grief. Families who believe that their loved ones did not suffer or die in vain but rather died fighting for a noble cause often have an advantage over those who cannot assign a purpose or "cause" to their loved ones' suffering. On the other hand, those who believe that their comrades or loved ones were victims of senseless violence or murder may be filled with rage, which will complicate their journey of grief.

WHAT IS BEREAVEMENT?

The word *bereavement* comes from a Latin word meaning to have been robbed, to have been ripped off. The Jewish mourning tradition of ripping, or rending, a garment over the heart is a powerful symbol of this literal definition of death-related loss. This practice is often modified by wearing a black ribbon pinned over the mourner's heart and then cut across its side by a rabbi. The tradition of wearing ribbons to signify particular causes, such as pink ribbons for breast cancer awareness, stems from this mourning ribbon tradition.

To experience bereavement, the state of having suffered a loss, one must first experience an attachment. Suffering does not occur unless there is a significant attachment, which may take many forms. Attachment may be to a person, place, or thing, as well as to a value, ideal, or belief system. The stronger the attachment to what was lost, the stronger the reaction to loss. War trauma bereavement may include all of these factors: loss of an attachment figure, loss of function (as in the case of losing a limb), loss of a sense of safety and security, and loss of home and/or country. It may also include conflict regarding previously held ideals, ethics, morals, and existential beliefs about humanity.

There is much written in grief and loss literature regarding challenges to one's **assumptive world** (Corr, Nabe & Corr, 2009), or the way one understands the order and fairness of the universe, in response to a loss. Rando (2000) describes the assumptive world as "the mental schema that contains all a person assumes to be true about the self, the world, and everything and everyone in it. Previous experiences in life form the basis for the person's assumptive world elements. These elements represent all of that person's assumptions, expectations, and beliefs, with most of these becoming virtually automatic habits of cognition and behavior" (p. 61). Mourners of any type of trauma typically describe inordinate challenges to their assumptive world and personal spirituality. The "why" questions may be extensive and complex for anyone bereft but are especially intense for mourners of war trauma.

Not everyone has a **religion**, defined here as a belief system that has been learned through culture and tradition, yet everyone has a personal **spirituality** that includes beliefs as well as nonbeliefs regarding existential matters. Spirituality involves core values and perspectives on meaning and purpose for life and living, as well as death and dying (Irish, Lundquist & Nelson, 1993). Being human, unlike other animals, which are predominantly instinctual, involves a spiritual quest for meaning. According to Ken Doka (1993), we are the only animals having to decide from moment to moment, who am I? What do I have to do? Spirituality includes philosophies and other movements in which persons find meaning in their lives. Doka asserts that we cannot escape from our spirituality (Doka, 1993).

LIFE REVIEW AND SPIRITUAL NEEDS OF OLDER VETERANS

I never talked about it until now, at 80 years old.
I've said more about it this year than I ever have my
whole life . . . . Why was I spared?

Joe Milich, WWII veteran

As they approach the ends of their lives, many veterans will share stories, search for meaning, and ponder their legacies. Doka and Morgan (1993) identified three major spiritual needs of those who are nearing the ends of their lives: (1) to find meaning in life, (2) the desire to die appropriately, and (3) to find hope that extends beyond the grave.

The search for meaning occurs because we wish that, in one way or another, our lives can be filled with purpose, significance, and meaning. Religious and spiritual belief systems can be important here to give one's life a sense of cosmic significance and to provide a sense of forgiveness of oneself and others for acts of commission and omission and for dreams not accomplished (Doka, 1993).

To die appropriately is described as dying in a way that is consistent with one's own self-identity (Doka, 1993). This typically means to die with dignity, as the individual would perceive it. Doka further defines dying appropriately as being able to have a framework to explain suffering. He suggests that caregivers explore with the dying their beliefs about pain and death.

The third spiritual need involves transcendence (Doka, 1993). We seek reassurance that spirits will live on or our legacies will continue. Legacies may include children, other creative works, accomplishments, and continued survival of whatever "group" we identify ourselves with. Such are the ways in which each life is extended beyond the grave.

Survival of the group, which is the mission of the soldier, is especially relevant for veterans and their families. Having served in a war to promote survival of the culture may fulfill this transcendental spiritual need. Dying for a "cause" is seen as noble throughout many cultures. The grief reaction multiplies when the cause was determined to be "unjust."

A Soldier Speaks At Last: 60 Years of Grieving

Joseph Milich, United States Army, World War II Veteran (Interviewed on January 26, 2010)

I was born in 1926, the only son of Croatian immigrants. My younger sister and I were raised in New York City's Washington Heights section of upper Manhattan. My family placed a high value on education, so I studied hard and did very well in school. I joined the United States Army because they offered an Army specialized training program where I would attend college for four years, get a degree, and then spend time in the Army.

I went to basic training. It was a coincidence that many of us ended up in the 94th division, Third Army. I was sent overseas the day after D-Day, as a replacement for someone who had gotten killed. I was sent to France and placed in Company A, 302nd Infantry, 94th Division, Third Army.

I left New York City on the Queen Mary, got to Glasgow in four days, was immediately put on a train to Southampton, put on a ferry to cross the Channel to Le Havre, then on a "40 and 8" freight car. That meant it could hold forty men or eight horses. We then got onto trucks, but we didn't know exactly where we were going. We got off the truck somewhere in France and were told what company we were in. We went into combat just eleven days after leaving New York City! I didn't have time to think about what was happening or where I was going.

The Battle of the Bulge was a big German breakthrough. The Third Army under Patton diverted and was sent north into the neck of the Battle of the Bulge. When we broke through and helped relieve the people in Bastogne, we were diverted to the Saar/Moselle Triangle (Bastogne). The German Zeigfried Line was broken through, and we were attacking a little town, Oberloken, where I was wounded.

We took off at 3:00 AM and proceeded up a small hill through machine gun and mortar fire. Only four of us made it to the top. I knew that I had to get off the hill, because the hill was zeroed in for

German mortars. The two men next to me were killed. Two of us were wounded. I don't know why I was saved. I had severe wounds on both legs, which ended any hopes that I had, like lots of kids do, for a career in sports. I may not have made it, but I would have at least wanted to try.

We were lying there, my fallen comrades and me, and by now it was high noon; nobody came. Then I looked over the hill and saw six Germans who surrendered to me. They were out of it, in a daze. They must have seen American troops close by. The troops came and the Germans carried us down the hill to a waiting jeep equipped with litters.

I went to a field hospital. The next day they flew me to a hospital in England. I was in the hospital for three months, had several operations, and then was put on a train to Scotland and flown home to the States in a hospital plane. I ended up in a hospital in Utica, New York, which was a temporary hospital where I had another surgery.

Sometime in October I was sent to Mitchell Field in Long Island for convalescence. I was honorably discharged from the Army on December 19, which was ten months to the day that I was wounded. I was just nineteen years old, so I was sent home to New York with my parents.

I got NO psychological counseling by the military upon returning home, and I never talked about it with anyone. What I did get was the GI bill, so my education and books were paid for, and I had a small pension. Since I was wounded, I also had some extra benefits.

I was able to perform during battle because it was all about survival. I didn't think; I just performed to save myself. But after, when it was all over, I'd shake. I never had a chance to grieve. When I was in the ambulance someone heard me talking and asked, "Is that you, Joe?" I said "Yes" and looked over at a friend who had both eyes bandaged. I don't know if he was ever able to see again. I couldn't keep track of everybody who was hurt and everybody who was dead. I saw a lot of things that you never want to see. We didn't have embedded news crews like they do today.

The grieving never goes away . . . . you just try to manage it. I have posttraumatic stress disorder. I have had trouble sleeping, nightmares, flashbacks. It came out when I was in the VA hospital. I only got four hours of sleep each night for the next fifty years! Now that I'm older, I get six hours of sleep per night. The PTSD got worse after retirement, maybe because I had more time to think. Plus, we've had the Gulf War, Iraq, Afghanistan, and my grandson went to Iraq. All of this has taken me back to my own experiences.

It wasn't until 1996 that I started going to annual reunions with other WWII veterans, but we NEVER talk about specifics. We don't have to. We were all there. I've made a lot of friends at the reunions, and it helps to be around people who know what you saw and what you went through. I've been grieving every day for 60-plus years. Not a day goes by that I don't think about what happened.

What has helped me to carry on? Activity saved me. I was fortunate to have a job that I liked. I also have a lot of hobbies like woodworking, golf, and photography, and I love walking in the woods.

What hasn't helped? More wars. Watching movies that were as real as you can get—for example, Robert Mitchum in *GI Joe* or *Saving Private Ryan*—because at the end of the movie I broke down. The movie *The Band of Brothers*, well that was also too real. Because I lost a lot of friends, war changed me. You can see it in the picture of me before going to war, and the self-portrait after the war. My wife got rid of one of the self-portraits because she said it bothered her too much. It didn't help that I had to grow up a lot, too fast, in a short time.

The advice I'd like to give to anyone joining the armed services: listen to all of the veterans and learn from us. I wish I had kept a diary and brought a camera. Put your thoughts down every day, because you won't remember everything. Listen carefully, pay attention, and learn all the lessons you can before you get into combat. Be alert, do your job, watch your buddy, and keep your head low.

I don't know why I was spared, but I guess that my legacy is that along with my wife, I raised four great kids.

I have an idea about Afghanistan. I'd like to trade places with a young recruit, with someone who has a family. There are a lot of us who were in WWII who are saying the same thing. There are men and women in the National Guard who are going over to the Middle East for the third or fourth time! The National Guard was not intended to be used as a regular army! Many of them have earned the Combat/Infantry badge. It's a rifle with a wreath. I saw some of them wearing it in the Memorial Day parade. Having that badge meant that they were in harm's way. Really, I would like to take their place. Let them live their life, raise their families. I've lived my life and I'm still healthy enough to do something over there so that someone else can stay home. Let me do it. I'm ready.

This is the most that I've ever said to anyone about my war experience. I hope it helps.

Lessons from Joe Milich

What can be learned from the stories of war veterans like Joe Milich? Grief does not vanish with time alone. More than sixty years later, he still grieves for his fallen comrades and friends. More than sixty years later, he still suffers from PTSD. According to the U.S. Department of Veterans Affairs, research addressing grief symptoms among war veterans is limited. A recent study of a sample of Vietnam combat veterans in a residential rehabilitation unit for PTSD indicates that unresolved grief can be detected as a distress syndrome, distinct from depression and anxiety. In this study, Dr. Ilona Pivar (2010) of the U.S. Department of Veterans Affairs, National Center for PTSD, reports that grief symptoms were detected at very high levels of intensity thirty years post loss. Joe Milich reports that his grief persists more than sixty years post loss and that his PTSD symptoms got worse when he retired from his career as an engineer. Grief support for veterans has been lacking, but stories from veterans and the existing research indicates that it should be a required component of postwar rehabilitation.

WHAT IS GRIEF?

The word *grief* comes from the Latin word *grave*, meaning heavy burden. Grief encompasses the mind, body, and spiritual *reaction* to loss, whereas bereavement is the state of having suffered a loss. Grief is much more than emotional responses. Rando (1988) discusses the many facets of grief reactions, including psychological (through feelings, thoughts, and attitudes), social (through behavior and connections with others), and physical (through health and body symptoms). Worden (1991) outlines and describes four general categories of grief: (1) feelings, (2) physical sensations, (3) cognition and (4) behaviors.

Grief is a reaction to all types of losses, not only death, and is based on the individual's unique, individualistic perception of the loss (Rando, 1988). The more significant the loss, the more profound the grief reaction will be. Many factors will influence an individual's grief, and not everyone will respond in the same manner to the same loss (Walsh & McGoldrick, 1991).

WHAT IS MOURNING?

Mourning involves the conscious and unconscious processes, rituals, and outward expressions of grief that help the bereaved adapt to the loss. Rando

(1988, 1993, 2000) developed what she outlined as the "6 R" processes of mourning:

1. **Recognize the reality.** View the deceased, an important component of this process. If viewing is not possible, collecting data that will confirm the death is imperative.
2. **React to the separation.** Allow for the affective reaction and expression of the loss. Suppressing feelings, tears, anger, guilt, or blame will impede this process.
3. **Recollect and reexperience the deceased and the relationship.** What is the legacy of the person who died? How did he or she contribute to your life and world view? Helping survivors develop rituals for this process may be helpful. Funerals, memorial services, and other significant dates may offer opportunities for this process.
4. **Relinquish the old attachments to the deceased and the old assumptive world.** This is a process of spiritual reappraisal and adjustment. Many people will resist the notion of relinquishing the old attachment, fearing they will lose their attachment if they move on with their life. This process is complicated further when there is guilt or blame.
5. **Readjust to move adaptively into the new world without forgetting the old.** This may be accomplished when the person who experienced the loss has come to terms with the new reality and is able to carry on without being overburdened with guilt or blame.
6. **Reinvest in new relationships and new pursuits.** In this process the individual is making choices based on the new reality and is no longer protesting their loss. He or she is carrying on and living in the present, while not forgetting the past.

COMPLICATED GRIEF

Complicated grief involves a significant disturbance in social or occupational functioning. Symptoms of grief may be identical to those for major depression. Grief counselors must learn and understand what may be considered normal for each individual's culture and tradition.

Rando (1988) asserts that complicated grief often develops when there is a problem in one or more of the "6 R" processes of mourning. For example, one method in which we recognize the reality of a death is to view the body. If there was no opportunity to do so, as in the case of a soldier's body that could not be recovered, or if the mourner did not take the opportunity to view the deceased, that becomes a risk factor for complicated grief. As sentient beings, we process our existence through our sense of sight, sound, touch, and taste. If we bypass sentient recognition of the loss, it will be more difficult to acknowledge the reality and proceed with the processes of grief and mourning. Many of the families who lost loved ones in the September 11, 2001, terrorist attacks were never able to recover their loved ones' bodies. For many, this complicated their grief, because the death was not confirmed through their physical senses.

Complicated Grief and the Body's Stress Response

Grieving a significant loss takes a toll on our physical bodies. The fight, flight, or freeze response is triggered, creating a cascade of autonomic responses that are evolutionary in nature. The result is that we experience a loss as a threat to our own survival, igniting our central nervous system. Basic functions such as sleeping, eating, and digestion are disturbed, and our immune system is compromised. When this reaction is prolonged and interferes with day-to-day functioning, such extreme symptoms are an indication of complicated grief. According to Dr. M. Katherine Shear, "This loop of suffering . . . . takes a person away from humanity and has no redemptive value. Simply put, complicated grief can wreck a person's life" (Schumers, 2009).

Current research defines complicated grief as persisting for more than six months, at least six months after a death. There is a persistent yearning for the deceased that is so intense that it usurps other interests or desires. The individual experiences no meaning or joy to life. There are often intrusive thoughts about death, uncontrollable bouts of sadness, guilt, and other negative emotions, as well as a preoccupation with, or avoidance of, anything associated with the loss. Dr. Holly G. Prigerson, associate professor of psychiatry at Harvard Medical School and director of the Center for Psycho-Oncology and Palliative Care Research at the Dana-Farber Cancer Insti- tute in Boston, asserts that there is a link between complicated grief and suicidal ideation, a higher level of substance abuse, and higher levels of cigarette and alcohol consumption (Schumer, 2009).

Treatment of Complicated Grief

Complicated grief may be difficult to treat, because those who suffer from this condition avoid recalling the events of the trauma. Moreover, they have difficulty finding the words to describe it (Bolte Taylor, 2006; van der Kolk, McFarlane & Weisaeth, 2007). Research indicates that the area of the brain that involves speech is shut down under extreme stress. If the individual does not feel "safe" in the therapeutic setting, talk therapy may be of no use.

Nonverbal therapies such as trauma-sensitive yoga, acupuncture, and massage may help to regulate the body's response. Once the body is relaxed, talk therapies, including eye movement desensitization and reprocessing (Shapiro, 2001; van der Kolk, McFarlane & Weisaeth, 2007) and cognitive behavioral therapy (van der Kolk, McFarlane & Weisaeth, 2007; Wilson, Fried- man & Lindy, 2001) may be employed to reprocess the trauma and re-establish functioning.

Complicated Grief and Suicide Among Veterans

Soldiers who survive combat remain at risk for war-related death when they come home. Kastenbaum (2007) reports that those who serve the nation in the armed forces are at heightened risk for suicide, both during and after their war experiences. Vietnam War veterans experienced the stress of engaging in a war in a remote land, followed by returning home to a nation that had become increasingly critical of the purpose and conduct of the conflict. Vietnam veteran Richard Darmofal recalls being shocked, upon his return from combat duty, to hear of veterans being called "baby killers," in stark contrast to the experience of veterans from WW II, who were regarded as heroes.

Other factors contributing to complicated grief and/or suicidal ideation and attempts include prolonged separation from family, inadequate preparation for the rigors of combat, inadequate preparation for return to family and community living, and insufficient resources for medical care and counseling (Kastenbaum, 2007).

Additional Risk Factors for Complicated Grief

1. Very significant attachment to whomever or whatever was lost
2. Very significant attachment to the deceased and not having seen the body after death
3. Sudden loss
4. Premorbid history: If the individual does not have a psychiatric diagnosis on Axis I or II, with grief education, support, and trauma intervention, the likelihood of complicated grief is less. If the individual does have a previous psychiatric diagnosis, the likelihood of complicated grief is high
5. Traumatic loss involving violence and/or trauma to the body
6. Loss of a spouse, loss of a child, loss of a parent during adolescence
7. Insufficient social support
8. Multiple losses within a short time

9. Self-medicating with alcohol, drugs, or ill-prescribed prescription drugs.
10. Self-blame or guilt, and the perception that factors exist that, if changed, would have prevented the loss.

GUILT AND GRIEVING

Guilt is intertwined with our need for a sense of control and a search for reasons behind the loss (Redmond, as cited in Doka, 1996, p. 60). Guilt also may create obstacles to moving on. Guilt is very common among those grieving any loss, but as with most issues having to do with war trauma, the response may be exaggerated and more difficult to overcome. Rando (1993) describes illegitimate versus legitimate forms of guilt. Unrealistic expectations and standards for assuming responsibility for someone's death that are out of proportion to reality can lead to illegitimate guilt. For example, a soldier may feel responsible for the death of a fellow soldier, believing that he "should have" been able to save his comrade, when, in fact, the soldier did the best that she or he could under the circumstances.

Francine Shapiro (2001), the originator and developer of eye movement desensitization and reprocessing (EMDR), tells the story of Eric, a veteran suffering with PTSD twenty years post combat. His most painful memories were not those in which his own survival was threatened by bombs and machine gun fire but, rather, the ones in which he had tried to save someone's life and failed or in which he believed he was responsible for someone's death. Eric went to war believing that life is sacred.

Soldiers are often unprepared for the reality that they may have to take the lives of others. One of Eric's most traumatic memories was of learning that the artillery fire he had to call in to protect the position of his platoon caused shells to land near a village, probably causing the deaths of many children (Shapiro, 2001).

Survivor guilt is a common type of illegitimate guilt. In such cases, the griever must be given ample opportunity to explore the events and circumstances of the event, rather than being cut off from such discussion by well-meaning family, friends, or therapists. Simply telling someone who feels guilty that they "shouldn't feel guilty... it's not your fault" will derail the natural process that needs to be explored by the griever. With optimum support and grief education, the grievers likely will reach the conclusion that they were not to blame for the catastrophic event. Support groups may be an especially powerful intervention for illegitimate guilt, because it is so universal. Hearing the stories of others with similar issues may pave the way for healing.

Illegitimate guilt, or self-blame, may serve the function of giving an individual a pseudo sense of control. If you were responsible for what happened, then you should find a way to stop it from happening again. This aspect of guilt serves as a defense against powerlessness. Clinicians and others must balance the need to help an individual get past guilt with sensitivity that guilt may be needed temporarily until the individual develops or redevelops a sense of control over her or his destiny.

Legitimate guilt occurs when there is a direct cause and effect relationship between what the griever did, or failed to do, and the serious harm or death that resulted (Rando, 1993). This type of guilt must be acknowledged and worked through by making restitution and attempting to develop strategies or programs for preventing such disasters from being repeated. Injuries and deaths resulting from "friendly fire" and the killing of civilians are two reasons for legitimate guilt.

Guilt, Blame, and the "Cave Man's" Atrocities in World War II

Father Edward McLean, a priest, known as "Father Ed" to his parish community, tells the following true story in his lecture series (McLean, 2008, tape 10, Forgiveness) of an elderly man who attended mass one Sunday. Later that same day, the man saw Father Ed at a local drugstore. The man called out to Father Ed, saying that he had heard Father Ed's homily that day. Father Ed turned to the man, expecting to hear something complimentary, smiled in anticipation and said, "Oh, you did?"

To Father Ed's surprise, the man growled back at him, saying, "You took too long! I missed the best play of the football game!" The man went on to say that Father Ed should spend less time talking; that people are in a hurry and need to get going, not to sit in church for so long. Father Ed, taken aback, paused for a moment and said, "I am interested in what you have to say. Would you be able to join me for a cup of coffee?" The man seemed surprised by this gesture but was willing to join Father Ed.

They discussed many things that day, and the conversation became relaxed and enjoyable for them both. Then, the man became teary eyed. He shared that he had been a "cave man" in World War II. It was his job to place explosives in caves where the enemy was thought to be hiding. The man was aware that there were also civilians—women and children, innocent people—hiding in the caves as well, and was riddled with guilt, shame, and fear. He was haunted by the acts of violence that he had committed, resulting in the deaths of hundreds of people. He was nearing the end of his life and was expecting to be punished after death for his sins. While in the military during the war, he was proud of himself and received accolades from superiors, so he thought of himself as a good soldier. As he grew older, however, he began to rethink his actions and was horrified by what he had done.

Blame may also be illegitimate or legitimate and just as powerful a psychological force as guilt. It may be directed toward an individual or group, as well as abstractly toward government and policies. Blame may become a strong motivator for social activism and change. It may also sow the seeds of retaliation in the form of war and militancy.

TASKS OF MOURNING: TIME ALONE IS NOT ENOUGH TO HEAL THE WOUNDS OF GRIEF

J. William Worden (1991) developed a task-based model of mourning and working through grief. He was among the first thanatologists to assert that one must take an active role in the process of adaptation to loss, challenging the notion that time alone will heal the wounds of grief. He believed that grief is not a passive process, it is work. Worden developed a task-based model of mourning that includes the following actions: to accept the reality of the loss; to experience the pain; to adjust to a new environment; to reinvest energy; to "relocate" the deceased; to reinvest energy that would have been expended toward the attachment; and to accept spiritual integration, which means adjusting one's assumptive world.

War trauma survivors may have little or no opportunity to process in the manner in which Rando, Worden, and other thanatologists outline. When survival is at stake, as in the case of a soldier or civilian in a combat area, there may be fewer, or no, opportunities for mourning than there would be under noncombat circumstances. Psychological trauma occurs when the brain is bombarded with more stimuli than it can reasonably handle, leaving the individual at risk for PTSD (Figley, Bride & Mazza, 1997). Trauma memories are stored in the brain and the body. Stress responses occur when the individual is exposed to stimuli that are perceived to be similar to the original trauma, thus complicating the mourning process (Kosminsky, 2007).

Traumatic grief, a condition that may result when unresolved grief and PTSD symptoms are present, is often accompanied by depressive symptoms. The trauma is experienced as if it is happening in the present moment, with accompanying physical distress. There is a movement among grief therapists to include a new diagnosis in the DSM-V recognizing the special challenges associated with prolonged grief (Prigerson et al., 2009), traumatic grief, and complicated grief.

HELPING CHILDREN OF MILITARY FAMILIES PROCESS GRIEF

Support and resources for children who are grieving were scarce twenty years ago. Thanks in part to Fred Rogers, who insisted that the death of a beloved character on his *Mr. Rogers* television program be acknowledged on the show, resources for children have become more available (Corr et al., 2009). Grief therapist Linda Goldman (2000, 2001) has written extensively on the grief of children and has also worked with many children who are dealing with the loss of their military parents. She asserts that children will be able to cope with adversity when they are given age-appropriate information. Her books offer specific language and discussion for adults to use when talking to children about tragic death.

The Good Grief Program (Fox, 1988) is a method developed by the late Sandra Fox, of the Judge Baker Center in Boston, for bereaved children. It involves four basic tasks that facilitate the process of working through grief: understanding, grieving, commemorating, and moving on. This paradigm was developed for working with children but may also be applied to persons of any age. The outline is uncomplicated and particularly useful as a model for therapists working in crisis situations.

The first step, understanding, refers to telling children in age-appropriate terms what has happened, then answering their questions regarding the circumstances of the death or loss of military family members. The second step, grieving, involves allowing for affective expression and processing reactions to the loss. The third step, commemorating, entails recalling memories and sharing stories. In the event of a death, this includes funeral and memorial rituals, allowing for personalization, and addressing the unique contributions of the deceased to their country, to the world, and to their legacy. Allowing children the opportunity to participate in military memorials gives them a sense of control over events that were out of their control. The fourth component, moving on, is not about forgetting their loved one but rather about continuing their life journey with a sense of hope and pride.

LEAVING FOR MILITARY DUTY: HOW TO SUPPORT YOUR CHILD

Children depend on their parents for their very survival. Separation for any reason is difficult and may be perceived by some children as a threat to their survival. The following is a list of phrases and topics that may be helpful to discuss with your children using age-appropriate terms. It is offered in the hopes of helping children and families cope and adjust to the extraordinary stress of separation due to military commitments.

I chose to enter the military, but I did not choose to leave you.

Of course you know that choosing to enter the military does not mean choosing to leave your child, but some children may experience your departure as abandonment. Let them know that they are the priority in your life and that if you had the choice, you would stay home to be with them.

There are lots of people who love you and will care for you.

There is no substitute for you, but while you are away from home, your children need to know specifically who will be there for them. Together, write a list of people who they can count on for love and support.

You will have a home with plenty of food, and clothes to keep you warm.

Basic needs for food, clothing, safety, and shelter usually are taken for granted, but children who must be apart from one or both parents will worry about their basic needs. Simple reassurance that they will be cared for, no matter what, will help them to feel more secure.

Are you worried that I might not come back? I will do everything I can to be safe and to get home as soon as possible.

If you are going into combat, this is the most difficult thing to verbalize because it acknowledges our greatest fears. To conquer any fear you must face it. If you have the courage to confront the possibility that you may be captured or killed, you will be giving them the greatest gift of all, the courage to face adversity. Acknowledge it and you will provide your family with a stronger foundation for the future.

STYLES OF GRIEVING

Styles of coping and adapting to bereavement and grieving are varied. Helping the bereaved involves understanding their patterns and styles of coping with stress, and understanding their attachment to the deceased. Misunderstandings of the nature of coping styles can lead to discord, dysfunction, and in extreme cases, dissolution of family relationships.

In their book *Men Don't Cry...Women Do: Transcending Gender Stereotypes of Grief,* by Kenneth J. Doka and Terry L. Martin (2000) challenge a gender notion of bereavement patterns. They offer definitions and descriptions of "instrumental, intuitive, and blended" styles of grief expression. Intuitive grief expression, in their definition, refers to persons with a predominantly affective domain with expressive response. Instrumental refers to persons with a predominantly cognitive domain with less-expressive response. Blended refers to combinations of instrumental and intuitive, but with greater emphasis on one or the other. The styles are on a continuum, with most people falling into the blended category.

ALCHEMY: A THERAPEUTIC TOOL

Through many years of journeying with those who are grieving and dying, the authors of this chapter have witnessed the value of alchemy. It is defined here as the purposeful, conscious, deliberate, method of working through trauma to transform it into something that will change someone's worldview for the better. In other words, to create changes that will be used for the greater good on both micro and macro levels. When a loved one dies suddenly, it is overwhelming. When he or she disappears, when the body cannot be recovered and he or she is presumed dead, the process of mourning is all the more complex (Manning, 2001). The following case history illustrates an extraordinary example of how purposeful alchemy can be an invaluable process for working through grief.[1]

Case History of Richard Keane and Judy Murphy Keane

Richard Keane, known as "Dick" to his friends and family, was the eldest of eight children. He served at Camp Pendleton in California and in Iwakuni, Japan where he served as a courier to Vietnam and provided drug counseling for Marines prior to returning to the United States.

Dick and Judy (Murphy) Keane were married before Dick's discharge from the Marines. On return to the states, he attended university, had a full time job, and enjoyed spending time with his five sons.

Dick was killed in the World Trade Center terrorist attack on September 11, 2001, along with 291 fellow employees who were on the 99th and 100th floor of Tower 1. (www.keanefoundation.org). He left for work that morning and disappeared.

Judy immediately went into action. This registered nurse and mother of five boys never imagined herself on an international stage, speaking to politicians and anyone within earshot, pleading for peace. "I don't want my children to have to go to war to avenge their father's death," she said passionately.

"We have an awful incident that should never have happened. And it is frightening and horrible. But we can stop it now. Anybody that thinks that terrorism is going to stop because we bomb Afghanistan is wrong." Judy then organized the signing of a banner by hundreds of local United States citizens that read, "Peace on Earth," which was sent along with a letter that she wrote to President George W. Bush.

Judy openly discussed her Catholic faith, reverence for life, and her memories of the horror of the Vietnam era. She said that she would lobby to avoid a war. She insists that she is not a pacifist. She describes herself as a mother whose husband has been murdered, and she wants the killing to stop.

An excerpt from the letter reads, "The recent events have overwhelmed many in the country with emotions of anger and frustration. Retaliation against another country for this horrendous crime is not the answer. We cannot be responsible for the suffering of innocent families in America and abroad. We cannot send loved ones off to war" (Green, 2001).

Although Judy's efforts were not successful in stopping the United States from bombing the Middle East countries, she redirected her energy. Her husband had a vision that she became determined to realize. Judy founded The Keane Foundation, a nonprofit organization that raised funds to bring Dick's vision of a Sports Center to their hometown of Wethersfield, Connecticut. She is a living example of a blended style of grieving. She went into action immediately and initiated a support group for families who lost loved ones in the September 11 terrorist attacks. She also participated in a support group for women whose husbands had died from a variety of causes. She surrounded herself with people who would support her need to be heard and to put her passion into action. She learned to manage her grief in a healthy manner, channeling her energy for the greater good.

The Grand Opening of the 9/11 Memorial Sports Center was held seven years later, on September 11, 2008. Judy selected several pieces of the World Trade Center ruins to be displayed at the Center.

Judy Keane was determined to harness her grief energy into building something positive and healing. She is engaging in the tasks of mourning and surrounding herself with a supportive group of family, friends, and community. She describes how the process of creating the center helped their family along their journey of grief. Her vision of her husband's worldview is realized, and his legacy is honored. Her ability to harness her grief and transform her loss from tragedy to triumph illustrates the concept of alchemy.

SUMMARY

Grief from war trauma is not resolved with time alone or without attention to bereavement issues, which are distinct from the trauma of war and PTSD symptomatology. Many bereaved veterans report that even thirty to sixty years post war, they continue to grieve and experience distress symptoms from unresolved loss. Bereavement research related to war trauma is limited, as are psychological services for this population.

Most individuals have remarkable resilience, even under the most inordinately tragic circumstances, yet there are certain conditions that may predispose an individual to complicated, prolonged grief. Survivors of war trauma tend to display greater resilience when they can attach meaning to their loss, rather than believing that their suffering was in vain.

The work of "alchemy" is emphasized in this chapter as an important component of healing war trauma and bereavement. Alchemy is a method of actively engaging in the process of transforming a tragic event, an event that at the outset appears to have no good purpose, into an event that serves as a catalyst for positive change for the greater good. The example of Judy Keane, whose husband Dick was a victim of the 9/11 terrorist attacks, illustrates how alchemy can be accomplished.

NOTES

1. Richard Keane's biography, from the Keane Foundation website, www.keane-foundation.org, describes a man who was lost in a terrorist attack and his family's conscious decision to carry on and work to create positive, peaceful change. His wife Judy appeared on the Oprah Winfrey show soon after his death, where she pleaded for peace and an end to violence and retaliation.

REFERENCES

Bolte Taylor, J. (2006). *My stroke of insight: A brain scientist's personal journey.* New York: Viking Penguin.

Corr, C.A., Nabe, C.M., and Corr, D.M. (2009). *Death and dying, life and living* (6th ed.). Belmont, CA: Brooks/Cole.

Doka, K. (Ed.). (1996). *Living with grief after sudden loss.* Bristol, PA: Taylor & Francis.

Doka, K., and Martin, T. (2000). *Men don't cry . . . women do: Transcending gender stereotypes of grief.* Philadelphia, PA: Taylor & Francis.

Doka, K., and Morgan, J. (Eds.). (1993). *Death and spirituality.* New York: Baywood Publishing.

Figley, C., Bride, B., Mazza, N. (Eds.). (1997). *Death and trauma: The traumatology of grieving.* Washington, DC: Taylor & Francis.

Fox, S. (1988). *Good grief: Helping groups of children after a friend dies.* Boston: The New England Association for the Education of Young Children.

Goldman, L. (2000). *Life and loss: A guide to help grieving children.* Philadelphia, PA: Accelerated Development.

Goldman, L. (2001). *Breaking the silence: A guide to help children with complicated Grief* (2nd ed.). Philadelphia, PA: Accelerated Development.

Green, R. (2001, September 21). Discovering a voice from within the sadness. *The Hartford Courant.* Retrieved from http://www.commondreams.org/headlines01/0921-04.htm

Irish, D., Lundquist, K., and Nelsen, V. (Eds.). (1993). *Ethnic variations in dying, death and grief: Diversity in universality.* Washington, DC: Taylor & Francis.

Kastenbaum, R. (2007). *Death, society, and human experience* (9th ed.). Boston: Pierson Education, Inc.

Kosminsky, P. (2007). *Getting back to life when grief won't heal.* New York: McGraw Hill.

Manning, D. (2001). *Please hear of my lost love: Dedicated to the families of the september 11 tragedy.* Oklahoma City, OK: In-Sight Books.

McLean, E. (2008). *A journey from head to heart (audiotape series).* Hartford, CT: CBS Lotus.

Pivar, I. (2010). *Traumatic Grief: Symptomatology and Treatment for the Iraq War Veterans.* United States Department of Veterans Affairs website, National Center for PTSD.

Prigerson, H., Horowitz, M., Jacobs, S., Parkes, C.M., Aslan, M., Goodkin, K., Raphael, B., Marwit, S., Wortman, C., Neimeyer, R., Bonanno, G., Block, S., Kissane, D., Boelen, P., Maercker, A., Litz, B., Johnson, J., First, M., Maciejewski, P. (2009). *Prolonged Grief Disorder: Psychometric validation of criteria proposed for DSM-V and ICD-11.* PLoS Med. 6 (8) e 1000121 published online 2009 August 4. doi: 10.1371/journal. pmed.1000121.

Rando, T. (1988). *How to go on living when someone you love dies.* Lexington, MA: Lexington Books.

Rando, T. (Ed.). (1993). *Treatment of complicated mourning.* Champaign, IL: Research Press.

Rando, T. (2000). *Clinical dimensions of anticipatory mourning.* Champaign, IL: Research Press.

Schumer, F. (2009, Sept, 29). *After a death, the pain that doesn't go away.* The New York Times. p. D-1, D-6.

Shapiro, F. (2001). *Eye movement desensitization and reprocessing* (2nd ed.). New York: Guilford Press.

van der Kolk, B., McFarlane, A., & Weisaeth, L., (2007). *Traumatic Stress: The Effects of Overwhelming Experience on Mind, Body, and Society.* New York: Guilford Press.

Walsh, F., and McGoldrick, M. (1991). *Living beyond loss: Death in the family.* New York: Norton.

Wilson, J., Friedman, M., and Lindy, J. (2001). *Treating psychological trauma & PTSD.* New York: Guilford Press.

Worden, J.W. (1991). *Grief counseling and grief therapy* (2nd ed.). New York: Springer.

Chapter 11

FORENSIC ASPECTS OF COMBAT TRAUMA AND PTSD: SPECIAL VETERANS' COURT, MALINGERING, AND CRIMINAL CONDUCT

JAMSHID A. MARVASTI AND JOSEPH E. PODOLSKI

INTRODUCTION

The consequences of war extend far beyond the battlefield. Although war and aggression may be evolutionary, they do not come without a cost. Among the most widely unreported casualties of war are those that involve criminal activity on the homefront.

It is not uncommon for veterans to have difficulty adjusting to civilian life. A number of returning combat veterans have been charged with criminal activity, and in many of these cases the charges involve felonies. Often these crimes take place years after the veteran's return. In January of 2008, *The New York Times* published a list of 121 veterans who were arrested and charged in homicide cases following their return from deployment in Iraq or Afghanistan (Sontag & Alvarez, 2008).

In this chapter, we present forensic cases of veterans who committed various felonies, including homicide. Defense attorneys have used war trauma, PTSD, and military training and indoctrination as mitigating factors during the penalty phases of trials. Attorneys have often blamed the military for their clients' actions, arguing that the Army and Marines train their personnel to become killers. Many feel that it is the military's responsibility to deprogram these individuals before returning them to the community.

MALINGERING

Malingering is not a recognized disorder but rather a condition that may be a focus of clinical attention. Malingering is not a modern phenomenon. One notable scientific reference is that of Galen's *On Feigned Disease and the Detection of Them*, published in the second century AD. This is the first documented scientific journal describing two patients who fabricated symptoms of medical illness for obvious secondary gain. One of Galen's patients simulated colic to avoid a public meeting. Galen's other patient feigned an injured knee to avoid accompanying his master on a long journey (Feldman, 2004).

The American Psychiatric Association (APA) defines the phenomenon of malingering as, "The intentional production of false or grossly exaggerated physical or psychological symptoms, motivated by external incentives" (1994, p. 638). External incentives include various forms of secondary gain, such as workers compensation or insurance benefits.

There are several entities commonly confused with malingering:

1. Factitious disorders involve conscious and intentional production of symptoms due to a psychological need to assume the sick role—the goal is to obtain emotional gain.
2. Somatization disorders involve recurrent physical symptoms that have no organic basis and are believed to be due to unconscious expressions of suppressed emotional conflict or stress.
3. Hypochondriasis involves the obsession with fears that one has a serious, undiagnosed disease.
4. Conversion disorders occur when an individual exhibits some physical symptom related to psychological stress. The symptoms are not intentionally produced or feigned (Diagnostic and Statistical Manual of Mental Disorders, [4th ed., text revision; DSM-IV-TR], 2000). An example would be fighter pilots who may develop "blindness" so they do not have to fly in combat.

Taylor (2008) divided malingering into three categories:

1. Pure malingering is the complete fabrication of symptoms and also fabrication of traumatic events.
2. Partial malingering is an exaggeration of existing symptoms and of the extent and intensity of a traumatic experience.
3. False imputation involves intentional and false attribution of symptoms to a traumatic incident (Taylor, 2008).

Rosenhan Experiment

One of the earliest landmark studies investigating malingering was by David Rosenhan, published in *Science* in 1973. Rosenhan developed this hypothesis to investigate the validity of psychiatric diagnoses given the subjective nature of criteria used to diagnose mental illness (Rosenhan, 1973). Dr. Rosenhan recruited eight individuals who had no history of mental illness and were called "pseudopatients" in this study, given that they were to feign mental illness when in fact they had none.

The instructions for the eight pseudopatients were simple. Each was to go to his or her local emergency department (each individual was from a different region of the United States) and complain of recurring phenomena that included hearing a voice saying "empty," "hollow," or "thud." The study protocol instructed the pseudopatients to express only this single complaint, and, if admitted, they were to experience complete resolution of this symptom. In other words, once they were admitted to the hospital, they were to act completely normal.

The results of the study were astounding. Each of the eight pseudopatients was admitted to a mental hospital. Furthermore, each individual was given the diagnosis of schizophrenia. The average length of stay in an inpatient unit was nineteen days, with a range of seven to fifty-two days. The average length of encounter with the psychiatrist was 6.8 minutes, with the range of 3.9 to 25.1 minutes (Rosenhan, 1973).

In response to the outrage over this study, Dr. Rosenhan conducted a follow-up experiment, wherein he gave the responsibility of identifying mental illness to health care providers. Dr. Rosenhan instructed staff to rate every patient admitted to the hospital on a scale of 1 to 10, where a patient rated 1 was highly suspected to be a pseudopatient (or a malingerer), and a patient rated at 10 was highly believed to be a true patient. The study was conducted over a three-month period, and in that time there were more than 193 admissions to the psychiatric hospital. Of those patients admitted, 41 patients (21%) were rated a 1 by at least one staff member, 23 patients (12%) were rated a 1 by at least one psychiatrist, and 19 patients (10%) were rated a 1 by one psychiatrist and one staff member. The shocking element of this study was the fact that Dr. Rosenhan did not recruit any "pseudopatients" for the study (Rosenhan, 1973).

"SYMPTOM EXAGGERATION" IN PTSD

PTSD is one of the few diagnoses in DSM which has, by definition, a direct "outside event" as the trigger. The fact that there are direct external elements as the cause means that issues of compensation and requests for reparation will also arise. As documented in the literature (Juven-Wetzler, Sonnio, Bar-Ziv & Zohar, 2009), most cases of compensation are connected to the level of disability. In cases involving PTSD, the severity of a symptom or constellation of symptoms, as well as the impact they have on a person's life (or the lives of his or her family members), is a determining factor in the assessment of compensation.

Some critics claim that a diagnosis of PTSD in veterans is more political and is used for secondary gain for disability and other forms of compensation. The psychiatric impact of war, however, which may become evident years after the end of combat, is real. In fact, it is a well-known contributing factor to self-destructive behavior. By 1998, more than 100,000 Vietnam veterans had committed suicide since the end of that war (Capps, 1982; Hallock, 1998; Tick, 2005). Obviously, there is no benefit or secondary gain for the individual in completed suicide, yet the incidence of suicide is almost twice the number of soldiers killed in combat during the entire Vietnam War.

Hickling, Blanchard, Mundy, and Galovski (2002) published an article titled "Detection of malingered MVA related PTSD: An investigation of ability to detect professional actors by experienced clinicians, psychological tests, and psychophysiological assessment." In this article the authors demonstrated the difficulty in recognizing symptom fabrication by professional actors, even when skilled clinicians were involved.

In PTSD litigation, symptom exaggeration, if any, should decrease after the compensation litigation has ended. However, as Juven-Wetzler and associates (2009) explained, there are several studies that failed to confirm an "improvement" in symptoms following finalization of compensation claims (Sayer, Spoont, Nelson, Clothier & Murdochs, 2008). The "unimproved" symptoms were thought to have different explanations. One possibility was that the individual who had exaggerated symptoms would continue them out of fear or paranoia that the "other side" might be watching him in order to find any basis or excuse for reversing the compensation that has been awarded. The other explanation is in the process of symptom exaggeration: a person may believe consciously or unconsciously in his exaggeration and develop or maintain it after the end of litigation.

Juven-Wetzler and colleagues (2009) explained that the phenomenon of symptom exaggeration is not harm free. After some time, the patient may "adopt" the symptoms and maintain them (a kind of "imprinting" of psychopathology). The authors bring up the issue of disuse atrophy as an analogy: if an arm is not used for some time, atrophy of muscles may develop, making it difficult to bring the arm back to full function.

PTSD IN COMBAT VETERANS AND CRIMINAL ACTIVITIES

In recent years, psychologists have tried to find a cause and effect relationship between PTSD in combat veterans and criminal behavior (Burchett, Ferreira & Sullivan, 2008). Some researchers have speculated that combat veterans may be more prone to entering a reactionary state, or a "combat mode," when confronted with perceived threats in their civilian life. Combat mode, which has also been described as a "survival mode," may include cognitive, behavioral, and psychological components that all transform to survival and combat strategies (fight or flight responses). Some clinicians wonder whether veterans with PTSD may misinterpret neutral events as threatening and then overreact to this misperception. In the U.S. military, combat mode means "Readiness to use total force without hesitation to destroy the source of a perceived threat" (Marvasti, 2010).

Other clinicians have focused on the elements of flashback and heightened startle reaction. Some wonder if at the time of the crime the veteran had a vision or a flashback, misperceiving a nonthreatening person as an enemy combatant. An innocent person may present frightening stimuli, prompting a startle reaction through a simple fast movement or rush toward the veteran.

These pathological symptoms (i.e., flashback, startle reaction) have been used in cases involving the special plea of not guilty by reason of mental disease or defect. In these instances it is important to determine if, at the time of the offense and as a consequence of acute emotional turmoil, the individual lacked substantial capacity to understand the wrongfulness of his or her acts and was unable to conform his or her behavior to the requirements of the law. Clinical literature indicates that there are historical precedents for these concerns. For example, the National Vietnam Veterans Readjustment Study warns of the potential for excessive aggression in response to perceived threats (Kulka et al., 1990). Other researchers have stated that there are higher rates of violence among combat veterans with PTSD compared to those without PTSD.

Psychiatric Symptoms in 121 Charged Veterans

Burchett and colleagues (2008) attempted to detect psychiatric symptoms in the 121 charged veterans. They were not able to arrive at any formal diagnoses, however, due to the anecdotal nature of the data they had obtained. They did detect significant psychiatric symptoms related to PTSD, drug abuse, antisocial personality disorder, and psychotic disorder in 94.2 percent of the cases. Only four cases (3.5%) had symptoms of psychotic disorder, and

70.2 percent were suffering from significant PTSD symptoms. During court proceedings, friends, defense attorneys, prosecutors, and judges referred to the defendants' symptoms of nightmares, sleep disorder, intrusive thoughts, survival guilt, hyperarousal, hypervigilance, intense anger, depression, and suicidal ideation.

Case History: Matthew Sepi

In 2005, twenty-year-old Iraq War veteran Matthew Sepi visited the 7-Eleven in a run-down section of Las Vegas. He was having problems with nightmares and had been abusing alcohol to cope with these experiences. According to a local homicide detective, the darkness and the litter surrounding the area made it seem "like Fallujah at night." A "gut feeling of lurking danger" compelled Sepi to stuff an AK-47 into his trench coat pocket. Detective Laura Anderson felt that this decision was mostly likely reflective of Sepi's military training "kicking in." She stated that he was frightened and, "In his mind he needed the weapon to protect himself."

Sepi was still too young to legally purchase beer, which may have been a distracting factor for him that night. As he hurried home he walked through a part of town that was purportedly gang controlled, ignoring warnings to avoid the area. Sepi explained during an interview that he was approached by two armed gang members, saw a gun, heard a boom, saw a flash, and "just snapped."

One gang member was left dead, and the other wounded. Then, in order to "break contact" with the enemy, as Sepi described it, he fled the scene. However, he remained in combat mode and went home to reload his weapon. When he was stopped by police, he asked them whom he had "taken fire from," as if he had been in a war zone rather than on a street in Las Vegas. By that time, he was crying and telling officers in military language that he had instinctively "engaged the targets" (Sontag & Alvarez, 2008).

In an unusual agreement with the court, Matthew Sepi was remanded to a treatment program for substance abuse in Prescott, Arizona, where he stayed for approximately three months. He was then allowed to enter a treatment program for a dual diagnosis of substance abuse and PTSD. In early 2006, he transferred to a PTSD treatment center run by the VA in Topeka, Kansas. Upon successful completion of the program all charges against him were dropped.

The courts were influenced by several factors in their decision to clear him after treatment, including the fact that Sepi received strong support from other veterans, whereas his victims were both drifters with no family to attend court and advocate for them. Another mitigating factor was that both of his assailants were gang members who were well-known for engaging in violent crime. Although it was unclear who fired first, other facts were apparent. Weighing 130 pounds, Sepi was much smaller physically than the 210-pound Crips gang member he wounded. The woman he killed was a convicted felon and a member of the Naked City gang; an autopsy showed alcohol, cocaine, and methamphetamines in her blood.

At the VA Center for PTSD in Topeka, Kansas, Sepi learned new ways to deal with anger, guilt, and sadness. He continues to deal with an occasional pathological reaction to loud noises and explained that sometimes a loud noise will incite racing thoughts and cause him to "break into a cold sweat, ready for action." (Sontag & Alvarez, 2008).

VETERANS IN THE CRIMINAL SYSTEM: IS THE VA HELPING?

The VA has initiated a veterans' justice outreach program to deal with returning soldiers who are arrested for various charges, including domestic violence, assault and battery, illegal gun possession, alcohol and drug charges, and homicide. The VA is training 145 specialists for its hospital network nationwide to help veterans who are either in prison awaiting trial or serving misdemeanor sentences. Other VA programs aim to assist in postincarceration adaptation in order to prevent unemployment and homelessness (Banda, 2009). However, as an old European proverb says, "Roman help always comes three days late." A number of veterans' advocates claim that, in this situation, help for these veterans is definitely a case of too little, too late.

In January 2010, Mimi Swartz wrote an article in *The Texas Monthly* about veterans who came back from combat in Iraq and Afghanistan and ended up in prison. She said that many returning soldiers were "left to fend for themselves." This disturbing situation is compounded by the fact that some of these soldiers entered the Army to escape poverty or other problems they had while growing up. Many of these individuals were the product of poor and dysfunctional families, hardly a nurturing and supportive environment to help a veteran survive combat stress. Even if they do manage to cope with it in the field, when they return home they are often unable to adjust to the stresses of the civilian environment. Swartz documented a statement from a Texas legislator who remarked that the skills that these soldiers have developed for their mission overseas–carrying weapons with them day and night, barreling through traffic intersections to avoid potential sniper fire–are not beneficial in civilian life. The Department of Justice has reported that 10 percent of all adults arrested in 2009 had served in the U.S. military. According to *The Texas Monthly*, the Harris County (Texas) jail takes approximately 300 veterans into custody each month (Swartz, 2010).

VETERANS IN THE DEPARTMENT OF CORRECTIONS

The United States prison system is the largest in the world. Despite the magnitude of our prisons, overcrowding continues to plague the system, which is riddled with substance abuse, violence, and suicide. There are nearly a quarter of a million veterans currently incarcerated. The various departments of correction struggle to provide basic healthcare as well as mental health services to inmates. Unfortunately, in the prison setting it is usually the behaviorally inappropriate and grossly psychotic individuals who receive mental health treatment. For these reasons, incarcerated veterans often do not receive the vital mental support they need to help them recover.

One veterans' advocate stated that jail is the absolute worst place for veterans with PTSD. Slamming doors, uniformed guards, shouting prisoners, gang violence, threats and riots, as well as seething hostility bring back their war memories, trigger startle reaction, and place them in "combat mode" or prompt them to prepare for fight or flight. This advocate even went so far as to suggest that "Combat would actually be a better situation for a lot of these guys" (La Plant, 2010).

SPECIAL TREATMENT COURTS FOR VETERANS

The VA is also helping to establish veterans' courts, modeled on drug treatment courts. The judge may order court-supervised treatment rather than prison, which the VA agent will arrange (Banda, 2009; Ruggeri, 2009). This is similar to a modified version of conditional release tailored to veterans.

Opposition to Special Veteran Courts

Hensley (2009) reported in the *Arizona Republic* that some state attorneys–especially those who objected to Arizona's specialty courts (such as a Spanish-language DUI court)–are opposed to a special court for veterans. One of their arguments is that "Justice should be blind." Others object to a special court for veterans because they feel it is unethical to make exceptions for veterans and not for other victims of trauma, such as those who were abused as children and later committed crimes as adults.

One opponent of the special courts is Connie Sponsler-Garcia, an advocate for battered women and sexual assault victims and military project manager for the Battered Women's Justice Project in Minneapolis, MN. She stated, "The reality is you have veterans who were using violence before they had PTSD." (Tabachnick, 2009) She and other victims' advocates believe that those veterans who are guilty of partner abuse should not get special treatment. In regard to sexual assault and rape, opposition to any special court is multiplied. In one study, almost 30 percent of offenders in military detention had been charged with sexual aggression and rape. In the civilian population, this rate decreased to 8 percent (Tabachnick, 2009).

The American Civil Liberties Union (ACLU) of Nevada objected to the creation of a special legal class of criminals based their status as warriors. They opposed veterans' courts because they would provide veterans with access to certain criminal defense rights that others may not have.

Some feel opposing veterans' courts may be misinterpreted as being unpatriotic. However, Mark Silverstein, legal director of the Colorado ACLU, explained in an interview his concern that if our county is finally doing away with "lock 'em up and throw away the key" justice for some criminals with psychiatric problems and addiction, should we not do the same for everyone? In answer, those who are for the veterans' courts argue that striving for this type of justice for all does not mean that one must oppose courts for veterans.

Many feel that this country's politicians should know that treatment works better than incarceration does when we are dealing with offenders who have psychiatric or drug problems. Logsdon and Keogh, two attorneys, wrote an article in *Arizona Attorney Journal* (2010) defending veterans' courts. They indicated that although veterans' courts would provide specialized services, this does not mean that those with PTSD, TBI, or any other war trauma should be given a "get out of jail free" card. In veterans' courts, a defendant may receive a conviction, incarceration, probation, or any other punishment that circumstances warrant. The primary focus of the veteran's courts is to identify and treat the underlying problems that contribute to crime, not to excuse inappropriate conduct.

Case History: David

David, a Phoenix Army Specialist, was suffering from PTSD and eventually turned to alcohol and drugs and even attempted suicide.

He was a model citizen before going to war. In Iraq, he was exposed to horrific events, such as his closest friend dying in his arms. He was assigned to clean up the mangled bodies of the victims of explosions. One of his most painful memories was seeing Iraqi prisoners "come back from interrogations with bloody, bruised, and tortured bodies." On February 13, 2008, he shoplifted beer from a local market. Police stopped him and tried to put him in handcuffs. As soon as the officer placed the first cuff around his wrist, he experienced a flashback to the zip ties he would put on the wrists of the Mujahideen detainees, and how they looked after they had been beaten. In his mind, he was back in Iraq.

In reaction, David wrestled the officer to the ground. Police were eventually able to calm him, and the state charged him with aggravated assault on a police officer, a charge to which he pled guilty.

The sentencing court was able to tailor David's probation to address the underlying issues of his PTSD. He was sent to the VA to undergo treatment, which has helped him to get his life back together. David is now sober and employed (Logsdon & Keogh, 2010).

Case History: Mark

Mark, a Marine with three tours of duty, was charged with assault, disorderly conduct, and failure to obey a police after he punched his girlfriend Julie in the face. He was exposed to devastating events in Iraq, which he relives over and over in his mind. One of his worst experiences occurred when he was assigned to work as a sniper in Ramadi, where he was expected to shoot at the enemy from long distances.

One night Mark was on a stakeout in near-total darkness, when he saw a man standing several blocks away. Looking through night-vision goggles, he was able to confirm that the man was an enemy; however, he was unarmed. The rules of engagement prevented him from shooting an unarmed man, so Mark waited, and soon a second figure approached. This second enemy was carrying a gun, which was all Mark needed to ascertain to fire. The enemy dropped dead instantly.

Mark watched as the unarmed man behaved in a manner that was not consistent with an enemy combatant. Instead of running for cover or taking an aggressive stance to retaliate, the man began to jump around, shouting in Arabic, banging his hands against his head, and drawing attention to himself. The man rushed to scoop up the dead body.

This gave Mark a perspective that he lacked before. Through night-vision goggles, with no reference point, it is difficult to judge a person's size. Now, Mark could see that the body of the gunman was that of a small child, no more than five years old. He could not believe his eyes. This is only one of many atrocities that Mark experienced or contributed to.

In the mainstream court system, someone like Mark would be required to attend anger management. However Logsdon and Keogh feel that Mark's case is appropriate for veterans' court, because he has no past history whatsoever of violence or criminal activity. Mark does not have an anger problem or a problem with domestic violence; he suffers from war-related PTSD (Logsdon & Keogh, 2010).

"WAR HEROES" VERSUS "WAR CRIMINALS"

There is also opposition to special veterans' courts from a number of anti-war activists. Although these activists agree that in every war there are "war heroes," they equally believe in the existence of their opposite, namely "war criminals." They consider this latter type as "criminal soldiers" who have committed crimes in foreign countries, only to employ those same tactics on their home soil. In their opinion, these soldiers do not need any special consideration, because they are not the victims; they are the victimizers who impose trauma on others (Marvasti, 2010).

Utilization of Combat Trauma by Defense Attorneys in Court

U.S. courts are revisiting the PTSD defense. In the recent past, many defense attorneys argued that their veteran client had been rendered temporarily insane due to flashbacks and startle reaction at the time the offense took place. Today, some defense attorneys take a more cautious approach, using war trauma and combat experiences to explain a state of mind at the time of the crime, rather than to disclaim their client's culpability. Many of these attorneys make statements such as "Were it not for my client's deployment to Iraq, he probably would never be in this court" and "He was in combat mode because the Army trained him to be a killer." They point out that, before deployment, their clients were not aggressive, jittery, paranoid, suspicious, suicidal, or explosive. They emphasize that before deployment their clients did not carry loaded guns with them day and night, never drank to excess, and never misread and misinterpreted others' actions as threatening.

A defense attorney may make claims such as, "When he returned from combat, the Army did not reprogram him for civilian life" and "Although his body was in the United States, his mind was still fighting in Iraq" (Sontag & Alvarez, 2008).

Case History: Oregon Jessie Lyn Bratcher

He was a "perfect boy," according to his family, was a B student, and had never been in trouble with the law before joining the Oregon National Guard and deploying to Iraq (MilitaryConnection.com). Surprisingly, although he served as a machine gunner in an armored division, Bratcher had a lifelong aversion to guns. However, he was poor, and his high school education in rural Oregon had not given him much in the way of career advantages in a difficult economy.

According to family and friends, Bratcher's behavior changed dramatically when he returned from Iraq. Once a "sweet, easy going boy," he became prone to outbursts of rage. He developed a severe sleep disorder, and when he did sleep it was with his AK-47. He spent days in the woods, sleeping, setting up perimeters, and designing fields-of-fire. Eventually his flashbacks and angry outbursts led him to a VA clinic in Boise, Idaho, for a checkup. He was diagnosed with PTSD, considered disabled, and started therapy (Militaryconnection.com). He was able to sustain a relationship with a girlfriend and some improvement was seen in his behavior. He was happy and excited when his girlfriend told him that she was pregnant, and he kissed the pregnancy test with joy (Murphy, 2009). They planned to get married, and he looked forward to being a father. Then, one night, his girlfriend explained to him that while he was in Boise for his therapy session, she and her girlfriend had gone out drinking and had met a Mexican man named Mr. Medina. She claimed she was raped by Medina and was not sure if Jesse was the baby's father. Bratcher went into the next room and put the barrel of an AK-47 into his mouth but then removed the weapon. Two days later, Bratcher and his girlfriend drove to the hardware store, where he purchased a gun. He asked her if she thought they should go find Mr. Medina or go to the police. She told him to go to the police; however, it was a weekend, and the police station was closed for the night. They then went to Medina's trailer. He denied the rape but did say that he and Jesse's girlfriend had had sexual intercourse, and he offered to take care of the baby. At this point Bratcher pulled out his gun. The horrific shooting was witnessed from the front porch by Medina's fourteen-year-old nephew.

Under most circumstances, Bratcher would have been charged with premeditated murder. But he was a combat veteran, and he confided to his attorney that he had felt as if he were in Kirkuk, Iraq, and that the fourteen-year-old had seemed like an Iraqi woman screaming (Murphy, 2009). Bratcher's attorney argued that his client was suffering from PTSD and was unable to keep himself from committing this act of violence. He said he was more than just "A furiously jealous boyfriend." He was a trained killer taught by the Army to mow down threats unhesitatingly. Sociologist William Brower, a former Army drill sergeant, testified that, "I only know of one cure for the experiences from these wars—that is a lobotomy." He also asserted that Bratcher was "A walking time bomb."

This soldier's war experience was used in his defense, and his attorney successfully claimed PTSD as a defense for murder. The public defender, Markku Sario, told the prosecutor in this trial that nobody had deprogrammed Bratcher when he returned from Iraq, and that he was the same "hair-trigger killing machine he had been trained to be" while in Kirkuk. He also raised questions about the way the military prepares soldiers for combat, saying the "One thing they always emphasized was instant reaction to threat. If there is a threat, eliminate it. Eliminate it now without thinking, with overwhelming force" (Murphy, 2009). The defense attorney's recommendation was that Bratcher be transferred to a state mental hospital.

The court agreed with Attorney Sario's reasoning; that Bratcher was suffering from a war flashback when he shot Mr. Medina.

CONCLUSION

Mental illness is a serious problem affecting our active duty soldiers and our veterans. PTSD, depression with suicidal ideation, and substance dependence are particularly problematic in this population. Although some argue that the relationship between PTSD and criminal behavior may be a sort of "chicken or the egg" scenario, where it is difficult to determine which came first, several models have been proposed to address this problem. Much attention has been given to this topic in recent years, but there is still much more that can and should be done to address this devastating issue.

The controversial subject of jail diversion programs and special treatment courts for veterans discussed in this chapter offers clear evidence of veterans with PTSD who commit crimes and who may get help through this type of court. One should differentiate between "war heroes" and "war criminals," because every war produces both. For these courts to work, the VA must have enough clinical resources for the purpose of rehabilitating soldiers.

REFERENCES

American Psychiatric Association. (1994). *Diagnostic and Statistical Manual of Mental Disorders* (4th ed.) (DSM-IV). Washington, DC: American Psychiatric Publishing, Inc.

Banda, P.S. (2009, August 5). V.A. works to prevent veterans from repeating crimes. *The Washington Post.* Retrieved on Nov. 13, 2011 from http://www.armytimes.com/news/2009/08/apvetvacrimes080509/

Burchett, K., Ferreira, D., and Sullivan, G. (Spring/Sumer, 2008). Postdeployment Homicide. *American Psychological Association,* Newsletter of Section VII, 13–14.

Capps, W.H. (1982). *The unfinished war: Vietnam and the American conscience.* Boston: Beacon Press.

Diagnostic and Statistical Manual of Mental Disorders. (4th ed., text revision) (DSM-IV-TR). Section 309.81: Posttraumatic stress disorder. Washington, DC: American Psychiatric Association.

Feldman, M.D. (2004). *Playing sick? Untangling the web of munchausen syndrome, munchausen by proxy, malingering, and factitious disorder.* New York: Brunner-Routledge.

Hallock, D.W. (1998). *Hell, healing and resistance.* Farmington, PA: Plough Publishing.

Hensley, J.J. (2009, January 6). New court is sought to aid vets charged with crimes. *The Arizona Republic.* Retrieved on Nov. 16, 2011 from http://www.azcentral.com/arizonarepublic/news/articles/2009/01/06/20090106veteranscourt1226.html

Hickling, E.J., Blanchard, E.B., Mundy, E., & Galovski, T.E. (2002). Detection of malingered MVA related posttraumatic stress disorder: an investigation of ability to detect professional actors by experienced clinicians, psychological tests and psychophysiological assessment. *Journal of Forensic Psychology Practice, 2,* 33–54.

Juven-Wetzler, A., Sonnino, R., Bar-Ziv, D., and Zohar, J. (2009). Symptom exaggeration in posttraumatic stress disorder. In D.J. Nutt; M.B. Stein, and J. Zohar (Eds.), *Posttraumatic stress disorder: Diagnosis, management, and treatment* (2nd ed.) (pp. 187–194). London, UK: Informa Healthcare.

Kulka, R.A., Schlenger, W.E., Fairbank, J.A., Hough, R.L., Jordan, B.K., Marmar, C.R., and et al. (1990). *Trauma and the Vietnam war generation: Report of findings from the national Vietnam veterans readjustment study.* Philadelphia: Brunner/Mazel.

LaPlante, M.D. (2010, April 25): From combat to lockdown. *The Crimes Report.* Retrieved on May 15, 2010; from http://thecrimereport.org/2010/04/25/from-combat-to-lockdown/#more-40415

Logsdon, C., and Keogh, M. (2010, November). Paid Twice: Homeland Justice for Veterans. *Arizona Attorney.* Retrieved on Nov. 14, 2011 from: http://azatty.wordpress.com/tag/asu-law-school/page/21

Marvasti, J.A. (2010). Combat trauma and PTSD in veterans: Forensic aspect and 12-step self-help program. *American Journal of Forensic Psychiatry, 31*(3), 5–30.

Military Connection.com (2009). *A groundbreaking court decision for vets with PTSD,* Retrieved December 13, 2009, from http://www.militaryconnection.com/articles/health/ptsd-groundbreaking-legal-action.asp

Murphy, K. (2009). Did the war make him do it? *Los Angeles Times.* Retrieved July 8, 2010, from http://articles.latimes.com/2009/nov/28/nation/la-na-soldier28-2009nov28

Rosenhan, D.L. (1973, January 19). Being sane in insane places. *Science, 179*(4070), 250–258, DOI: 10.1126/science.179.4070.250

Ruggeri, A. (2009, April 3). New courts give troubled veterans a second chance: Th e system can better take account of a veteran's physical and emotional condition. *U.S. News and World Report.* Retrieved on Nov. 15, 2011 from http://www.usnews .com/news/national/articles/2009/04/03/new-courts-give-troubled-veterans-a-second-chance

Sayer, N.A., Spoont, M. Nelson, D.B., Clothier, B., & Murdoch, M. (2008). Changes in psychiatric status and service use associated with continued compensation seeking after claim determinations for posttraumatic stress disorder. *Journal of Traumatic Stress, 21*(1), 40–48.

Sontag, D., and Alvarez, L. (2008, January 27). Across America, deadly echoes of foreign battles. *The New York Times,* Retrieved January 15, 2008, from http://www.nytimes.com/2008/01/13/us/13vets.html

Swartz, M. (2010, January). Home front lines: Will Iraq and Afghanistan be the wars that teach us how to take better care of our returning warriors? *The Texas Monthly.* Retrieved May 15, 2010, from http://www.texasmonthly.com/2010-01-01/btl.php

Tabachnick, C. (2009, November 10). From the battlefield to prison. *The Crime Report.* Retrieved May 15, 2010 from http://thecrimereport.org/2009/11/10/from-the-battlefield-to-prison-troubled-soldiers-and-the-u-s-justice-system/

Taylor, S. (2008). Malingering. In G. Reyes, J.D., Elhai, & J.D. Ford (Eds.), *The Encyclopedia of Psychological Trauma* (pp. 399–400). Hobokem, NJ: Wiley.

Tick, E. (2005). *War and the soul: Healing our nation's veterans from post-traumatic stress disorder.* Wheaton, Illinois: Quest Books.

Chapter 12

VETERANS' EXPERIENCES OF WAR

Valerie L. Dripchak

INTRODUCTION

*Any soldier worth his salt should be anti-war. And yet there
are things still worth fighting for.*
General Norman H. Schwartzkopf, U.S. Army (Ret.)

Most military personnel return to their homes from combat zones and
readjust successfully without problems (Tanielian, Jaycox, Schell, Marshall & Vaiana, 2008, p. 433). Nevertheless, data indicate how service members tend to experience a variety of effects, which are often categorized as
either positive or negative. Some discuss the positive impressions of serving
in a militarized area, such feelings of pride, accomplishment, and a sense of
honor (Armstrong, Best & Domenici, 2006). However, a smaller, yet significant, number return from war with mental health issues such as PTSD,
depression, and substance abuse (Karney, Ramchand, Osilla, Caldarone &
Burns, 2008). This chapter presents a qualitative study about a wide range of
reactions experienced by war veterans that sometimes changed during different stages of their lives.

STAGES OF DEPLOYMENT

*One of the many casualties of war's devastation [is] the
illusion of manly honor and glory in battle.*
Judith Herman

Slone and Friedman (2008) discussed the impact of three distinct stages that a military person experiences as she or he is sent to war: predeployment, deployment, and postdeployment. The predeployment stage is the period between the day that the service member receives orders for deployment and the day she or he leaves for the post. According to these authors, military personnel may experience different feelings in this stage, from anticipation and even excitement about departure to distress over the disruption and physical separation from family. During the deployment stage, the soldier is sent to a war zone and is required to carry out specific tasks. There is a wide range of emotions felt by service members who experience war.

The final stage is postdeployment, when the soldier has returned home from the war. It begins with the "honeymoon" period, followed by a time of readjustment and reintegration. This time involves first an acceptance (or, in some cases, a rejection) of changes that have been made by the war veteran's experiences, as well as changes made at home during deployment. Expectations may need to be reexamined, and new roles and responsibilities need to be recognized and integrated into one's life. The achievement of this balance is no easy task for some veterans, and it may be a time of great emotional stress, according to some individual traits that are discussed later. Some of these experiences are discussed in the following narratives by the veterans who agreed to share their stories.

Research in the Stages of Deployment

The stages of deployment, as well as demographic characteristics, have significant impact on how the soldiers experience war. For example, researchers (Yerkes & Holloway, 1996) found that a younger returnee who was drafted out of school is viewed differently by society than is the older veteran, who had established a place in society before war. The unmarried veteran lacks the support of a spouse, but the married returnee may have immediate responsibilities to provide economic securities to others or return to a previous role of parent, and so on. The career military veteran returning to a highly structured military life may receive more emotional support than does the reservist who, in the absence of a support network, may return to a less than caring and understanding group and may even encounter some criticism if the war is controversial in nature. It was further noted that postdeployment is influenced by the circumstances at home at the time of deployment and is further shaped by the quality of communications during deployment.

Ursano and Norwood (1996) indicated that, during postdeployment, the response by returning soldiers is influenced by the role and status of the soldier in the military and the status granted the veteran in society. They noted that members of the "privileged" sector in the United States historically were deferred from combat zones, and the nonprivileged achieved positions of responsibility that were unavailable to them in civilian life. Therefore, some of those individuals, who did find status, respect, and enhanced self-esteem through the military, were disappointed when they were not afforded this same recognition when they returned to civilian life. It further was suggested that the quality of demobilization is often the first indication of how society will welcome home the returning soldier.

ALL WARS ARE NOT THE SAME

The distinction between a hero and a failure is not an objective one. Rather it is based on political and ideological factors in the receiving social group.

Yerkes & Holloway (1996, p. 33)

In the twentieth and twenty-first centuries, there has been no generation without war. Yet, all wars are not the same. War is often "measured" by its duration or the numbers of soldiers and civilians killed or injured. There is more to war than what these figures demonstrate, however. The personal stories shared in the following pages demonstrate different reactions to the different stages of deployment. The experience of these stages may have unique meaning to each veteran, yet some of what was shared was validated and confirmed by other veterans. These are real people who gracefully, emotionally, and courageously told about a critical point in each of their lives that has had and will continue to have great impact on their lives.

Eighty-two service members completed questionnaires for this study, seventy of whom were interviewed in focus groups. They served various times from World War II to the current conflicts in Iraq and Afghanistan. The narratives that are contained in the subsequent pages are a collection of representative experiences from the focus groups that were held. No actual names or other identifying data are used. It is important to further state that this writer took away much more from these war heroes than can be articulated adequately on these pages. As a daughter, wife, and sister of war veterans, the encounters with the service men and women brought a new understanding of what these heroes faced.

World War II: "The Good War"

The United States entered into World War II after the bombing of Pearl Harbor on December 7, 1941. Although it lasted less than four years, it was the largest conflict, involving over 16.1 million American military personnel (Sollinger, Fisher & Metscher, 2008). Eight men who had been in combat during World War II completed questionnaires. Lou is an eighty-six–year-old veteran of World War II, who served as a Marine staff sergeant in the Philippines. This was his second enlistment in military service.

> After high school, enlisting in the military service was a good option for those of us who were not able to get a decent job. The service was a way to learn a skill. When the war broke out, I reenlisted, because I already had some training in the Army. I would be assigned a higher rank and pay scale in the Marines. My friends and relatives were also going to war. After all, World War II was known as a "good war."
>
> What do I remember about the war? We were in the jungle and it was hot. I did kill enemy soldiers; it was "kill or be killed." I don't feel guilty about killing; that is why we were there. I have felt a lot of anger all of my life. I don't attribute that to the war, however. I just have a short fuse. We did drink and smoke some marijuana; nothing big. We played cards, saw movies, read, waited for the mail, and talked. There wasn't much else you could do in the camp.
>
> When I did get out of the Marines, I was treated differently–free drinks and food, good job, and a kind of respect from people that I never had before. I got married a year later, and we had five kids. I went to school and became a draftsman. I worked all my life for an aircraft company that made planes for the military.
>
> I have grandchildren and great grandchildren now. If there is something that I can't forgive, it is those lousy "Japs" bombing us in the first place. Well, we got even with them! But it is still difficult for me today to deal with any of those people.

Lou's story suggests that the military may have some informal ways of perpetuating hatred toward a group by portraying them as the enemy that must be killed if necessary. It is known, however, that the United States has a history of policies that openly target specific racial or cultural groups during these crises, which are reinforced in the military in informal ways. According to Straussner and Phillips (2004), the United States detained 77,000 Japanese and Japanese-Americans in internment camps in the United States following the attack on Pearl Harbor in an effort "to protect the country."

Although Lou's account was the only one of these narratives to openly include anger, it appeared as an underlying issue for many of the veterans who participated in the focus groups. Anger was expressed as a reason for engaging in combat and, in some cases, for killing the enemy, who were also viewed as "killers." This paradox seemed to be rationalized through their military training, because a number of these combat veterans discussed that their training taught them to redirect their feelings in a way that helped to "preserve" or "defend" the United States. Although anger is a common emotion for everyone, it can vary in intensity, duration, and frequency. It may also be used as a mechanism to cover up feelings and to avoid dealing with events (Dripchak, 2010).

Many people viewed World War II as less controversial than other conflicts that the United States has been involved in, as indicated by an airman who sent a letter to his mother that contained the following statement: "We are faced with the greatest organized challenge to Christianity and civilization that the world has ever seen and I count myself lucky and honored to be the right age and fully trained to throw my weight into the scale." However, critics of this war included American war veteran and literary critic, Paul Fussell, who said, "There has been too much talk about the Good War, the Justified War, and the Necessary War. It was war and nothing else and this was stupid and sad" (Shephard, 2000, p. 325).

Korean Conflict: "The Forgotten War"

The Korean War came as a "terrible bombshell" to the United States, in response to the North Korean invasion of South Korea in June 1950. According to Shephard (2000), the U.S. government sent to Korea "one of the least professional, least motivated armies America had ever sent to the field" (p. 341). A stalemate developed and peace talks began as early as June 1951, but it was not until two years later that an armistice was signed. Soldiers experienced two years of static trench warfare with a mixture of coldness, boredom, bad food, fear, and endless patrolling.

No veterans who served during the Korean War participated in these interviews; however, the following is a portion of a letter that was sent by an Army soldier serving in the Korean War to his sister.

Dear Katherine,

I am writing you to let you know that I am doing alright. I don't want to worry mom and dad with anything, so please screen what I am telling you when you talk to them. Being here is not at all what I expected. The cold weather conditions are unbelievable; we are told that our bodies will adapt to the weather, but none of us have experienced that yet. We heard from some of the guys who left today to return stateside that we should prepare for even worse temperatures and heavy rains.

I am getting use to the gunfire at night. It is not so bad when I am on patrol, but I have begun to have problems sleeping even when there is no noise. We hear talk about peace being discussed yet we hear the gunfire. It doesn't make sense. Some of the guys are really afraid, so they just hide for cover. At first, I was angry at these guys for not getting into it, but now I don't blame them because it might be me doing the same thing someday soon . . . .

Vietnam: "The Jungle War"

Vietnam was a different war. The U.S. military was not there because of our country's national survival, as in World War II, but initially to resist the spread of communism. According to Shephard (2000), Vietnam was a "guerilla war" that was fought without clear military objectives and no front line. The soldiers who fought there were on a thirteen-month tour of duty with a five-day R&R. Furthermore, it was fought surrounded by the civilian population. Most of the fighting took place at night in small-scale actions in which the "enemy" could not be seen because they were in the depths of the jungle. Many of the war veterans who participated in the author's study were Vietnam veterans. Below are two personal accounts: one from Martin, who was drafted into the Army, and another from Mike, who enlisted in the Marines.

Martin is sixty-two–year-old army veteran who served in Vietnam from 1967 to 1968.

> I grew up in a family that stressed the importance of being a part of our family. We hung out with our cousins and were close to our aunts and uncles. I was always told that "family comes first"—before friends, et cetera. When I was drafted at twenty years old, I felt that it was my duty to serve. My dad served in World War II, so I knew about duty. I say all of this because after I went to Vietnam, all of this changed. After putting up with the heat, bugs, endless nights of patrols, walking through thick jungles, my unit became my family in a way that was deeper than blood bonds. We had a very important thing in common and that was we were all scared...I mean really scared. We didn't say this to each other, but we knew it.
>
> When I got out of the service, it seems that people were tired of hearing about Vietnam. I think that Americans were embarrassed by this war. Everyone was talking about our "drug use." Well, when I was there I did smoke marijuana and did a little drinking, but no more than I did before I was drafted, and no less since I returned home. Some of my friends were even called "child killers" after they returned home. You have to understand that we were being told that anyone,

even a child, could be carrying an explosive, so you have to watch out. However, to the best of my knowledge no civilian was intentionally killed by our unit.

After returning home, it was difficult to adjust to civilian life again. My friends had moved on and seemed more settled. It was as if time had given me an experience that I could not use or share. Time also had shifted other people who I knew before going into the Army to different places. I was left alone in my own limbo. That was the hardest part of this experience for me. Today, when I look back on the war, I wonder why we were even there. And yet, I am grateful for those deep bonds that I experienced. I can go almost anywhere and connect with a Vietnam veteran. My long-term relationships have come through other veterans. It is just like being in the war: we don't have to talk about what we experienced if we don't want to talk. It is something that I don't even talk about with my own family and why I am so active in the VFW [Veterans of Foreign Wars].

Martin brings up some interesting issues that were conveyed by other Vietnam veterans. Most of the negative references about the Vietnam War reflected the news media coverage of the war. Up until 1967, the war had been strongly supported by the media, Congress, and the American public. During the Tet Offensive[1] in January 1968, however, television journalists reported the fighting in graphic images as a brutal defeat for the United States. In fact, while the North Vietnamese soldiers moved through more than 100 southern Vietnamese cities, they suffered a large number of casualties (Hallin, 1986). After that, Walter Cronkite[2] made his famous statement on a CBS news special that helped to perpetuate the idea that the United States was not able to win the war, and journalists began to show a negative shift in their coverage. Negative media attention included stories about low morale, drug use among the soldiers, racial conflict, and disobedience (McLaughlin. 2008).

Although two of the forty-three Vietnam veterans who were interviewed by the author acknowledged a drug problem, the majority openly admitted to alcohol use and, to a lesser extent, marijuana use before, during, and after the war. They related that during the war it helped to relieve tensions and was a way to bond with fellow soldiers. Shephard (2000) found that support troops were the heaviest users, although combat units smoked marijuana between battles. Shephard also wrote, however, that although soldiers have always used drugs, mainly alcohol, it was heroin that became the drug of choice during the Vietnam War because it was readily available and difficult to detect. It was suggested that approximately 20 percent of the Army was addicted by the late 1970s, an idea that surprised all of the veterans who were interviewed.

Michael is a sixty-three–year-old, married Vietnam veteran who enlisted for four years in the Marine Corps and served thirteen months in Vietnam. He was a staff sergeant who commanded a thirteen-man unit to help the South Vietnamese rebuild their villages after the invasion of North Vietnam.

> I enjoyed the Marine Corps. I didn't know what I wanted to do after high school and didn't think that I was ready for college. How can a seventeen-year-old make that kind of decision about what they want to do as a profession at that age? I learned a lot about the trades in the military. Although I am not in these professions today, I am able to do my own plumbing and electrical work in the homes that I own. My unit moved four or five times during our deployment, which included the Tet Offensive. Although we patrolled our camp, we did not sustain any real action. There were lots of units like mine, but no one ever talks about them.
>
> I am surprised to learn that heroin was used so much in Vietnam. When I was there, no one in our unit even used drugs or alcohol. It just would not have been a smart thing to do. Now, many of us did drink a lot during R&R, but that was it. Rest and relaxation was a five-day leave to Hong Kong, Malaysia, or someplace, often described as a "vacation." When I returned home, I decided to start college. I was met with a lot of ridicule from students who were not in the military, particularly because I enlisted in the service. The university that I went to did nothing really to support the veterans; in fact, it seemed that this university supported the dissention. I eventually got my degree after six years of going to school part-time.

During postdeployment, the veterans were often met with negative or even hostile homecomings. McLaughlin (2008) noted that, for many veterans, any discussion about the experiences of Vietnam was not encouraged by family members or friends. She noted that many Vietnam veterans were stereotyped during and after the war as "baby-killers," "drug-taking soldiers," or "crazy vets." All of the Vietnam veterans, who were interviewed had similar experiences.

Another issue raised about the Vietnam War by veterans in this sample was that their views of the war had changed over the years, especially because many of them were approaching retirement age. Previous to this stage, they were busy "getting back their lives." During postdeployment, they were involved in a variety of areas, such as trying to find jobs, resuming or initiating relationships, raising families, or deciding to continue their education. As their busy lives began "to slow down," however, they started to think about the "traumatic" period of their lives when they served in the Vietnam

War. Some reported that they began to have nightmares about the war. For this reason, some of the veterans who completed questionnaires opted not to participate in the focus groups.[3]

On the other hand, some Vietnam veterans feel that the tide has turned regarding the public perception toward the soldiers who fought in Vietnam. One veteran commented, "There seems to be less dissention today than forty years ago . . . . not for being in Vietnam, but more for who was to blame about being there." However, the struggle to achieve this different sentiment was not attributed to the military or to the media or to the government. It was emphatically stated that it had been accomplished by veterans caring for themselves and each other. One may conclude that the Vietnam Veterans Memorial Wall is a visual representation of this achievement.

The Gulf War: "Desert Storm"

In August 1990, Iraqi leader Saddam Hussein invaded Kuwait. This act of aggression against an oil-rich neighbor resulted in the United States, along with Great Britain and Canada, sending troops to assemble in Saudi Arabia. In early 1991, General H. Norman Schwartzkopf, the American commander in the Gulf, launched an intensive thirty-nine–day air campaign, followed by his ground offensive on February 24, 1991, to liberate Kuwait. This military strategy, considered to be a "model of efficiency," involved a total of 697,000 U.S. troops. The fatalities included 148 soldiers killed in action. An additional 35 soldiers died from "friendly fire," and 145 soldiers were killed in noncombat accidents (Shephard, 2000).

In Desert Storm, there was a "new military" that was different from the soldiers who served in Vietnam. The changes that took place between the two wars included the shift from a draft to an all-volunteer force, which included activating the reservist force. This resulted in more women in the military serving in a variety of jobs. In fact, mobilization for the Gulf War included an unprecedented proportion of women, with 7 percent coming from the active forces and 17 percent from the reserve and National Guard (Norwood & Ursano, 1996). Other changes included more service members with children, more working spouses outside the home, and more dual-career military couples. The military force also was better educated (Norwood, Fullerton & Hagen, 1996). It was interesting to note that most service members who were deployed reservists and National Guard soldiers never expected to have to deal with deployment to a war zone when they enlisted, even though they were aware that going to war was a possibility as part of the enlistment (Slone & Friedman, 2008). This was the case for Wanda.

Wanda is a forty-one–year-old divorced woman who has four children. She was twenty-two years old and married with two children when she was deployed to Kuwait. She had been in the U.S. Army Reserves for three years.

> I was surprised . . . . even shocked when I received my orders for de- ployment. My husband at that time was a truck driver and did a lot of traveling, so I tried to appeal them. In the end, I was told that I had to go because my mother was available to take care of my children. The military is different for women than for men. Initially, we were sent to Saudi Arabia, where having females in combat was a sensitive issue. During our predeployment exercises, we were told that women would not be involved in the ground patrols. However, once we were deploy- ed, there were no differences between men and women; we were all soldiers!
>
> I remember that our unit moved around a lot. The desert was difficult, and there were no amenities, not even for basics like showering. You had to rely on and trust each other in a way that was new for me. It was just what you had to do. Whatever we did, it had to remain in the desert. When I returned from combat, I was a different person. I did not know it, though, until I returned home. My babies got so big; my younger one did not recognize me at first. Both children were more attached to their grandmother than to me.
>
> It was different between me and my husband too. At that time, I saw his traveling as a way for him to escape his family responsibilities. We divorced two years after I came home. I wanted to have another baby after all of this occurred, but I also knew that soldiers were getting sick. I thought about the possibility of passing on some type of birth defects to my baby, even though I did not have any symptoms of Gulf War Syndrome. I found myself pregnant anyway. I guess I wanted to feel life inside of me again. She is fine so far, but it is still a worry for me.

The Gulf War Syndrome to which Wanda referred began to emerge almost immediately during and after the conflict. It included chronic complaints ranging from headaches and fatigue to motor neuron diseases, heart conditions, and forms of cancer. However, in a report released by the Presidential Advisory Committee on Gulf War Veterans in 1996, the committee concluded that there was no evidence that the long-term effects reported by these veterans could have been related to the "low-level exposure" to toxins. Instead, they were attributed to the effects of stress. Nevertheless, the Department of Veteran Affairs declared 183,000 United States veterans of the Gulf War "permanently disabled" in the year 2000. This is more than 25 percent of the U.S. troops who participated in the war. Approximately 30 percent still suffer from a variety of symptoms, whose causes are not fully understood (Shephard, 2000). The ten service members from this conflict who filled in surveys expressed concerns about this issue.

Afghanistan and Iraq: "War on Terror"

The invasion of Iraq began in March 2003, when there were allegations that Iraq was in possession of materials of mass destruction. It was later discovered, however that Iraq had ended its nuclear, chemical, and biological programs in 1991 (Shrader, 2006). The two areas that have been specifically identified in this part of the chapter, Afghanistan and Iraq, represent the war zones of veterans who participated in the focus groups and are continuing today. A perspective that seemed to be typical of the twenty-one veterans from this era was provided by Tony.

Tony is a twenty-four–year-old enlisted in the Army and a veteran of Operation Iraqi Freedom. He has volunteered to be redeployed.

> Why did I volunteer to be redeployed to Iraq? Lots of soldiers do the same thing. Once you have been over there, it is something that you just have to do. I want to do something that is meaningful—not necessarily in a big way, but in some way. Most of the people that I went to high school with are in routine jobs, married, and have a couple of kids. I am married and we have a baby on the way, but the difference between them and me is that I am doing good for my family and my country. I am doing something meaningful! Do I worry about dying? I sure do, especially now that I am married and about to have a family. I try to avoid thinking about it, though. People don't understand that more of us return home from fighting than don't. We take care of each other; we are closer to each other than most family members are. As far as drugs are concerned, I don't use them. I do drink some, so I don't have to think about what I don't want to, but who doesn't? If something does happen to me, my wife will be ok; she will get a good pension.
>
> It is important to provide a better life for my family. That is one of the reasons that I take these college courses, too. I want my children to be proud of their dad. In this way, they will always know who I am even if I do die.

According to Slone and Friedman (2008), a unique consideration regarding the conflicts in Iraq and Afghanistan is that many soldiers experience multiple deployments. One may expect that with each deployment the stages of the emotional cycle may become easier, because the expectations are cushioned by experience. Each deployment may yield more difficulties, however, particularly if issues remained unresolved in the previous deployment cycle. Time has yet to share the types of future reactions that service members like Tony will encounter. There may be reasons to expect both delayed and long-term reactions.

DISCUSSION

Keep silent about war . . . . about what you have seen and suffered.
America cannot stand to hear what you have to say and the nation
isn't strong or healthy enough to cope with your truths, let alone
help you through your anguish to a healthier way of being

Trimm, 1993, p. XVII

The survey tool used in this study asked respondents to identify from a list of descriptors what they experienced before, during, and after being in a war zone. These participants pointed out more positive views (e.g. pride, self-respect, stronger bonds) during their time in the war zones than negative responses (e.g. anxiety, depression, chemical dependency) by a ratio of two to one. A high number of respondents (80%) indicated that overall they have mixed feelings, however. Many of these war veterans (68%) who did identify negative issues upon homecoming or since homecoming also identified that these problems existed prior to their deployment. Although none of the individuals who were interviewed defined their responses along particular pathologies, they each clung to certain coping mechanisms. Some of these strategies were expressed in ideals or values; others resorted to use of chemicals, divorces, hatred, and so on.

How did their experiences in war result in these varied responses? Kendler, Gardner, and Prescott (2002) present an interesting hypothesis that Karney and associates (2008) suggest is applicable to war veterans. They discussed the stress-diathesis model, because the presence of a diathesis, or vulnerable area, is by itself not sufficient to result in pathology. Individuals who have such susceptible areas will be more likely to experience mental health issues when they are confronted by some additional stressor. Otherwise, they may function in a healthy way. In applying this model to service members returning from combat who have particular vulnerabilities, it is more likely that they will experience negative consequences of that condition, to the extent that the service member had predisposing factors and encountered stressors that were significant enough to ignite these areas. The resulting conditions also may have cumulative effects with long-term consequences, as is being seen today in the Vietnam veterans. Therefore, it is imperative to provide early intervention strategies for veterans who have served in a combat zone. More research is needed to study the various kinds of effects and what kinds of services are needed.

CONCLUSION

It seems that some war veterans seek to establish a sense of identity through the military. Erikson (1963) suggested that as human beings we need to establish a sense of identity as something that is necessary for the ego. In order to do this, we all need to be subjected to experiences in our environments that offer continuity and sameness and to act accordingly. Viktor Frankl (1984) also affirmed our need to seek out meaning and purpose even under horrific circumstances. He suggested that "We cannot change the horror to which we are condemned. But we can to a large degree, respond even to the worst circumstances with transcendent meaning and loving responsibility." He wrote these words while he was in a Nazi concentration camp (Tick, 2005, p.206).

We must be aware that although seeking identity may be a goal for some, war veterans also need help piecing together what they witnessed through the horrors of combat. This is an important task that may challenge the veteran and her or his family. It may also challenge the clinician, who wants to provide services to assist them. Understanding the story from the service member's view is a beginning in this critical process.

NOTES

1. The Tet Offensive was a military operation that occurred during the Vietnam War. The National Liberation Front and the People's Army of Vietnam launched their largest wave of attacks against the Republic of Vietnam, the United States, and their allies since the beginning of the conflict (Halin, 1986).
2. Walter Cronkite (1916–2009) was an American broadcast journalist and anchorperson on *CBS Evening News* for nineteen years. In February 1968, he traveled to Vietnam to report on the aftermath of the Tet Offensive. Upon his return, he stated the following:

To say that we are closer to victory today is to believe, in the face of the evidence, the optimists who have been wrong in the past. To suggest we are on the edge of defeat is to yield to unreasonable pessimism. To say that we are mired in stalemate seems the only realistic, yet unsatisfactory, conclusion. On the off chance that military and political analysts are right, in the next few months we must test the enemy's intentions, in case this is indeed his last big gasp before negotiations. But it is increasingly clear to this reporter that the only rational way out then will be to negotiate, not as victors, but as an honorable people who lived up to their pledge to defend democracy, and did the best they could. (*Wikipedia Encyclopedia*, 2010)

3. In this study, focus groups were used as a form of qualitative research in which a group of veterans were asked about their perceptions, opinions, beliefs, and attitudes toward their deployment and homecoming from their participation in war. The questions were asked in an interactive group setting where participants were free to talk with other group members.

REFERENCES

Armstrong, K., Best, S., and Domenici, P. (2006). *Courage after fire.* Berkeley, CA: Ulysses Press.

Dripchak, V.L. (2010). Dealing with anger as a trauma-related issue. *The Forensic Therapist, 9,* 18–19.

Erikson, E. (1963). *Childhood and society.* New York: Norton Books.

Frankl, V. (1984). *Man's search for meaning.* New York: Washington Square Press.

Hallin, D.C. (1986). *The uncensored war: The media and Vietnam.* Los Angeles, CA: University of California Press.

Karney, B.R., Ramchand, R., Osilla, K.C., Caldarone, L.B., and Burns, R.M. (2008). Predicting the immediate and long-term consequences of post-traumatic stress disorder, depression and traumatic brain injury in veterans of operation enduring freedom and operation Iraqi freedom. In T. Tanielian and L.H. Jaycox (Eds.), *Invisible wounds of war* (pp. 119–166). Santa Monica, CA: Rand Corp.

Kendler, K.S., Gardner, C.O., and Prescott, C.A. (2002). Toward a comprehensive developmental model for major depression in women. *American Journal of Psychiatry, 159,* 1133–1145.

McLaughlin, E. (2008). Television coverage of the Vietnam War and the Vietnam veteran. Retrieved on September 6, 2009 from http://www.warbirdforum.com/media.htm.

Norwood, A.E., Fullerton, C.S., and Hagen, K.P. (1996). Those left behind: Military families. In R.J. Ursano and A.E. Norwood (Eds.), *Emotional aftermath of the Persian Gulf War* (pp. 163–196). Washington, DC: American Psychiatric Press.

Norwood, A.E., and Ursano, R.J. (1996). The Gulf War. In Ursano, R.J. & Norwood, A.E. (eds.), *Emotional aftermath of the Persian Gulf War* (pp. 3–21). Washington, DC: American Psychiatric Press.

Shephard, B. (2000). *A war of nerves.* Cambridge, MA: Harvard University Press.

Shrader, K. (2006, June 22). New intel report reignites Iraq arms fight. Washington Post. Retrived on Nov. 15, 2011 from: http://www.washingtonpost.com/wp-dyn/content/article/2006/06/22/ar2006062201475.html

Slone, L.B., and Friedman, M.J. (2008). *After the war zone.* Philadelphia: Da Capo

Sollinger, J.M., Fisher, G., and Metscher, K.N. (2008). The wars in Afghanistan and Iraq–An overview. In T. Tanielian and L.H. Jaycox (Eds.), *Invisible wounds of war: Psychological and cognitive injuries, their consequences and services to assist recovery* (pp. 19–31). Santa Monica, CA: Rand Corporation.

Straussner, S.L.A., and Phillips, N.K. (2004). *Understanding mass violence.* Boston, MA: Pearson.

Tanielian, T., Jaycox, L.H., Schell, T.L., Marshall, G.N., and Vaiana, M.E. (2008). Treating the invisible war wounds: Conclusions and recommendations. In T. Tanielian and L.H. Jaycox (Eds.), *Invisible wounds of war: Psychological and cognitive injuries, their consequences and services to assist recovery* (pp. 431–453). Santa Monica, CA: Rand Corporation.

Tick, E. (2005). *War and the soul.* Wheaton, ILL: Quest Books.

Trimm, S. (1993). *Walking wounded.* Norwood, NJ: Ablex Publishing Corporation.

Ursano, R.J., and Norwood, A.E. (1996). *Emotional aftermath of the Persian Gulf War.* Washington, DC: American Psychiatric Press.

Wikipedia Encyclopedia. (2010). Walter Cronkite [Online]. Retrieved on June 1, 2010. Available: http://en.wikipedia.org/wiki/Walter_Cronkite

Yerkes, S.A., and Holloway, H.C. (1996). War and homecomings: The stressors of war and of returning from war. In R.J. Ursano and A.E. Norwood (Eds.), *Emotional aftermath of the Persian Gulf War* (pp. 25–42). Washington, DC: American Psychiatric Press.

Chapter 13

THE BATTLE AFTER THE WAR: CULTURAL CHALLENGES FOR THOSE COMING HOME

Claire C. Olivier

Disabled American Veterans say the PTSD rate in modern wars is 100 percent. It's not whether you get PTSD, it's how severe your case is.

Edward Tick (Kupfer, 2008, p. 8)

INTRODUCTION

They have come home. They rush to embrace their families and loved ones who are so thankful they are back, possibly wounded but alive. However, countless veterans carry home more than physical wounds. A significant number of veterans carry the symptoms of war trauma, (e.g. PTSD or its comorbidities). Yet, how does American culture challenge those living with the emotional aspects of war trauma and PTSD? How are these men and women integrated back into society when they may not be who they were before going to war? What added challenges does our "quick fix" culture add to their already difficult path of healing?

WHAT HAPPENS TO COMBAT VETERANS AFTER RETURNING HOME?

We may divide veterans into several categories. The quantity and percentage of veterans who end up in each category are unknown, because some of these categories (e.g. becoming homeless or addicted) may materialize years after the war has ended. Most research is done on military personnel upon returning to the United States or shortly after. In general, one could categorize those returning in the following ways:

• Some return to their previous life, changed, but able to readapt to society without demonstrating any overt clinical symptoms.
• Some readapt with the help of alcohol/drugs. After some years, however, "the solution" (intoxicants) becomes a problem itself.
• Some struggle with having PTSD and work to find their place once again in society and to life before war.
• Some become "soldiers of fortune" or "forever warriors" who remain permanently in combat mode (Marvasti, 2011, personal communication). They cannot live without war, because that is how they have been trained to live, so they may seek out other paid positions and may join private armies. Certain soldiers have commented that it is easier for them to live "over there" and fight, than to remain "home" where they do not know who they are, what to do, or how to be.
• Some become peace activists or conscientious objectors.
• Some end their lives in suicide.

"You're In Therapy, Why Aren't You Better?"

Although the idea of going to therapy for a mental health disability has become more normalized in U.S. culture, there may still be some misguided ideas regarding what the therapeutic process can be like for someone with PTSD. Some professionals even consider the term disabled, when referring to veterans with PTSD, to be a misnomer. Edward Tick, a psychologist who has worked with veterans since the 1970s, states that veterans are not disabled citizens simply because they do not meet a civilian norm (Kupfer, 2008). As he clarifies, "They are war-wounded soldiers and have different values and expectations about life. When we require that they get on with 'business as usual' now that they are home, we put the blame on them for having broken down in the first place" (Tick as quoted in Kupfer, 2008, p.6).

There can be the assumption that a person suffering with PTSD or war trauma will become "better" at one specific point in time and will go back to being how they were before, as if their traumas never occurred. Furthermore, some people may believe that as soon as a person begins therapy, she or he should automatically start to feel better. As Jasmin Cori points out, however, there are two types of pain experienced with trauma (Cori, 2008). The first is from the actual traumatic event or events that occurred; the second occurs as one enters the healing process. This is something one may have blocked off during the actual event itself because it was too much for one's psyche to handle. During the healing process is when certain losses are felt and grieved (Cori, 2008). Delving deep into the issues of PTSD that arise can often be painful and may bring up other traumas one has experienced earlier in life. Therefore, it is not uncommon for therapy sessions to seem emotionally intense. Although one might wish to come out of each therapy session feeling completely *healed*, it is the commitment to exploring the "dark emotions" of one's trauma that can bring lightness back into one's life. One veteran explains how, through therapy, he was able to recognize certain issues as being actual symptoms of PTSD. Previously, he had not thought they were out of the ordinary because he had had them for so long (Sample Stressor Letter, 2011).

Do Heroes Have Nightmares?

If you ask the average person about nightmares, chances are they will refer back to their childhood and images of monsters in the dark. If you ask that same person about heroes, they might conjure up images of strength and valor, a person fearlessly saving others from trouble. What happens, however, when our heroes have nightmares and feel fear? Do we still see them as heroes when their supposed invincibility wears off, when cultural expectations of what a veteran hero should be clashes with reality? Whereas, physically, these men and women are no longer at the battle site, their minds may wander back during the day or night and reconnect with horrors they experienced there. In an attempt to "fit in" and be "normal" again, many veterans experiencing nightmares may not share this truth with anyone and instead continue to suffer alone. The desire to feel accepted by one's peers and society can be intimidating or even prevent people from reaching out to receive help.

Am I "Going Crazy?"

Many who experience the symptoms of PTSD, without knowing what they are, may feel that they are "going crazy." This may be compounded by a cultural expectation of quickly returning to the person one was before the war. Unless someone is a therapist or has studied the topic of trauma, the various stages one experiences can feel very shocking and unexpected. Anger or stress may arise faster, and the sufferer may not feel as if he or she can control it. Individuals with PTSD may feel shame because of who they feel they have become. As Cori points out, they may connect with the label of being a "highly sensitive person" (2008, p. 56). They might be triggered while walking down the street and begin to cry or become full of rage. Not only might they feel embarrassed and confused by this but also, they now have strangers witnessing this behavior. Maybe someone will ask if they are okay, but others may look at them strangely or move to avoid them.

Certain groups have stereotyped Vietnam veterans as being strange, labeling certain behavioral tendencies as "freaking out." The result was a shunning of these veterans. Although the type of societal reaction a veteran with PTSD receives may vary, what is important to note is that there usually is a reaction. Therefore, the veteran may suffer not only from the symptoms experienced, but also from the continuous response to them. In part, this may be a result of living in a culture that does not allow expression of "hard" or "negative" emotions easily. This resistance can be felt as early as childhood. Psychotherapist Miriam Greenspan relates the frustration of one of her clients, who as a child cried to her mother, "I feel like I was sent to the wrong planet. I can feel everything, and everyone acts like you're not supposed to" (Greenspan, 2003, p. 19). What can provide relief is an appropriate, "well-functioning support group" in which members' feelings can be normalized (Maxmen, Ward & Kilgus, 2009). Through sharing in such a setting, one can learn how to handle one's range of emotional responses and learn coping skills.

Pretending I Am "Normal"

How do cultural assumptions affect veterans with trauma? Veterans may already be putting pressure on themselves to "be normal" again. Having the added pressure of friends and family and society expecting it to happen quickly may push them to only skim the surface of what is happening internally in an effort to speed up the process. This fast-paced cultural healing expectation is not universal. Tick points out that the aboriginal Tohono O'odham (Papago) people of southeastern Arizona offer a nineteen-day ceremony of ritual healing and support to a warrior upon his return from his first experience in battle (Kupfer, 2008). What is offered by the rest of U.S. culture?

The Dilemma of Invisibility

It can be difficult for those who have not experienced PTSD or war trauma to understand those who have. Often, the traumatized person is responding to something invisible to anyone but himself or herself. Neither a friend nor the person experiencing PTSD knows exactly what will be a trigger. Dr. Jonathan Shay, a clinical psychiatrist, has stated that some veterans may isolate themselves because they view themselves as toxic. They may believe they could harm others with their knowledge of the atrociousness of war. Inside their heads they may be thinking, "If you knew what I know it would destroy you" (Shay as cited in Mat- sakis, 2007). The idea of invisibility has two sides. On one hand, it represents the "invisible triggers" that may occur at any time. The other side refers to how any mental illness or "warrior wound" can be invisible to outsiders. A veteran's family or friends may not be able to conceive that their beloved soldier is suffering or has anything wrong with them because, visibly, they appear to be fine (Tick interviewed by Kupfer, 2008).

PSYCHOEDUCATION FOR FAMILIES AND FRIENDS: PROBLEMS AND POTENTIAL

Research has illustrated that family support can specifically assist the healing process of trauma survivors (Sherman, Blevins, Kirchner, Ridener & Jackson, 2008). A study in Cambridge involving people with PTSD and one self-identified key relative revealed the impact one's positive social surrounding can have on treatment response (Tarrier, Sommerfield & Pilgrim, 1999). Additionally, a lack of positive relationships can hinder one's healing. Despite the positive response with family support, there have been low rates of family involvement in the cases of people with serious mental illnesses, especially those recovering from PTSD (Sherman et al., 2008).

One concern with this topic is a lack of specific definition and clarity regarding terms such as family involvement, family or spousal support, and psychoeducation. Psychoeducation is a term that includes various therapeutic and consultative aspects, in addition to overlapping with other family styled interventions (Dixon et al., 2001). A study regarding family involvement for clients of the VA system identified nine groups of issues related to lack of involvement. In the just-mentioned study, reasons for lack of family involvement included but were not limited to (a) concerns of confidentially, (b) fears of exposure, (c) apprehension, and (d) the lack of ability or desire of the survivor to talk directly to his or her family about the experiences. These reasons are related to the fact that, in this study, the definition of family involvement included therapy sessions where the veteran and family members were present together in the process. It is possible, however, that psychoeducation sessions specifically for the family and friends of trauma survivors, where the survivor is not present, could relieve some of the previously mentioned concerns. In these sessions, families and friends would be able to mention their own concerns without worrying about offending their loved one. Additionally, they would be able to learn about the process their loved one is going through and ask questions freely. In addition to the barriers mentioned in the earlier study, there are others that would need to be addressed as well. Concerns such as availability of facilitators, time, transportation, and stigma are only a few of the many possible issues (Dixon et al., 2001).

Additionally, psychoeducation studies with veterans have focused on the soldier's biological family (Sherman et al., 2008). Therefore, it is unknown how close friends and one's "chosen family" would respond to psychoeducation and what effect they would have on the healing of a trauma survivor. It is important to extend studies beyond biological family and spouses, because trauma survivors may be single, without biological family, or live far away from biological family. Therefore, support networks may include various nonbiological relationships.

THE OTHER WAR: FIGHTING THE VA HEALTH SYSTEM

An e-mail from a VA mental health integration specialist in Temple, Texas, in 2008 became notorious after it was revealed that a military physician seemed more concerned about financial constraints than proper diagnostic procedure for soldiers. Dr. Norma Perez directed staff to "refrain from giving a diagnosis of PTSD straight out" and to "consider a diagnosis of adjustment disorder, instead." In the same e-mail she mentioned the problem of "more and more compensation-seeking veterans" (Malbran, 2008, p. 1).

One trained in psychopathology would know that it is vital not to confuse PTSD with an adjustment disorder. "Adjustment disorders are triggered by more ordinary stressors (e.g., exams to graduate from college, a court hearing, or divorce)" (Maxmen et al., 2009, p. 279). These men and women have been through a much greater trial. Perez later apologized once her statements were made public; however, her actions, which resulted in a lack of proper treatment for soldiers, seems to warrant something more significant than an apology.

The news media demonstrate multiple incidents of soldiers who have become frustrated when trying to deal with the system in order to get treatment. One soldier (Sergeant Chuck Luther) reported that he had survived dangerous missions in the Middle East but then became desperate after being denied help when he knew he needed it. He was promptly criticized and portrayed by his superior as trying to evade duty (Kors, 2010). The military discharged him with a diagnosis of personality disorder. Later however, he was diagnosed with TBI and PTSD by a private psychologist, Troy

Daniels, who told the media that Luther was like hundreds of other soldiers he had treated who had all been similarly misdiagnosed. Daniels confirmed that "None of them actually had personality disorder" (Kors, 2010, p. 8).

A backyard conversation with U.S. President Barack Obama got emotional when the son of a U.S. veteran spoke up about the VA's lack of care for his father (Korte, 2010). He told the President, "Well, unfortunately, at the VA sometimes he doesn't get the care and the services that he should. I mean, he sacrificed his body." The father, Andy Cavalier, was a staff sergeant in the Marines for thirteen years. Cavalier has had twenty-five surgeries for problems with his feet, ankles, knees, and sinuses and is also in treatment for PTSD. Cavalier complained about the way the VA doctors seem to hurry him through the process, saying, "Sometimes they cut you off, tell you there's not enough time. I had a few doctors rush me through it to get me in and out. There's a lot of issues you've got to take care of when you only see them for a month, three months, six months" (Korte, 2010, p. 10). There is no shortage of complaints from our wounded warriors in regard to their medical care.

ARMY CULTURE VIEWS ON MENTAL HEALTH

The November 2009 shootings at Fort Hood, where an Army psychiatrist killed multiple people including other mental health workers and soldiers, prompted intense scrutiny of the Army's capacity to provide adequate mental health care (Stahl, 2009). The general consensus is that the Army is faced with a major deficiency in mental health staffing, not just at Fort Hood but across the board. The current number of psychiatrists in the U.S. Army is around 400; the same number as before the wars in Iraq and Afghanistan began. According to Stephen M. Stahl (2009, p. 684), "There are fewer psychiatrists in the entire U.S. Army today than there are in San Diego. There are ten times more psychiatrists in Manhattan than there are in the army." This is despite the Army's own admission that they are short about 800 mental health care professionals and at least 300 substance abuse counselors (Stahl, 2009). Without the proper amount of mental health providers, the providers themselves suffer and are unable to give quality care to clients when their caseload is too high. Additionally, one can likely assume there is a waiting list for people requesting services; therefore, soldiers are not able to be seen when needed. What kind of message does this send concerning the importance of a soldier's mental health condition? Does it have a negative impact on how a veteran views his or her own experience with PTSD when the Army, an organization in which one has dutifully served, does not prioritize mental health?

Personal Visit to VA Medical Center: VA Giving Reassurance

The VA, however, is working on new programs to take care of veterans. Upon a recent visit to the VA Medical Center in San Francisco (2011), the author was in audience with several staff members discussing current and upcoming programs. They explained their plan to meet the various health care needs of returning veterans by offering primary care, mental health services, and social work services, all in the same location for easy access (OEF/OIF Veteran Program, 2010). In terms of establishing combat veteran eligibility, the Department of Veterans Affairs has changed its eligibility rules so that they now "provide active component and reserve component personnel who served in designated combat zones (since November 11, 1998) with five years of free care from the date of separation from active duty" (San Francisco VA, 2010). Furthermore, "free care refers to all services related to the veteran's combat experience, even if there is insufficient medical evidence to conclude that such a condition is attributable to such service" (San Francisco VA, Rev. 2010). There may be cause for concern regarding any time limit for mental health and social work services, however, because there is no time limit on when, or for how long, PTSD can affect someone. Additional VA services are offered at the Psychosocial Rehabilitation and Recovery Center (PRRC) (PRRC classes/appointments offered at the San Bruno VA clinic in California include Interpersonal Therapy Workshop, Reducing Isolation, Depression Support Group, Music Over Mood, Creative Art, Mindfulness, Anger Management, Doc & Peer Talk, Spiritual Support, etc. [San Bruno VA, 2011]). Because it may be difficult for veterans to travel to a clinic where these classes are offered, certain PRRCs are offering video conferencing for greater accessibility.

Foreshortened Future and Fatalism

Researchers have documented that during and after exposure to trauma, the victim's sense of time is altered. Victims are often more oriented toward the present than the future. Alterations in time may influence his or her capacity to set goals and make long-term plans, due to a foreshortened sense of the future. It is speculated that rehabilitation and therapy intervention may be impeded by this foreshortened sense of the future. As explained by the American Psychiatric Association (2000), a foreshortened sense of the future is defined as a lack of ability to make plans or to imagine having a job, family, or marriage after experiencing a severe trauma. A normal life span is not easily imagined by the victims.

A sense of fatalism may develop in some combat veterans caused by a sudden puncture to their "bubble of invulnerability." When soldiers are involved in a close encounter with death, they can no longer deny its existence or remain at a distance. PTSD victims may take on a belief that sooner rather than later their life will end (Stahl & Grady, 2010).

Employment Struggles

Trauma can seriously affect ones' ability to become and stay employed. A soldier in his late twenties returned home after active duty in Iraq and began working at a factory (Maxmen et al., 2009). His adjustment to his life was interrupted when Fourth of July fireworks triggered him. Memories resurfaced of being the target of enemy fire, witnessing exploding grenades, and carrying the bodies of those who had died. He became withdrawn from his family and friends and experienced nightmares and extreme emotional states. He began receiving multiple treatments, such as cognitive-behavioral therapy and psychiatric medications, however, and was able to reduce his symptoms and their severity within a couple months, enabling him to work again (Maxmen et al., 2009).

Cori gives some insight regarding the reintegration. "The damage to relational life is not a secondary effect of trauma, as originally thought. Traumatic events have primary effects not only on the psychological structures of the self but also on the systems of attachment and meaning that link an individual and community" (2008, p. 51).

INTIMATE VIOLENCE

According to Stacy Bannerman, author of *When the War Came Home: The Inside Story of Reservists and the Families They Leave Behind*, the connection between postwar trauma and veteran domestic violence has been extensively documented in earlier wars. Veterans with PTSD are two to three times more likely to commit intimate partner violence than are veterans without the disorder, according to the Veterans Administration (Bannerman, 2009). There have been cases of murder committed by veterans in their civilian life, particularly in the special forces community (Moore, Hopewell & Grossman, 2009). Warriors are taught that aggression and the capacity to kill without doubt, delay, or hesitation are essential to their work. Literature illustrates the difficulty of transitioning from a trained killer in war to an ordinary citizen in civilian life where killing is considered unthinkable or criminal at the very least. Their actions and abilities to kill are celebrated on the battlefield, yet back home, these reflexes and abilities could land them in jail. Unanticipated by many soldiers, there are emotional and cognitive side effects affecting one's social and moral understanding that comes from carrying out killing orders (Moore et al., 2009).

Although warriors may have gone into their training knowing that killing the enemy (and not a family member) is what they have to do, this is not the only perspective to consider. As Bannerman states, "The men who enlisted knew that putting on a uniform meant being willing to die for their country. But as a military wife, I can assure you that not one of us took an oath at the altar saying that we were willing to die for our country at the hands of our husbands" (2009).

HOMELESS VETERANS

The speed at which veterans are becoming homeless is changing, and the problem becoming more prevalent. The Iraq and Afghanistan veterans of America reported that Vietnam veterans who became homeless utilized shelters five to ten years after their term of service, whereas veterans from current conflicts are homeless within 1.5 years (Healing our troubled vets, 2009).

"Roughly 56 percent of all homeless veterans are African American or Hispanic, despite only accounting for 12.8 percent and 15.4 percent of the U.S. population respectively" (National Coalition for Homeless Veterans, 2011). As reported by the VA in January 2008, 130,000 veterans were without a place to sleep. This number is double that of the average American (Healing, 2009). Statistics show that California hosts the largest number of homeless veterans, with approximately 20,000 in Los Angeles alone. Problems that plague people across the nation, such as high rent costs and high unemployment, however, also affect the high numbers of veterans in this state. These stressors can sometimes be too much for those already dealing with war trauma (Healing, 2009). The San Francisco VA does have a Healthcare for Homeless Veterans Program. Services include individual psychosocial assessments; information and referrals to medical, mental health, and substance abuse treatment facilities; information and referrals to agencies providing benefits, disability, and vocational assistance; and assistance with housing applications (Healthcrae For Homeless Veterans Program, 2011).

WARRIORS FOR PEACE

Whether or not it is because they were able to receive help when needed, some veterans have gone in a different direction after returning from war, becoming human rights activists, religious believers, and peace advocates. Although certain groups would criticize veterans who demonstrate against the war as being unpatriotic, has not each veteran earned the right to define patriotism in whatever way he or she sees fit? As one Marine who participated in the antiwar movement stated, "I am more the patriot today as I march in protest and dissent than when I wore the uniform of a United States Marine, nor am I less the warrior, armed with a bullhorn rather than a sawed-off shotgun" (Bica, 2008, p. 2).

Repairing the Destruction

Certain veterans may harbor deep feelings of guilt regarding atrocities they feel they have committed. Various Vietnam veterans returned to Vietnam to rebuild schools and villages they had bombed. This, along with apologizing to civilians they had harmed can be a powerful tool in their own recovery process (Tick interviewed by Kupfer, 2008). To offer support in the healing of another may be the gateway to one's own healing. Although it may be tempting for people to encourage veterans to "let go of the war" and move on with their lives, this may not be possible if trauma has a tight grip. As has been stated when working with hard times, sometimes "the only way out, is through."

Moving Forward

The struggle continues to exist for veterans with PTSD or war trauma. U.S. society at times prefers to see things as black or white, and PTSD is consistently varying shades of gray. Although trauma is something that can be recovered from, it may not be linear, or necessarily logical, in how it unfolds. As far as what may offer relief or support to those suffering, Tick suggests that instead of simple parades or fireworks, we listen to them, listen to their stories (Kupfer, 2008). Instead of labeling any veteran as "fully disabled," we revisit what these men and women can offer, such as visiting other vets and going to inner city schools. Finally, we, as a culture, should take some responsibility for what they are going through now. As Tick states, "it's not enough just to 'bring the boys home,' because they aren't boys anymore, and getting them home physically does not do it. We need to help them heal and help shoulder their burden" (Kupfer, 2008, p. 7).

Many Americans may be unsure of the difference between Veterans Day and Memorial Day (Healing, 2009), however, it is important to acknowledge the distinction. Memorial Day honors soldiers who served this country and have died. Veterans Day is for acknowledging those who are still living with us. We honor those who have passed by making certain that veterans who are living today receive the support and services that they need and deserve (Healing, 2009).

REFERENCES

American Psychiatric Association. (2000). *Diagnostic and statistical manual of mental disorders* (4th ed.). Arlington, VA. American Psychiatric Publishing, Inc.

Bannerman, S. (2009, April 13). Veteran domestic violence remains camouflaged. *Women's E-News.* Retrieved from http://www.womensenews.org/story/military/090413/veteran-domestic-violence-remains-camouflaged.

Bica, C. (2008, March 14). Thoughts of an Ex-Marine Officer Turned Peace Activist. t r u t h o u t | Perspective. Retrieved from http://www.truthout.org/docs_2006/031408K.shtml

Cori, J.L. (2008). *Healing from trauma: A survivor's guide to understanding your symptoms and reclaiming your life.* New York: Marlow & Company.

Dixon, L., McFarlane, W., Lefley, H., Lucksted, A., Cohen, M., Falloon, I., Mueser, K., Miklowitz, D., Solomon, P., and Sondheimer, D. (2001) Evidence-based practices for services to families of people with psychiatric disabilities. *Psychiatric Services, 52*, 903–910.

Greenspan, M. (2003). *Healing through the dark emotions.* Boston, Massachusetts: Shambhala Publications, Inc.

Healing our troubled vets: Suicide, homelessness, stress disorders–caring for today's veterans will be a long-term and costly commitment. [Editorial] (2009, November 11). *Los Angeles Times.* Retrieved from http://latimes.com/news/opinion/editorials/la-ed-veterans11-2009nov11,0,4186443.story

Healthcare for Homeless Veterans Program. (2011). San Francisco, VA Medical Center Publication

Kors, J. (2010, April 8). Disposable soldiers. *The Nation.* Retrieved from http://www.thenation.com/print/article/disposable-soldiers .

Korte, T. (2010, September 29). Obama gets earful about problems at VA during backyard conversation. *Journal Inquirer*, p. 10.

Kupfer, D. (2008, June). Edward Tick on how the U.S. fails its returning soldiers. *The Sun*, pp. 4–12.

Malbran, P. (2008). VA Staffer to Testify Over PTSD E-Mail: Veterans Affairs Coordinator Suggested Staff "Refrain" From Diagnosing PTSD To Save Money. *CBS News.* Retrieved July 8, 2010, from http://www.cbsnews.com/stories/2008/06/03cbsnewsinvestigates/main4147898.shtml

Matsakis, A. (2007). *Back from the front: Combat trauma, love and the family.* Baltimore, MD: Sidran Institute Press.

Maxmen, J.S., Ward, N.G., and Kilgus, M. (2009). *Essential psychopathology & its treatment* (3rd ed.). New York: W.W. Norton & Company, Inc.

Moore, B., Hopewell, C., and Grossman, D. (2009). After the battle: Violence and the warrior. In S.M. Freeman, B.A. Moore, and A. Freeman (Eds.). *Living and surviving in harm's way: A psychological treatment handbook for pre- and post-deployment of military personnel* (pp. 307–327). New York: Routledge.

National Coalition for Homeless Veterans. (2011). Frequently Asked Questions About Homeless Veterans. Retrieved from http://www.nchv.org/background.cfm#questions.

OEF/OIF Veterans Programs. (2010). San Francisco, VA Medical Center Publication.

Sample Stressor Letter for the Department of Veterans' Affairs. 2011, April 14. Retrieved from http://www.ptsdsupport.net/stessor.html

San Bruno VA Clinic. (2011). *Psychosocial Rehabilitation and Recovery Center (PRRC), San Bruno V.A. Clinic–Winter Schedule.* Obtained from San Francisco VA Medical Center.

San Francisco VA Medical Center. (2010). *OEF/OIF veterans programs.*

San Francisco VA Medical Center. *Healthcare for homeless veterans program.* (2011).

Sherman, M.D., Blevins, D., Kirchner, J., Ridener, L., and Jackson, T. (2008). Key factors involved in engaging significant others in the treatment of Vietnam veterans with PTSD. *Professional Psychology: Research and Practice, 39*(4), 443–450.

Stahl, S. (2009). Crisis in Army psychopharmacology and mental health care at Fort Hood. *CNS Spectrums, 14*, 12, 677–684.

Stahl, S.M. & Grady, M.M. (2010). *Stahl's Illustrated: Anxiety, Stress, and PTSD.* New York: Cambridge University Press.

Tarrier, N., Sommerfield, C., and Pilgram, H. (1999). Relatives' expressed emotion (EE) and PTSD treatment outcome. *Psychological Medicine, 29*, 801–811.

Chapter 14

THE EFFECT OF PARENTAL DEPLOYMENT ON CHILDREN IN MILITARY FAMILIES

Nina M. Dadlez

INTRODUCTION

A staggering number of American children have been affected by the current wars in Iraq and Afghanistan right here on the homefront. Based on 2005 data, more than 2 million children have had a parent deployed to Iraq or Afghanistan (Chartrand, Frank, White & Shope, 2008; Department of Defense [DoD], 2005). Overall, there are 1.1 million children younger than age eighteen in U.S. military families (Levin, 2007). In 2007, 479,115 active duty members were married to a civilian and had children, 39,045 active duty members were dual military parents with children, and 70,583 active duty members were single parents with children (DoD, 2007). Of the active duty members with children, the average number of children was two. The largest percentage of minor dependents of active duty members were between birth and five years old (41.0%). The next largest percentage was six to eleven years of age (31.4%). Almost one quarter (23.8%) of minor dependents were twelve to eighteen years of age.

In military families, when a parent is deployed to war, the whole family is symbolically deployed and greatly affected by the consequences. Children whose caregiver is sent to war have increased emotional stress, and greater responsibilities and exhibit a sense of loss of the absent parent. In a 2006 survey of at-home caregivers, 20 percent of parents reported that their children coped poorly during their spouse's deployment (Gorman, Eide & Hisle-Gorman, 2010).

CHILDREN'S ADJUSTMENT TO DEPLOYMENT

Flake, Davis, Johnson, and Middleton (2009) report a series of child reactions during a parental deployment cycle. Initially, when the children learn of the deployment and prior to parental departure, they exhibit emotional withdrawal, apathy, and regressive behaviors. Early in the deployment phase, Flake and colleagues report, children are characterized by depressive, anxious, and clingy behaviors. They may report increased somatic complaints and be increasingly aggressive with peers and siblings. The children may then readjust, and their maladaptive behaviors diminish as they develop new routines without the absent parent. They may become increasingly independent. Upon the return of the deployed parent, there is a sense of relief and excitement but also stress of reintegration (Flake et al., 2009).

What happens to children who do not adapt to the absence of their deployed parent and continue to exhibit depressive or aggressive behaviors? What are the long-term effects of multiple cycles of deployment on children throughout the developmental spectrum as they grow and learn to explore their surroundings in a state of heightened stress? It is known that many children exhibit long-term academic and behavioral consequences as a result of military deployments.

Effects on Children by Age Group: Increased Psychosocial Morbidity

Prenatal

Research has shown that even unborn children are not protected from the effects of deployment. A study of 503 military spouses showed that when their husband was deployed, women had a harder time accepting their pregnancies. This can lead to weaker formation of maternal identity and identification with the fetus (Weis, Lederman, Lilly, & Schaffer, 2008).

Three to Eight Year Olds: Developmental Tasks

In these preschool years, children start to have curiosity and interest in people and objects that are not directly present. They begin to engage in group play with their peers and to develop an understanding of rules. Language development is an important task as they move from using three-word sentences to speaking intelligibly.

A study examining the effects of deployment on the youngest group of children demonstrated that children in the three to five-year-old age group showed increased internalizing and externalizing symptoms by a standardized parental assessment tool completed by both parental caregivers and daycare providers (Chartrand et al., 2008).

G. H. Gorman and colleagues (2010) demonstrated that there was an 11 percent increase in number of outpatient visits for mental and behavioral health complaints in children age three to eight years old during a parent's military deployment. In addition, pediatric behavioral disorders increased by 18 percent and stress disorders increased by 19 percent. They noted that there was an 11 percent decrease in overall visits to a primary care provider during the deployment period, perhaps due to the fact that it was harder for a single caregiver to take children to medical appointments (Gorman, Eide, et al., 2010).

Five to Twelve Year Olds

As children move through this stage of life they are evolving from what Piaget would call the "pre-operational stage," characterized by imaginative play and egocentric thinking, to the "concrete operational stage," where they are able to appreciate the perspective of others and understand laws of conservation and serial ordering. Children in the concrete operational stage have rigid problem-solving skills and only see one way to approach a task (one-dimensional thinking).

Flake and associates studied a group of children five to twelve years of age by use of a parental report scale during a 15-month deployment and concluded that one in every three children was at "high risk" of psychosocial morbidity. In addition, over a third of parents reported that their children were more anxious, worried more, or were crying more frequently. Approximately two thirds of parents whose children were identified as high risk recognized the need for mental health treatment (Flake et al., 2009).

Eleven to Seventeen Year Olds

Adolescents are in a constant battle to separate themselves from their parents and develop their own identity. There is an emphasis on association with a peer group and they often feel insecure about self-image. They are in Piaget's "formal operational" stage, where they are cognitively capable of hypothesis testing, idealism, and metacognition. Adolescents are able to engage in "abstract thinking" and often are "philosophers" because they are able to challenge adults as their intellectual equals through complex reasoning.

The oldest group of military children studied was a group of 1507 adolescents age eleven to seventeen. This study showed that military children had more emotional difficulties than did children in national samples. Additionally, female and older adolescents in the study reported more school, family, and peer-related problems with parental deployment (Chandra, Lara-Cinisomo, et al., 2010).

Mediating Factors Across Age Groups

Research has demonstrated that in all age groups, children's ability to adapt to the stress of parental deployment is mediated by their home caregiver's level of anxiety, depression, and stress (Chandra, Lara-Cinisomo, et al., 2010; Flake et al., 2009; Houston et al., 2009). It appears that children are an extension of their parents in regard to their emotional reactions. This is quite significant when one considers the fact that nearly 50 percent of spouses report depression and anxiety during military deployments (McFarlane, 2009; SteelFisher, Zaslavsky & Blendon, 2008). Increased behavioral problems, depressive symptoms, and academic troubles also correlated with increased length and frequency of deployments (Chandra, Lara-Cinisomo, et al., 2010).

Gender

School teachers and counselors who were interviewed about students from military families felt that there were gender-specific reactions to deployment. Boys exhibited more externalizing behaviors, such as anger and aggression. Girls demonstrated more somatic complaints and depressive symptoms. Additionally, adolescent girls were reported to engage in cutting and promiscuous sexual behaviors (Chandra, Martin, Hawkins & Richardson, 2010). A study of adolescents eleven to seventeen years of age demonstrated that girls had more problems with the reintegration period after deployment than boys did. This was postulated to be secondary to the difficulty of teenage girls relating to their father and issues in connecting emotionally to an absent parent (Chandra, Lara-Cinisomo, et al., 2010).

Academic Performance

Research has shown that children's reading and math scores are lower during parental deployment. Additionally, a study of standardized test scores in schools run by the DoD between 2002 and 2005 found that parental deployment was associated with lower test scores. This was most significant when the parent was deployed during the testing month. Interviews with school staff identified student uncertainty about length of deployment, fear of death of the parent, increased stress in the home, and perceived mental health issues of the home caregiver as significant contributors to difficulty functioning in school (Chandra, Martin, et al., 2010).

CHILD MALTREATMENT

A large-scale study by Gibbs and colleagues published in the *Journal of the American Medical Association* in 2007 noted that 1858 parents in 1771 families had substantiated cases of child maltreatment from 2001 to 2004. In those families, rates of child maltreatment were highest while the soldier-parent was deployed, and rates of neglect doubled during deployment. Specifically among female civilian spouses of deployed parents, rates of maltreatment were three times greater, rates of neglect were four times greater, and rates of physical abuse were two times greater during deployment. They did not find the same increases in male civilian parents when their wives were deployed. When looking at both parents collectively, rates of physical abuse were greater when the soldier-parent was at home, indicating that they were the most common perpetrators of physical abuse. Researchers found similar increases in maltreatment rates in both lower and higher enlisted pay grades. Rates of maltreatment were higher for non-Hispanic whites than for blacks or Hispanic whites (Gibbs et al., 2007).

A second study by Rentz and colleagues (2007) looked at the rates of maltreatment in Texas from 2000 to 2003. They compared 1399 children in military families with 146,583 children in civilian families. The authors demonstrated that since the one year anniversary of the September 11 attack, the rate of child maltreatment has doubled in military families but has not changed in nonmilitary families. This reversed a decade-long downward trend of child abuse and maltreatment in military families (Newhouse, 2008). Additionally, they found that child maltreatment rates in military families as a whole increased by 30 percent for each 1 percent increase in the number of soldiers departing for or returning from deployment. The authors concluded that the circumstances concerning both departure and reintegration from deployment produced strain on the family that caused more abusive and neglectful behaviors. They also noted that in the majority of cases the perpetrator of maltreatment was the nonmilitary spouse (Rentz et al., 2007).

Child maltreatment has been shown to have lasting negative effects on psychological and physical health. Both of these studies highlight the need for additional family support during deployment. Because most substantiated child maltreatment is at the hands of the home caregiver and occurs during the deployment period, steps must be taken to support both the mental health of these individuals and to help with the responsibilities of child rearing. Community resources for military families are essential.

NATIONAL GUARD AND RESERVISTS

According to 2007 data, more than 450,000 National Guard and reserve troops had been deployed to Iraq and Afghanistan (Houston et al., 2009). Deployments for these soldiers are typically longer than the reported twelve to fifteen months because they require several months of training prior to deployment, increasing their time apart from their families. Houston and colleagues (2009) point out that the impact of deployment on National Guard families may be exceedingly challenging due to the fact that they are usually living in communities, as opposed to bases, and may not be integrated into military life. In a study of eleven to seventeen year olds, home caregivers who lived in military housing during deployment reported that their children had fewer difficulties than did parents who lived elsewhere during the deployment period (Chandra, Lara-Cinisomo, et al., 2010).

A 2010 study gaining the perspectives of school staff on the social and emotional functioning of children in military families reported that students in reservist or National Guard families lacked a support network in school of people who understood their experience during deployment. Staff reported having only one or two students in school in reserve families, and most of them did not know other children of military families. The authors quote a counselor as saying, "They feel like they are the only ones . . . [parental deployment] needs to be normalized . . . . I think that is the key thing that's missing. It is an issue with the National Guard because [the families] are all spread out" (Chandra, Martin, et al., 2010).

Not only is being the only child of a deployed parent in a school extremely isolative during a vulnerable time, but also children are subject to the comments of insensitive peers. Hearing classmates question or denigrate the war can challenge their view of their parents as heroes. Many children need this perception of their deployed parent as a person fighting for their rights and serving their country to help them cope with his or her absence. A challenge to this thought construct by peers, or even the news media, can be quite unsettling.

"UNJUST" WARS

In both National Guard and Reservist families and enlisted families, criticisms of war can be confusing and stressful for children. During the Vietnam,

Iraq, and Afghanistan Wars, some soldiers or their families developed the idea that they were or are fighting "unjust wars" (Marvasti & Dadlez, 2011). The family no longer views the mission as heroic and may have moral questions associated with the deployed parent's role in it. This can be a strong dividing factor if the family does not have a common ideology. Additionally, if a veteran regrets his time in combat, his pain may be reflected in his interactions with his family when he returns home.

FEAR OF DEATH OF A PARENT

Many children are worried about the safety of their deployed parent and are haunted by a sense of uncertainty about their return. Cozza, Chun, and Polo (2005) feel that children have a disproportionate fear of the risk of death of their parent compared to the number of deployed service men killed and that this fear is fueled primarily by the media. Of twenty-four children of deployed members of the National Guard interviewed, eleven said that their biggest worry about deployment was their father getting hurt, and four replied that they were concerned about their father dying or not coming back (Houston et al., 2009). A six-year-old girl told Houston and colleagues that, "My daddy sometimes has to kill people and run away from their bullets."

Children living on military bases are in an environment where knowledge of the death of an unknown soldier spreads through the community quickly through informal communications and community activities. Cozza and associates (2005) note that this unofficial notification of the death of a service member causes an overwhelming sense of fear in a child until confirmation is received that the deceased is not that child's parent. This can create a disruptive and stressful environment for children, leading to significant anxiety.

PARENTIFICATION OF CHILDREN

Children in military families are increasingly experiencing role confusion as they take on tasks in the home that are often outside their developmental stage. Houston and colleagues (2009) shared a quote from a six-year-old girl who said that she learned, "Now I have to be big and help my mommy more with [her five-year-old brother and eight-month-old sister] so mommy doesn't cry." Overall, five children out of the twenty-four they interviewed said that what they learned from deployment was that they had to help their mom around the house. Reasons cited included avoiding maternal stress or to make their mother's life easier. Although children said the hardest part of deployment was missing their absent parent, they reported that the biggest change was increased responsibility (Houston et al., 2009).

Chandra, Lara-Cinisomo, and colleagues (2010) reported that the older adolescents in their study of eleven to seventeen-year-olds reported more problems with parental deployment and reintegration. The authors attributed this to greater assumption of responsibilities in the household due to their age, leading to increased role shifting during deployment and reintegration. McFarlane (2009) highlights adolescents with deployed parents as having increased uncertainty, boundary ambiguity, and emotional conflict. He notes that adolescents often must take on and relinquish certain roles in family life, causing confusion about how they fit into the family system.

In a series of twenty-four focus groups with teachers and counselors, half of them raised concerns over increased responsibilities carried by children during deployment. Many are caring for younger siblings and essentially becoming a coparent. Chandra, Martin, and colleagues (2010) included a story of a young girl who woke her siblings in the morning; fed them breakfast; dressed them; prepared them for school, including packing their backpacks; got herself ready for school; and then walked them to school. She told her teacher that she was just too tired to do her homework and succeed academically (Chandra, Martin, et al., 2010).

Another concern voiced by school staff in 42 percent of the focus groups was that many children became the emotional partners of their home caregiver (Chandra, Martin, et al., 2010). It is well-documented that at-home spouses of deployed soldiers often experience depression and anxiety. For children to carry the burden of parental depression and the constant pressure to lift their parent's spirits in addition to their own fears and concerns is quite stress provoking. Additionally, school staff in the study reported that depressed parents missed meetings with their child's teachers, did not bring them to their school activities, and did not follow up on their school assignments. They also state that some parents kept their children home from school during the deployment as a source of personal support and comfort (Chandra, Martin, et al., 2010). Gorman, Fitzgerald, and Blow (2010) point out that children growing up with depressed parents are at increased risk for mental health issues themselves because they try to manage their parent's emotional state and do not have enough psychic energy left to manage their own.

Big Man or Big Woman Syndrome

Wolfelt (2004) describes a syndrome termed "big man" or "big woman" syndrome in which children have an accelerated pseudomaturity in the absence of one of their caregivers. This may be facilitated by comments made by a deployed parent before his or her departure, such as a father telling his eight-year-old son to take care of the house while he is gone. He may use a phrase, such as "You are the man of the house now" or "Take care of your mother while I'm gone." In this way, the child may feel that he has to assume the role of the father during the deployment period (Solt & Balint-Bravo, 2008; Wolfelt, 2004).

REINTEGRATION AND ITS DIFFICULTIES

Although the deployed parent's return is much anticipated by all members of the family, three out of four families report that the first three months after the service member's homecoming are the most stressful part of a deployment (Flake et al., 2009). A deployed parent must shift paradigms from spending more than a year in a combat zone to rejoining family life. Reintegration can be difficult as reassigned responsibilities are reclaimed, and the parentification of children cannot be reversed so easily.

A study of recently returned veterans found that two thirds of veterans referred to the VA for behavioral health counseling reported family adjustment problems (Newhouse, 2008). Additionally, 56 percent described domestic disputes that included shouting, pushing or shoving. The rates of infidelity among returned veterans increased from 4 percent in 2003-2005 to 14 percent in 2006 and 15 percent in 2007. Divorces rates have been climbing as well from 11 percent of veterans planning divorce in 2003 to 2005 to 15 percent in 2006 and 20 percent in 2007 (Newhouse, 2008). With the family unit threatened by domestic violence, infidelity, and impending divorce, military children are not immune. This turmoil creates a toxic environment for a developing child who desperately needs stability.

In addition, more than 30 percent of veterans returning home have PTSD, TBI, and/or depression (Gorman, Fitzgerald, et al., 2010). The emotional numbing, irritability, and social withdrawal can be internalized by children who do not understand that these personality changes are not a result of their personal behavior (Gorman, Fitzgerald et al., 2010; McFarlane, 2009).

CHALLENGES OF "URBAN" WARFARE

U.S. military conflicts over the last five decades are different from previous wars, in that conflicts take place within city limits and often within civilian homes as opposed to classic wars, which were fought on the battlefield. In this "urban warfare," the distinction between armed combatants and civilians is murky. One cannot differentiate friends from foes. This causes increased numbers of atrocities and "collateral damage" that are carried out by veterans. The result is increased shame, remorse, and confusion on the part of the soldiers that causes tremendous pain. This will eventually affect veteran's interactions with their family and transfer psychic pain to their children as well (Marvasti & Dadlez, 2011).

PARENTAL PTSD

The challenge of interpreting parent's invisible injuries as returning veterans struggle with PTSD is difficult for children. They may feel a sense of rejection that lowers their self-esteem. The reverse may also be true because veterans may be unaware of their altered personality and unable to perceive their changed intrafamilial relationships (Gorman, Fitzgerald, et al., 2010). Additionally, the stigma associated with mental illness creates a barrier that may keep veterans from getting much-needed treatment. If children experience a lack of emotional support from their withdrawn veteran parent and often overwhelmed nonmilitary parent, they are at risk for disorganized attachment, decreased emotional response in relationships, developmental delays, lack of interpersonal growth, and poorer health outcomes (Gorman, Fitzgerald, et al., 2010).

Parents experiencing flashbacks and hyperresponsiveness to neutral stimuli as part of PTSD are often quick to anger and may be violent in the home. Children may witness domestic violence and find themselves in a hostile home environment. The unpredictable, erratic behavior of the returned parent is disruptive to established routines, which maintain order in childhood. In addition, studies have demonstrated that offspring of individuals suffering from PTSD have a greater chance of developing PTSD themselves if exposed to traumatic situations. This is thought to be secondary to heritable genetic modifications leading to biological changes in their hypothalamic-pituitary stress hormone axis secondary to trauma. This has been demonstrated in the offspring of Holocaust survivors with PTSD (Yehuda et al., 2007).

Research of children of Vietnam veterans with PTSD found that these children suffered from high levels of anxiety, nightmares, aggressiveness, and preoccupation with the specific traumatic event that the parent actually lived through. These children's therapists indicate a kind of association between child and parent in terms of PSTD symptoms, which is called "secondary traumatization," by Rosenheck and Nathan (1985).

Clinicians have developed several theories to explain the transference of trauma from parent to child. The first is "direct specific transmission," whereby children learn to behave and think and feel in traumatic stress–related ways, similar to those of their parents. This is learned dysfunctional behavior due to parental modeling. This would result in higher rates in the children of the same disorders of the traumatized parent.

A second theory is labeled "non-direct-general transmission." In this kind, the children's difficulties are due to the long-term effects of their parent's extreme traumatization, which causes difficulty and impairment in the capacity for parenting. This leads to a variety of emotional problems in the offspring, but not necessarily the psychiatric disorders from which the parents themselves are suffering (Wiseman, 2008).

On the basis of the attachment theory principle, parents who were traumatized may display frightened or frightening behavior, leading to failure in adequate responsiveness to the child's needs. This would cause the child to develop a feeling or fear about being unprotected (Scharf, 2007).

PTSD IN VETERANS' FAMILIES

A recent study presented at the annual meeting of the International Society for Traumatic Stress Studies by Nash and colleagues established that rates of PTSD in family members of war veterans were actually higher than rate in veterans themselves (McNamara, 2010). The investigators found that 56 out of 273 partners, parents, and siblings of veterans who had been deployed to Iraq, Afghanistan, Vietnam, Korea, and WW II have PTSD, a rate of 21 percent. This contrasts with studies showing a 6 percent prevalence in Afghanistan veterans and 13 percent in Iraq War veterans. Nash stresses that this indicates a lack of support for the veterans families during deployment and upon their return. Nash states, "We prepare our troops before they leave, but we do not prepare their families" (McNamara, 2010).

Communication About the Injury

Ideally, communication with children about parental illness is an ongoing process geared towards the child's developmental stage in an open environment where questions are allowed. Children should be prepared for sights, smells, and sounds that they will experience during a visit to the parent at the hospital (Gorman, Fitzgerald, et al., 2010). Unfortunately, interactions between parents and children may not be constructive and may be driven by parental anxiety rather than the needs and fears of their children (Cozza et al., 2005).

There are several dysfunctional styles of communication between parents and children that fall into the following categories:

1. Parents who in an effort to protect their children from stress or worry withhold information about serious injuries from them. This promotes

increased catastrophizing by children, causing them to fear the worst, and sets up a lack of trust between the parents and children in which children wonder what other secrets are being kept from them.

2. Parents who provide too much exposure to the injury and may actually demand that a child look at a graphic, disfiguring injury in order to fully appreciate the nature of the injury sustained. This is fueled by the parent's need for acceptance and personal anxiety, but can lead to undue stress for their children.

3. Parents who, due to their own grief about their injury, distance themselves from their children and set up a barrier that leads to feelings of rejection on the part of the child. Parents may feel disempowered and unable to effectively parent their child due to limitations and push away good faith efforts to help them by their children.

4. Parents who hide the circumstances of their injury if it happened in a routine part of military service in an effort to preserve an image of themselves as war heroes. This puts a strain on their relationship with their child because they must work to maintain the façade. (Cozza et al., 2005)

5. Parents who are injured may regress emotionally (due to injuries) and a role reversal in their relationship with the child may develop. In this situation, parent depends on child for nurturing, support, and dependency needs and emotional safety.

6. Parents who return from war with TBI or PTSD may have damage in executive functioning; the result may be inappropriate behavior and judgment which is embarrassing to the child in latency or adolescent period.

At times there can be a complete lack of communication. When the returning parent has severe injuries or is disfigured, in a semi-coma, or suffering from brain damage (can not recognize people), the reaction of children may at times be an extension of the other parent's reaction. In some cases, they may not understand why their comatose parent is not responding to their attempts at interaction. A child who constantly was told his father is "a hero" whenever he is asked about him, eventually he said, "I want my daddy, not a hero."

Experiential Empathy

It is important to respect the children's wishes and capacity to understand their parent's injury. For example, when children have a parent blinded during combat who has difficulty ambulating, the children may blindfold themselves and navigate around the room to see how their parent deals with their physical environment. This allows them to empathize and connect with their parent in a unique way. Similarly, children may engage in play with their parent's crutches or imitate an injury when playing with peers. Parents may become angry and discourage this out of their own anxiety when this inno-cent play may be a coping mechanism for their child and a kind of "play therapy" that the child created for the purpose of integration of a traumatic event.

Parent–Child Relationship

The parent–child relationship may be challenged by extended separations due to rehabilitation, hospitalizations, surgeries, and doctors visits that take away both the injured parent and the noninjured spouse. This can cause inse-cure and disorganized attachment in children and a lack of social and emo-tional support for their development. Parents may also miss key events in the children's life, such as sporting events, school awards, and performances, and may not be available to provide academic support for projects and home-work.

Injured parents may also be struggling psychologically with disfiguring and painful injuries leading to altered body image, low self-esteem, feelings of failure due to inability to provide for their family and social stigmatization producing depression (Cozza et al., 2005). They may be so invested in deal-ing with their own psychic pain that they are not able to provide emotional support for their children. Physical pain may also prompt injured parents to take narcotic medications that may prompt mood swings or somnolence when approached by their children. Additionally, the spouse may be so invested in the physical and emotional needs of their partner that he or she has little time and energy left for the children.

Family Responsibilities

Gorman, Fitzgerald, and colleagues (2010) suggest that parents and chil-dren are empowered when the injury is framed as a family issue. This avoids blame or resentment of the injured parent by redistributing responsibilities and bringing the family together as a team. Although some would deem this parentification of children as they take on increased chores in the home, oth-ers would argue that taking on age-appropriate tasks enables children to feel as if they are contributing positively to the family. This can encourage resilience and cooperation (Gorman, Fitzgerald, et al., 2010).

CONCLUSION

Children's interactions with their parents are multifactorial. They are greatly influenced by their environment, amount of time and attention they receive from their parents, and their parent's mental health. Although each child is unique, there are some common reactions among children according their age and developmental stage. Support for military families would help to prevent children from assuming overwhelming responsibilities and being forced into the role of a second parent while a military parent is deployed. Children are extensions of the parents, and the reactions of the home caretaker to deployment greatly influence their response and resiliency in the absence of the military parent. Additionally, upon return and reintegration of a veteran into the family, parents need to be sensitive to children's attempts to empathize with their deployed parent's psychic and physical injuries.

REFERENCES

Chandra, A., Lara-Cinisomo, S., Jaycox, L.H., Tanielian, T., Burns, R.M., Ruder, T., and Han, B. (2010). Children on the homefront: The experience of children from military families. *Pediatrics, 125*(1), 16–25. doi: peds.2009-1180 [pii] 10.1542/peds. 2009-1180

Chandra, A., Martin, L.T., Hawkins, S.A., and Richardson, A. (2010). The impact of parental deployment on child social and emotional functioning: perspectives of school staff. Journal of Adolescent Health, 46(3), 218–223. doi: S1054-139X(09) 00598-9 [pii]10.1016/j.jadohealth.2009.10.009

Chartrand, M M., Frank, D.A., White, L.F., and Shope, T.R. (2008). Effect of parents' wartime deployment on the behavior of young children in military families. *Archives of Pediatrics & Adolescent Medicine, 162*(11), 1009-1014. doi: 162/11/1009 [pii]10.1001/archpedi.162.11.1009

Cozza, S.J., Chun, R.S., and Polo, J.A. (2005). Military families and children during operation Iraqi freedom. *Psychiatric Quarterly, 76*(4), 371–378. doi: 10.1007/s11126-005-4973-y

Department of Defense (DoD). (2005). 2005 *Demographics Profile of the Military Community.* Washington DC: DOD. Retrieved from http://cs.mhf.dod.mil/content/dav/mhf/QOL-Library/PDF/MHF/QOL%20Resources/Reports/2005%20 Demographics%20Report.pdf

Department of Defense (DoD). (2007). *Demographics 2007: Profile Of The Military Community.* Washington DC: DoD Retrieved from http://militaryonesource. mmidevsite.com/Portals/0/Content/Service_Provider_Tools/2007_Demographic s/2007_Demographics.pdf

Flake, E.M., Davis, B.E., Johnson, P.L., and Middleton, L.S. (2009). The psychosocial effects of deployment on military children. *Journal of Developmental and Behavioral Pediatrics, 30*(4), 271–278. doi: 10.1097/DBP.0b013e3181aac6e4

Gibbs, D.A., Martin, S.L., Kupper, L.L., and Johnson, R.E. (2007). Child maltreatment in enlisted soldiers' families during combat-related deployments. *JAMA, 298*(5), 528–535. doi: 298/5/528 [pii] 10.1001/jama.298.5.528

Gorman, G.H., Eide, M., and Hisle-Gorman, E. (2010). Wartime military deployment and increased pediatric mental and behavioral health complaints. *Pediatrics, 126*(6), 1058–1066. doi: peds.2009-2856 [pii] 10.1542/peds.2009-2856

Gorman, L.A., Fitzgerald, H.E., and Blow, A.J. (2010). Parental combat injury and early child development: A conceptual model for differentiating effects of visible and invisible injuries. *Psychiatric Quarterly, 81*(1), 1–21. doi: 10.1007/s11126-009-9116-4

Houston, J.B., Pfefferbaum, B., Sherman, M., Melson, A., Haekyung, P., Brand, M., and Jarman, Y. (2009). Children of deployed National Guard troops: Perceptions of parental deployment to Operation Iraqi Freedom. *Psychiatric Annals, 39*(8), 805–811.

Levin, A. (2007, September 7). Military deployment stress tied to child-abuse increases. *Psychiatric News*, 42(17), 8.

Marvasti, JA., and Dadlez, N.M., (2011, March). U.S. military families: Unrecognized casualties of modern warfare. *Clio's Psyche, 17*(4), 300–303.

McFarlane, A.C. (2009). Military deployment: The impact on children and family adjustment and the need for care. *Current Opinion in Psychiatry, 22*(4), 369–373. doi: 10.1097/YCO.0b013e32832c9064

McNamara, D. (2010, March). PTSD rates in army families surpass those of veterans. *Adult Psychiatry*, (38)12.

Newhouse, E. (2008). *Faces of Combat PTSD and TBI.* Enumclaw; WA: Idyll Arbor.

Rentz, E.D., Marshall, S.W., Loomis, D., Casteel, C., Martin, S.L., and Gibbs, D.A. (2007). Effect of deployment on the occurrence of child maltreatment in military and nonmilitary families. *American Journal of Epidemiology, 165*(10), 1199–1206. doi: kwm008 [pii]10.1093/aje/kwm008

Rosenheck, R., & Nathan, P. (1985). Secondary traumatization in children of Vietnam veterans. *Hospital and Community Psychiatry, 36*, 538–539.

Scharf, M. (2007). Long-term effects of trauma: Psychological functioning of the second and third generation of Holocaust survivors. *Development and Psychopathology, 19*, 603-622.

Solt, M., and Balint-Bravo, S. (2008, September). Children Adjusting to Military Deployment of a Caregiver. *Play Therapy*, (17)20–21.

SteelFisher, G.K., Zaslavsky, A.M., and Blendon, R.J. (2008). Health-related impact of deployment extensions on spouses of active duty army personnel. *Military Medicine, 173*(3), 221–229.

Weis, K.L., Lederman, R.P., Lilly, A.E., and Schaffer, J. (2008). The relationship of military imposed marital separations on maternal acceptance of pregnancy. *Research in Nursing Health, 31*(3), 196–207. doi: 10.1002/nur.20248

Wiseman, H. (2008). Intergenerational Effects. In G. Reyes, J.D. and Elhai, J.D., Ford (Eds.), *The Encyclopedia of Psychological Trauma* (pp. 358–363). Hoboken, NJ: Wiley.

Wolfelt, A.D. (2004). *A child's view of grief: A guide for parents, teachers, and counselors.* Fort Collins: Companion Press.

Yehuda, R., Teicher, M.H., Seckl, J.R., Grossman, R.A., Morris, A., and Bierer, L.M. (2007). Parental posttraumatic stress disorder as a vulnerability factor for low cortisol trait in offspring of holocaust survivors. *Archives of General Psychiatry, 64*(9), 1040–1048. doi: 64/9/1040 [pii]

Chapter 15

FAMILIES OF VETERANS: THE FORGOTTEN WAR FRONT

VALERIE L. DRIPCHAK

If the military had wanted you to have a
family, they would have issued you one.

Military saying

W hen a service member is deployed to a war zone, she or he usually leaves behind a family. Often, the family members are required to make sacrifices for war but are not given the choices to do so. They do not enlist or volunteer for this duty, nor are they compensated for the changes that they must make when their family member is away. Family members never receive medals or other honors for their sacrifices This chapter reviews how the stages of war are also fought by the family members of veterans.

STAGES OF EMOTIONAL IMPACT ON FAMILIES

When a soldier receives his orders for deployment, more
than just the soldier prepares to go to war.

Anonymous

The emotional impact of sending military personnel into combat areas has been divided into three phases: (1) predeployment, (2) deployment, and (3) postdeployment (Amen, Jellen, Merves & Lee, 1988). Predeployment is the period of time between when orders are received for deployment and the day the soldier leaves for his or her post. This may last from six to eight weeks or longer. The phase of deployment is the separation period when the service person is sent to a location outside of the United States, which may include combat areas. The length of deployment varies according to military orders. The postdeployment or reunion phase is when the soldier returns home. Although these phases are focused on the experience of the service person, they may also be adapted to the emotional experiences that family members endure, because both parties are undergoing changes. A failure to adequately negotiate these areas in healthy ways may lead to problems.

Predeployment

This stage creates a "double bind" for spouses: the desire to be close, but also the need to begin the distancing process as a defense against the pain of separation. It is further characterized by alternating between anticipation and denial. The soldier usually has augmented field training that entails many hours away from home. There also is an increased bonding for military personnel to the assigned unit and a focus on the upcoming mission. These activities often result in a growing sense of physical and emotional distance for the spouses,which reportedly begins earlier for wives than for their deploying husbands. In regard to children of service members, it was noted by Amen and colleagues (1988) in their study of offspring of 13,000 troops that some parents try to protect their children from their own fears of having their loved ones injured or killed in battle by having little or no discussion of the impending departure with them. This behavior may result in guilt feelings by some of the sons and daughters.

As the pragmatic issues of deployment are realized, specific tasks of how to deal with such issues as finances, home repairs, child care, and so on are addressed. In the time left before deployment there also begins the "countdown," which may lead to additional pressure as preparations are made for the "best" birthday, anniversary, or other holiday celebration before the service member leaves (Pincus, House, Christenson & Adler, 2008).

Another common occurrence within the stage of predeployment described in the literature (Black, 1993; Pincus et al., 2008) is the tendency for the service member and spouse to have a significant argument before separation. It was suggested that, from an emotional perspective, it is easier to be angry with another person than to confront the pain of saying goodbye to that loved one for an extended period of time.

Deployment

The deployment period is a time of adjustment for the families of military personnel, who may be filled with a variety of emotional responses. The initial responses usually last from one to six weeks and may include a sense of abandonment, loss, disorganization, emptiness, fear, and anger. Slone and Friedman (2008) examined responses of family members of soldiers who were deployed during the Gulf War and found that partners, parents, and other family members were angry about a number of issues. These included anger with the government or military for "forcing" the separation and placing loved ones in danger, as well as anger toward the service member, who, in their absence, seemed to be placing family responsibilities entirely on them. The family members reported a constant fear for the safety of their loved ones and also listed other worries about their children, as well as their family finances. Some experienced "anticipatory grief" as they tried to emotionally prepare for the possibility that their loved one would not return alive.

After the initial responses, a period of sustainment is maintained until postdeployment. Norwood, Fullerton, and Hazen (1996) found that adult family members experienced both relief and anxiety during this stage. Depressive symptoms in the form of being tearful, withdrawal, sleep disturbances, and physical complaints initially were reported. There also was an increase in busy activities and a need to fit into new roles that helped to increase the adjustment to the separation but could become problematic after the service member returned. Following the initial responses, adult family members experienced the establishment and maintenance of new routines, promoting self-growth, feelings of hope, and a decrease of anger and loneliness.

As the service member's deployment nears its end, the family may be planning for homecoming. While there is anticipation, there can also be a rush of conflicting emotions such as excitement and apprehension. Some of the questions that family members have experienced include *Is my spouse changed by war? Will she or he agree with the changes that were made during the months of absence? Will we still get along? How will the children react to everything?* (Norwood, et al., 1996; Pincus et al., 2008).

Postdeployment

According to Mateczun and Holmes (1996), the postdeployment stage of the service member's reunion with his or her family is marked by three important areas: (1) return, (2) readjustment, and, (3) reintegration. The initial *return*, however, may bring some disappointment or frustrations, because the date of return may change or the soldier is not welcomed back in the manner that she or he thought was deserved. Once the service member is reunited with his or her family, there is a period usually referred to as the honeymoon. Sex is an important part of return for couples. This is a time when couples reunite physically, although not necessarily emotionally (Pincus et al., 1996).

The *readjustment* phase of this stage involves the veteran's desire to reassert his or her role within the family. This process can lead to new stressors, however. The returning soldiers who present the most problems in readjusting to their families are those who may feel some pressure to take back their roles and execute them in exactly the same way as they had before deployment. They may not take the time to acknowledge the changes that were made during their absences. According to Zeff, Lewis, and Hirsch (1997), some spouses reported distress and a loss of independence during this time. They may feel resentment at having managed the home and family during the deployment of their spouses but not being recognized for these "heroic acts." This is a time when previous responsibilities need to be reexamined and changes recognized and either integrated or set aside. It is in this way that the goal of *reintegration* can be achieved.

REVIEW OF RESEARCH ON DIFFERENT WARS: CHANGING DEMOGRAPHICS-DISTINCTIVE STRESSORS

> *No story is ever told in its entirety—too much goes on during wartime. Sometimes we censor ourselves unconsciously.*
>
> (Trimm, 1993, p. xv)

World War II: 1939–1945

Early studies reported by Hill (1949) and Boulding (1950) examined World War II veterans and their families. They found that good marital adjustment and the degree of family affection before deployment predicted good reunions. Families that only partially "closed ranks" (i.e. kept the absent parent's role and its importance a focus in the family emotional environment yet went on with their routines), however, suffered more during the separation. These families did better at reunion, however, than those families that fully closed ranks (as if to block the reality of the absence of the parent) at the time of the parent's deployment. The study also noted exceptions within their findings that supported the idea that parental absence during wartime may have a variety of outcomes that are not always harmful.

Vietnam Conflict: 1955–1975

The terror of war was brought into people's homes for the first time by way of the television news during the Vietnam conflict. The media coverage had a great deal of impact on the families of soldiers, who were eager for information. It also affected society with its changing views of the war. The coverage was generally positive regarding the United States' involvement in Vietnam prior to 1967. During this time the soldier was portrayed as a *hero* fighting the spread of communism (Wyatt, 1995). Following the Tet Offensive in January 1968, however, CBS journalist Walter Cronkite made his well-known statement in a television special: "To say that we are closer to victory today is to believe, in the face of the evidence, the optimists who have been wrong in the past. To say that we are mired in a bloody stalemate seems the only realistic, yet unsatisfactory conclusion" (Hallin, 1986, pp. 161–162). From that point, combat scenes on television were more graphic, and films of civilian and military casualties increased. Many U.S. soldiers were depicted by television journalists as drug abusers who were involved in racial conflicts. Unfortunately, much of the growing dissent about the United States' military role in Vietnam was misplaced onto the veterans, and this issue had ramifications on their families.

Many families of service members reported heavy consumption of news stories, which produced nightmares, depression, and fears regarding death, injury, or capture of their loved ones. Some family members would not seek mental health care because there was a perception that it might do some harm to their spouses' careers or anger them (Scurfield & Tice, 1992). Other studies done during the Vietnam conflict documented the significant effects, both positive and negative, of fathers' absences that were particularly noted on their male children. For example, Hillenbrand (1976) found that there were higher IQ scores in the soldiers' first-born sons but increased aggression and dependency needs as well. The research also revealed higher math scores for boys who had older siblings, than in the control group.

Persian Gulf War (Operation Desert Storm): 1990–1991

In order to understand what families go through when their loved ones are deployed, one must consider the changes in military life for the soldier. There have been some significant transformations in all branches of the armed forces since the Vietnam conflict. Norwood and colleagues (1996) suggested that the changes are reflected in the current military and include the following: all volunteer force, more women, wider range of occupational specialties for military women, more dual-career couples, more married service members, more service members with children, more military wives working outside the home, and higher education levels. These changes have brought about some added stressors for families. For example, single parent households were especially vulnerable to the stress of deployment during the Gulf War. There were concerns raised about the effects of war on the children when their primary caretakers, either through deployment of both parents or those from single-parent families, were absent for a period of time. There were approximately 22,895 single parents deployed, and it is estimated that 32, 048 children were affected by the deployment. Additionally, joint service marriages, in which both parents were deployed, were estimated to involve 5706 couples and 4656 children during Desert Storm (Norwood et al., 1996). Hardaway (2004) reported that many soldiers in Desert Storm were not adequately briefed before returning to their homes. Some also developed a sense of entitlement as "returning victorious warriors" but were not treated as such by their families. In some instances, there was an increase in reported spousal and child abuse rates.

In another study, Rosen, Westhuis, Teitelbaum (1993) described the results in which adults were asked to rate children's reactions to their parents' deployment during Desert Storm. The most common complaint was sadness for both boys and girls. The researchers found that 42 percent to 64 percent of the children between the ages of three and twelve years old were described as being tearful or sad. In addition, discipline problems at home were reported to occur frequently with male children, but infrequently with female children. It is important to note that both genders demanded more attention from the nondeployed parent.

The media coverage that brought the battle into the living rooms of Americans as it was occurring was reportedly an additional stress factor for family members during the Gulf War (Slone & Friedman, 2008). While it provided up to the minute news for some people, it added to the concerns for families of deployed soldiers who were fighting in the war zone when accurate information from the military was slower in reaching families. According to Norwood and colleagues (1996), families identified that the most important aid was accurate information from formal sources of the military. On the other hand, family members who did not receive formal information and relied on rumors and misinformation, reported more stress and anxious feelings.

LESSONS LEARNED?

*The ability of humans to understand and organize their
experiences is directly related to a tendency to construct
world views or perspectives from which each life
experience is assessed, understood and then acted upon*

(Greene, 2007, p. 161).

There are many lessons that can be learned from the research that has already been done with families of war veterans; understanding their changing needs is an ongoing endeavor. Families of soldiers have changed since the Vietnam conflict because the texture of the American family has changed. Some of these changes include more single-parent households, dual-career military couples, the impact of the female soldier's absence on her children, repeated terms of deployments, and so on.

Mental health clinicians must also keep in mind that some of the services seem to stigmatize or pathologize individuals who do seek help and may therefore serve to dissuade others. Military culture needs to make it acceptable to seek mental health services. According to the Department of Defense Task Force on Mental Health (2007), the results of four surveys of service members deployed to Iraq and Afghanistan indicated that 59 percent of the Army and 48 percent of the Marines perceived that they would be treated differently by leadership if they sought counseling (p.15). This stigma is subsequently passed along to their families, causing individuals who are in need of mental health services to not seek them out. According to this same report, psychological concerns among family members have yet to be quantified. Although the report proposes a campaign towards decreasing this stigma, prejudice of this nature is very difficult to fight against.

The DoD (2007) report further identified significant geographic variability in the provision of psychological health services to spouses and children, in spite of the fact that the need for such services did not seem to match any geographical differences (p. 27). More specifically, the task force found that children had limited access to clinical treatment services. It was noted that teenagers who had substance abuse problems had constrained access to intensive outpatient programs for treatment. This issue often required families to send their children two to four states away for appropriate services. Children with special needs also had limited access to psychological health services (DoD, 2007, p. 28). According to some veterans' advocates, we can no longer afford to have services for veterans and their families be viewed in terms of a medical model, which tends to pathologize people who are in need of services (Wheeler & Bragin, 2007). Instead, there needs to be a seamless continuum of services that incorporates all three levels of intervention:

primary, secondary, and tertiary. Furthermore, the services need to ensure that mental health professionals apply evidence-based clinical practice guidelines.

On a final note, it is clear that the country cannot continue to provide its veterans and their families with inadequate mental health services. The evidence suggests that there are growing issues of concern. According to the DoD Task Force (2007), despite the restraining effects of stigma, more than one third of active duty military and one half of the reserves self-reported psychological health problems in the months following deployment. The problems are compounded and the numbers escalate when family members are added to the count. If we do not act, we can look forward to increased numbers of incidences of domestic violence, traumatic family disruptions, divorces, suicides, chemical and behavioral addictions, and child abuse.

REFERENCES

Amen, D.G., Jellen, L., Merves, E., and Lee, R.E. (1988). Minimizing the impact of deployment on military children: Stages, current preventative efforts and system recommendations. *Military Medicine, 153,* 141–146.

Black, W.G. (1993). Military-induced family separation: A stress reduction intervention. *National Association of Social Workers, 38,* 277.

Boulding, E. (1950). Family adjustments to war separation and reunion. *American Academy of Political and Social Science Annals, 272,* 59–67.

Department of Defense (DoD) Task Force on Mental Health. (2007). *An achievable vision: Report of the Department of Defense on mental health.* Falls Church, VA: Defense Health Board.

Greene, R.R. (2007). *Social work practice: A risk and resilience perspective.* Belmont, CA: Thompson Brooks/Cole.

Hallin, D.C. (1986). *The uncensored war: The media and Vietnam.* Los Angeles, CA: University of California Press.

Hardaway, T. (2004). Treatment of psychological trauma in children of military families. In N.B. Webb (Ed.), *Mass trauma and violence: Helping families and children cope.* New York: Guilford Press.

Hill, R. (1949). *Families under stress.* New York: Harper & Row.

Hillenbrand, E.D. (1976). Father absence in military families. *The Family Coordinator, 25,* 451–458.

Mateczun, J.M., and Holmes, E.K. (1996). Return, readjustment and reintegration: The three R's of family reunion. In R.J. Ursano and A.E. Norwood (Eds.), *Emotional aftermath of the Persian Gulf War* (pp. 369–392). Washington, DC: American Psychiatric Press.

Norwood, A.E., Fullerton, C.S., and Hazen, K.P. (1996). Those left behind: Military families. In R.J. Ursano and A.E. Norwood (Eds.), *Emotional aftermath of the Persian Gulf War* (pp. 163–196). Washington, D.C.: American Psychiatric Press.

Pincus, S.H., House, R., Christenson, J., and Adler, L.E. (2008). The emotional cycle of deployment. *HOOAH4Health.com.* Retrieved from http://hooah4health.com/pageprinter.asp?f=/deployment/familymatters/emotioanlcycle.htm&1=3

Rosen, L.N., Westhuis, D.J., and Teitelbaum, J.M. (1993). Children's reactions to Desert Storm deployment. *Military Medicine, 158,* 465–469.

Scurfield, R.M., and Tice, S.N. (1992). Interventions with medical and psychiatric evacuees and their families: From Vietnam through the Gulf War. *Military Medicine, 157,* 88–97.

Slone, L.B., and Friedman, M.J. (2008). *After the war zone.* Philadelphia: DaCapo.

Trimm, S. (1993). *Walking wounded.* Norwood, NJ: Ablex Publishing Corporation.

Wheeler, D.P., and Bragin, M. (2007). Bringing it all back home. *Health and Social Work, 32,* 27–31.

Wyatt, C.B. (1995). *Paper soldiers: The American press and the Vietnam war.* Chicago, IL: University of Chicago Press.

Zeff, K.N., Lewis, S.J., and Hirsch, K.A. (1997). Military family adaptation to United Nations operations in Somalia. *Military Medicine, 162,* 384–38.

Chapter 16

VETERAN'S SUICIDE: PREVALENCE, CONTRIBUTING FACTORS, AND PREVENTION

Jamshid A. Marvasti and Kenneth A. Fuchsman

INTRODUCTION

They survived the war zone and the hazards of fighting in foreign lands. Now, soldiers are coming home to face long battles with combat PTSD; struggles that all too often end in self-destructive behaviors and suicide. Although these suicide victims die at their own hands, they are no less casualties of war than the soldiers who are killed on the front lines. Suicide is a multidisciplinary, multifactorial, and complex phenomenon that cannot be comprehended from a one-dimensional point of view. Although PTSD and war trauma appear to bring suicidal behavior to the surface, other elements such as childhood adversity, cultural factors, religious beliefs, and the ego structure of a veteran may all play a role. Nevertheless, the element of war has been the most significant contributing factor in PTSD and self-destructive behavior.

Psychological reactions to war experiences could cause depression, guilt, shame, and/or ruminations on existential fears as a reaction to symbolic and/or real losses (Conesa, 2010).

Suicide can be described as a process that starts with ideation, shifts to attempt, and may eventually lead to completed suicide. In any case, it needs to be looked at as a personal intent to alleviate or end an unbearable suffering. This intense pain and suffering exceeds the individual's capacity to formulate any other response besides suicide; an indication of hopelessness and helplessness. Regardless of the situation, suicide is "a permanent solution to a temporary problem."

DEFINITION OF SUICIDE

The word *suicide* is derived from the Latin, *sui caedere*, which means "to kill one's self." We can divide suicidal and parasuicidal phenomenon into several groups (Dripchak, 2008):

1. *Suicidal ideation*: when an individual is thinking about ending his or her life.
2. *Suicide threat*: when a person verbalizes thoughts of suicide but has yet to act on them. The threat may include a plan, but no act has taken place. This phase is considered "potentially dangerous" (Roberts, 1991).
3. *Attempted suicide*: when one attempts to take his or her life and survives.
4. *Completed suicide*: when an individual concludes the act of suicide and dies. Completed suicide often depends on the lethality of the method used, as well as the opportunity for possible rescue.
5. *Parasuicidal behavior*: described as nonfatal but intentional self-inflicted injurious behavior that may result in injury, illness, or death (Kreitman, 1977). Parasuicidal behavior is different from suicide because there is no intention to cause death.
6. *Assisted suicide*: the completion of suicide by a terminally ill or suffering individual with the help of a second person. Assisted suicide also may be referred to as "euthanasia," the act of ending the suffering of a human or animal when there is no hope for healing.
7. *Cluster suicides*: defined as the occurrence of multiple completed suicides within a given geographical area. These may be sensationalized by the news media, often resulting in further suicides that are deemed "copycat" acts. Questions may be raised concerning whether the high numbers of suicide cases among military personnel in the same unit can be categorized as cluster suicides.
8. *Inviting suicide*: the act of placing oneself in such a dangerous position that grievous bodily harm or death may occur. This is also referred to as indirect suicide. Demonstrations of this behavior can be more subtle, such as walking in a bad neighborhood or dangerous part of a war zone, or more aggressive, such as approaching a police officer in a threatening manner, which then prompts the officer to shoot.
9. *Kamikaze and suicide warriors*: suicide intended to harm the enemy. With this type of suicide, the main goal of the perpetrator is not to cause his or her own death, but rather to inflict damage on the enemy. Suicide is forbidden in many religions, including Islam. However, Islamic warriors who approve of suicide missions justify that these missions are not acts of suicide, but that the suicide bomber is merely a vehicle of transportation. A warrior is assigned to carry a bomb from point A to point B, using his body as a vehicle, because he does not have a missile, helicopter, or F-16 (Marvasti, 2008, 2009).

FACTORS CONTRIBUTING TO SUICIDE

In general, motivational factors for suicidal acts are specific, individualized, and multidimensional. For one person, a suicidal act may be designed to send a message; for another, the motivation may be to cause a change in environment. Buddhist monks, for example, self-immolated as a protest against the Vietnam War. Often, the goal of suicide is to end long-term emotional and spiritual pain and frustration. Suicidal acts and ideation may also be expressions of rage, guilt, self-punishment, or frustration at seemingly impossible situations.

Case of Chuck Luther

U.S. soldier Chuck Luther reported that he thought of committing suicide in front of his commander as a way to communicate feelings of anger and frustration about the treatment he received after seeking help with war trauma (Smith, 2009). The military discharged him with a diagnosis of a personality disorder. Later, however, he was diagnosed with TBI and PTSD by a private psychologist, who told the media that Luther was like hundreds of other soldiers he had treated. They had all been similarly misdiagnosed. "None of them–actually had a personality disorder" (Kors, 2010).

Those who have severe PTSD, which some clinicians have labeled as an "identity disorder," experience profound change in their identity and may harm themselves as a rejection of the new self. One needs to differentiate between the precipitating factors for suicidal actions and the main element that initially caused the suicidal ideation. For example, the element of rejection by a partner or family member (i.e. receiving a "Dear John" letter) is considered a precipitating factor, not a cause of suicide. Attention should be given to the horrors of war that led to the state of mind of these soldiers, not to isolated incidents they may otherwise have handled appropriately.

PRIMARY RISK FACTORS OF SUICIDE IN VETERANS

Severe PTSD and TBI

The combination of PTSD and TBI should always raise a red flag for the risk of aggression toward self (suicide) or others (homicide). TBI, especially damage to the frontal lobes of the brain, is considered to increase suicidal risk (through both neurobiological and psychosocial mechanisms). A rigorous risk assessment for those veterans with such brain injuries and comorbidity of PTSD is strongly recommended (Gutierrez, Brenner & Huggins, 2008).

Severe PTSD and ADHD

The combination of PTSD with childhood or adult attention-deficit/hyperactivity disorder (ADHD) increases the risk of self-destructive behavior. A person with ADHD exhibits impulsivity, is easily frustrated, and may not think about the consequences of his or her behavior.

Anxiety, Depression, and Previous Suicide Attempts

Those veterans who screened positive for PTSD and two or more comorbid mental disorders were significantly more likely to experience suicidal ideation in comparison with veterans with PTSD alone (Jakupcak et al., 2009). Army researchers suggest that veterans need at least two years of noncombat time before the signs and symptoms of anxiety and depression decrease; therefore, multiple combat tours are cumulative and detrimental to mental health. Research revealed that reintegration to civilian life can be a time of elevated risk for self-harm. "They [veterans] have this high adrenaline from being in the theater [combat], and they don't know what to do with it. They take out a motorcycle and drive it at 120 miles an hour" (McNamara, 2010).

Side Effects of Medication

Akathisia (restless leg syndrome), which can be a side effect of antipsychotic and SSRI antidepressants, may be associated with suicide. Additionally SSRIs are known to cause suicidal ideation in some young people. Any young soldier on an SSRI should be assessed frequently, especially in the first few months of pharmacotherapy, for any indication of suicidal ideation. Other medications, such as mood stabilizers, anti-malarial treatments, and the antismoking medication varenicline (Chantix®) carry warnings for risk of suicide.

Multiple Deployments

According to *The Wall Street Journal*, "Army officials say the strain of repeated deployments with minimal time back in the U.S. is one of the biggest factors fueling the rise in military suicides" (Dreazen, 2009, p. A-4). In these situations there are also questions of medical ethics to be raised. If evidence shows that soldiers with multiple deployments are at high risk for suicide, should the military continue to repeatedly deploy these soldiers?

Researchers have been warning of the dangers of extended time in the midst of combat since WW II, when psychiatrists Appell and Beebe (1946) reported psychiatric breakdowns among men with a total of 200 to 240 days of combat. A recent military report states, "It has long been recognized that mental health breakdown occurs after prolonged combat exposure. During World War II, entire units were withdrawn from the line for months at a time in order to rest and refurbish. Even during the Vietnam War, week-long combat patrols in the field were followed by several days of rest and recuperation at the base camp" (MHAT IV, 2006, p. 76). This has not been the case in the current wars in the Middle East. A "considerable number" of American military in Iraq have been "conducting combat operations every day of the week, 10–12 hours per day, seven days a week for months on end. At no time in our military history have soldiers been required to serve on the front line for periods of six months to a year, without a significant break in order to recover from the physical, psychological, and emotional demands that ensue from combat" (MHAT, IV, 2006 p. 76).

Stress and Guilt Regarding Combat Actions

Those who participated in activities that they saw as amoral, such as the killing of civilians, executing or torturing prisoners, or other atrocities, may develop multiple symptoms, including acute shame, remorse, and guilt. They are also prone to developing psychiatric symptoms such as PTSD, depression, and suicidal ideation.

In a study of U.S. veterans published in 1991 in the *American Journal of Psychiatry*, Hendin and Haas studied 187 Vietnam veterans, 19 of whom had committed suicide. They found that PTSD emerged as an emotional disorder among combat veterans with high risk for suicide. They also concluded that intensive combat-related guilt feelings were found to be the most significant explanatory factors. For a great number of suicidal veterans "such disturbing combat behavior as the killing of women and children took place while they were feeling emotionally out of control because of fear or rage" (Hendin & Haas, 1991, p. 586).

Hendin and Haas also looked at the capacity of the veteran's war experience to produce guilt feelings later on in their lives. These combat actions included inadvertent or deliberate killing of civilians, mutilation of the enemy, torture of the enemy, the wounding or killing of fellow soldiers, and rape. It also included the passive witness of nonmilitary action by fellow soldiers, such as manipulating civilians in the war zone into selling drugs, or other corrupt activities. Among the nineteen suicide victims, 68.4% had killed civilians. This percentage was slightly higher than it was for the non-suicidal veterans, 57 percent of whom report having killed civilians (Hendin & Haas, 1991).

The following are two case histories that indicate the depth of the emotional pain felt by these soldiers in relation to their combat activities.

Case History of Jeffrey Lucey

One highly publicized case involved a Marine reservist named Jeffrey Lucey, who served for five months in Iraq. When he returned home, he began drinking heavily and was diagnosed by physicians as having PTSD, depression, and suicidal ideation.

Jeffrey Lucey suffered war-induced rage so intense that his parents needed to physically rock him in their laps to calm him. On July 22, 2004, at age 23, Jeffrey was no longer able to handle the intensity of his emotions and their effects—the daily vomiting, the feeling that he was a murderer, the fear that none of his military higher-ups even cared. Jeffrey's father came home to find that his son had wrapped a garden hose around his neck and hanged himself. On his bed he had placed the dog tags of two unarmed Iraqi prisoners he said he had been ordered to shoot (Srivastava, 2004).

Six weeks before his death, Jeffrey Lucey paid his last visit to the VA clinic and was admitted for a three-day stay in the hospital psychiatric ward. He was prescribed a number of antipsychotic drugs and tranquilizers, such as Haldol® (haloperidol), Klonopin® (clonazepam), and Ativan® (lorazapam), and was given warnings not to drink alcohol. Two days after his release from the hospital, he destroy- ed his parents' car in an apparent suicide attempt. A little more than a month before he killed himself, he told his parents that he had been refused mental health treatment by the VA because he was drinking. His parents insist that the VA focused on a symptom, his drinking, rather than the cause of his mental deterioration, PTSD due to combat. In January 2008, Jeffrey's parents were awarded a $300,000 settlement from the VA, although they admitted no wrongdoing in his suicide (Notte, 2009).

Case History of Ken Dennis

Corporal Ken Dennis, of Renton, Washington, had been a rifleman in a special operations unit. In 2004, he was sent into intense combat duty during the invasion of Iraq. At 22 years of age, he had already been deployed to Pakistan, Somalia, and Afghanistan. He committed suicide two months following the completion of his enlistment period. Right before his death, he confessed to his father, "You know, Dad, it's really hard–very, very hard–to see a man's face and kill him" (Lyke, 2004). His father told reporters that although his son was a "tough kid," scenes from Iraq haunted him. Ken had described an event that occurred when he was at a checkpoint in Iraq. A van tried to approach, and soldiers commanded the driver to stop, in English. When he did not comply, Marines opened fire at the van. After the shooting, they discovered that they had killed an entire family of innocent civilians, including a mother, father, and two young children. Ken's father explained, "That kind of disgusted him–he always questioned, "did I shoot a Fedayeen, or did I shoot a civilian?" (Lyke, 2004).

PREDICTING SUICIDE: MISSION IMPOSSIBLE

Predicting suicide is nearly impossible in many cases; however, researchers have indicated several characteristics, or red flags, that may correlate with suicide. These characteristics typically fall into one of three categories: (1) of and relating to loss, (2) affective and emotional states;, and, (3) attitudes, behavior, mental states, and mindset.

Loss can be described as:

- Isolation or lack of a support system. This includes the loss of an intimate friend, comrade, close family member, or confidante. It may be enhanced by a history of loss of a parent or caretaker in early childhood, which may prompt feelings of abandonment or of having been deserted.
- Lack of strong attachment, bonding, affiliation or association with another person, group or organization. Life can be defined as a chain of interpersonal connections, attachments, and bonding. Those who attempted suicide felt, at the moment of their decision, disconnected from the world, and believed no one would feel a loss from their death. Those who survived explained that at the last moment they were able to reconnect, in some cases by thinking about a family member who would suffer if they died.
- History of suicide by family members or friends. This can serve as an example and make suicide seem more like a viable option. In the case of family members, one may wonder if there is a genetic element, or identification with the lost object.

Affective and emotional states may include:

- Feelings of hopelessness, helplessness, worthlessness, or humiliation. Also, presence of suppressed rage, free-floating hostility, and anxiety.
- Unresolved guilt feelings, such as survivor guilt or shame, guilt and remorse in regard to participation in atrocities, or guilt from involvement in amoral or illegal acts.
- Feelings of being trapped.
- Having a self-image of being dirty and sinful.
- Increase in chronic physical pain of old injuries or new ones; heavy reliance on pain medication, which sometimes the victim feels is not working.
- Existence of psychiatric disorders such as PTSD, TBI, severe depression, paranoid disorder, or addiction to alcohol and drugs. In addition, research reveals a significant association between the presence of manic/hypomanic symptoms and the likelihood of suicidal ideation or attempted suicide in those with PTSD (Dell'Osso et al., 2009 May).

Attitudes, behaviors, mental states, and mindset may include

- Previous suicide attempts and previous high-risk reckless behavior, for instance, driving a motorcycle without a helmet.
- Having a mindset and ideology of violence as a solution to life's problems (Matsakis, 2007). Also, having an overall negativistic or pessimistic attitude toward the world.
- Conflict with authority figures; a feeling of being deceived or betrayed by governments, commanders, family, partner, and the VA system.

Clinicians report that most suicides happen after some kind of warning signal. The patient will often give clues regarding intentions and suicidal preoccupation, although, in some cases, even the patient was not aware of his or her intention until the hour of action. In addition, many clinicians report false positives or false negatives with regard to the diagnosis of suicidal intention.

WAR TRAUMA AND SUICIDE

Suicidality is a concern for individuals with PTSD, both veterans and civilians. Suicide attempts have been identified in 25 percent of cases where PTSD is present. This rate may become higher when a comorbidity of bipolar disorder is present. Dell'Osso and colleagues (2009) suggest that subtle bipolar disorder, which is defined as the presence of manic/hypomanic symptoms, in PTSD patients may be a potential predictor of suicidality. They strongly recommend that even subthreshold manic/hypomanic features in PTSD patients be considered a red flag.

Veterans who screened positive for PTSD and two or more comorbid mental disorders were significantly more likely to experience thoughts of suicide relative to veterans with PTSD alone (*Science Daily*, 2009).

Clinical literature reveals a strong relationship between combat experiences, such as being shot at, handling dead bodies, or killing the enemy combatant, and the prevalence of PTSD (Kaplan, 2006). Scientific studies also have established PTSD as the top risk factor for suicidal ideation in veterans (Jakupcak et al., 2009). Army officials now recognize that the seemingly endless deployments may be one of the largest risk factors contributing to the rising numbers of military suicides (Dreazen, 2009). It is documented that when trauma and victimization occur in less personal circumstances (e.g. hurricanes, tornados, or instances of burglary without direct confrontation), there may be a lower risk of suicide than when traumas are interpersonal, such as in the cases of war, abuse, or sexual assault (Desai, 2008).

For a combat veteran, a lowered frustration tolerance mixed with a familiarity and possession of firearms is a deadly combination. As psychologist and Army Reserve Lieutenant Colonel Kathy Platoni puts it, "When you are used to using a weapon, or dealing with problems with a weapon, or killing people with weapons, you are desensitized. In this sense it is not terrifying to think of using a weapon or having it in your home in civilian life" (DeBrosse & Srivastava, 2010).

POSTTRAUMATIC MOOD DISORDER AND SUICIDE

Sher (2009) proposed that some of the soldiers who are diagnosed with comorbid PTSD and major depressive disorder (MDD) may have a separate psychobiological condition that may be called post traumatic mood disorder (PTMD). Studies suggest those who are suffering from comorbid PTSD and MDD differ clinically and biologically from individuals with PTSD or MDD alone. This new category of PTMD includes those patients who have greater severity of symptoms, increased suicidal ideation, and a higher level of social or occupational disorder, in comparison to individuals with either one of these disorders alone. There is some neurobiological evidence supporting the concept of PTMD obtained from neuroendocrine challenge tests, analysis of cerebrospinal fluid, neuroimaging, and sleep studies (Sher, 2009).

ATROCITIES, MORAL INJURY, AND SUICIDE

Besides extended exposure to physical danger in heavy combat, there are other wartime stressors that increase the likelihood of PTSD. Judith Herman reports that it is "the participation in meaningless acts of malicious destruction that rendered men most vulnerable to lasting psychological damage" (1992, p. 54). She cites a study of Vietnam veterans, in which about 20 percent admitted to having witnessed atrocities during their tour of duty in Vietnam, and another 9 percent acknowledged personally committing atrocities (Herman, 1992).

In an insurgent war, where the enemy blends with the civilian population, service members may easily mistake innocent civilians for enemy combatants. They are more likely to unexpectedly encounter human remains, to be exposed to injured women and children, and to be directly involved in the deaths of their victims. These factors contribute to moral injury, a malady that is only just beginning to be recognized as a war wound. According to Bill Rider, counselor and president of the American Combat Veterans of War, formally recognizing moral injury as an issue and a precursor to PTSD is long overdue (Walker, 2010). Edward Tick, who facilitates a series of healing retreats for veterans, discusses our need for modern rituals as a way to heal our psychologically wounded warriors. He describes PTSD as, in part, the tortured consciences of good people who did their best under conditions that would dehumanize anyone. He states his belief that war is inherently a moral enterprise, and that "healers and communities must walk with them" (Tick, 2005).

IRAQ WAR ATROCITIES AND SELF-DESTRUCTIVE BEHAVIOR

The MHAT IV survey of American military in Iraq found that approximately "10% of soldiers and Marines report mistreating non-combatants" (2006, p. 4). The frequency of these destructive actions increases the likelihood of trauma for the perpetrators. A July 2004 study published in the *New England Journal of Medicine*, revealed that 28 percent of Marines in Iraq reported they were responsible for the killing of civilians; twice the number of Army soldiers who answered yes to the same question (Hoge et al., 2004).

Case History of Jeans Cruz

Jeans Cruz was one of the Army soldiers who captured Saddam Hussein. After his tour of duty in Iraq, he came back to the Bronx to be with his son and was treated as a war hero by the mayor of New York, the borough president, and officials in his parents' native town in Puerto Rico.

He says, "I've shot kids. I've had to kill kids. Sometimes I look at my son and am like, 'I've killed a kid his age.' At times we had to drop a shell into somebody's house. When you go to clean up the mess, you had three, four, five, six different kids on these. You had to move their bodies." A counselor wrote in his military medical record, "He sees himself in his dreams killing or strangling people . . . . he is worried about controlling his stress level. He stated that he is starting to drink earlier in the day." The Army gave him a medical discharge declaring him unfit for military service due to a preexisting personality disorder.

Back home in the Bronx, Cruz is stressed out. He says, "My son's out of control. There are family problems . . . . I start seeing these faces. It goes back to flashbacks, anxiety. Sometimes I've got to leave my house because I'm afraid I'm going to hit my son or somebody else" (Priest & Hull, 2007). On July 25, 2007, Cruz told CNN about serving in Iraq, "mentally I died, but I'm here" (Zahn, 2007). Emotionally, Cruz was traumatized. He heard voices, was haunted by visions of dead Iraqi children, smelled blood, and eventually slashed his forearms.

VIETNAM WAR ATROCITIES AND SUICIDE

The response Cruz had to the Iraq War is reminiscent of a particular Vietnam veteran:

Case History of Varnado Simpson

Varnado Simpson is an African-American who in 1967, at the age of 19, entered the U.S. Army. He was trained as an Infantryman and sent to the American Division Eleventh Light Infantry Brigade in South Vietnam. On March 16, 1968, his company, under the command of Captain Ernest Medina, went into the village of My Lai and killed more than 500 people. Simpson later told Army investigators, "I killed about 8 people that day" (Olson & Roberts, 1998, p. 89). Twenty years later, he confessed to having killed about 25 Vietnamese at My Lai (Bilton & Sim, 1992, p. 7). Before the Army panel, he said, "I would like to stress that everyone was ordered by Medina to kill these people, that the killing was done on his orders" (Olson & Roberts, 1998). At first, Simpson had refused to murder the residents of the village. He later stated, "If you don't follow a direct order you can be shot yourself" (Bilton & Sim, 1992, p.7). Following a directive from his platoon leader, he shot a woman (Olson & Roberts, 1998, p. 89). "I went to turn her over and there was a little baby with her that I had also killed. The baby's face was half gone. My mind just went. I just started killing," Simpson recalled. "Old men, women, children, water buffalos, everything. I cut their throats, cut off their hands, cut out their tongues, their hair, scalped them. I did it" (Bilton & Sim, 1992, p. 7).

As Judith Herman stated, "Years after their return from the war, the most symptomatic men were those who had witnessed or participated in abusive violence. A study of Vietnam veterans found that every one of the men who acknowledged participating in atrocities had post-traumatic stress disorder more than a decade after the war" (Herman, 1992).

Simpson told a reporter that he had killed innocent civilians in My Lai. People on the street began calling him a baby killer. Simpson had to quit his bank job. He had recurring nightmares that the people he had massacred would return to life and murder him. Then, in 1977, his ten-year-old son was accidentally killed by a stray bullet from two neighboring teens who were fighting. Simpson recalled, "He died in my arms, and when I looked at him, his face was like the same face of the child that I had killed. And I said 'This is the punishment for me killing the people that I killed'" (Bilton & Sim, 1992).
"I can't forgive myself for the things I did. There's more wanting to kill or hurt than to love or care. I don't let anyone get close to me. That was caused by My Lai, the war. I'm ashamed, I'm sorry, I'm guilty. But I did it. It can happen to you if you go to war." (Bilton & Sim, 1992) In 1997, Simpson killed himself.

For a small number, the desire to kill and mutilate others in war is consistent with their superego, and for others it is a violation of all they believe in. The intensity of combat can activate dormant unconscious needs for severe self-punishment, resulting in the development of psychiatric disorder, including self-destructive action. For those who feel justified in killing and mutilating an enemy, they may come out of war feeling emotionally entitled. War is the ultimate sadistic and masochistic enterprise (Fuchsman, 2008).

DEMOGRAPHIC AND EPIDEMIOLOGICAL ASPECTS OF SUICIDE IN U.S. VETERANS

Veterans make up 6 to 7 percent of the American population. Yet, year after year, according to the Secretary of Veterans' Affairs, around 20 percent of the suicides in this country are by military veterans (Maze, 2010). In 2007, the findings of a twelve-year study of suicide rates of 320,000 American men over eighteen were released. "Male veterans are twice as likely as their civilian counterparts to die by suicide," said study author Mark Kaplan (Reinberg, 2007). Among Vietnam veterans with PTSD, the risk of suicide is seven times higher than that of the general population (Bullman & Kang, 1996). Older veterans are also at risk. One veteran of WW II reported that since he has retired he is more likely to have flashbacks (Glantz, 2010). The impact of being in the military, and especially at war, can pose dangers to individuals that can affect them from their time of enlistment through old age.

A Pentagon report released in July 2010 notes that more soldiers die by suicide than during combat (Bumiller, 2010). More than 6000 veterans from various wars commit suicide every year, an average of eighteen veterans per day (Miles, 2010). In January 2009, the number of suicides surpassed the number of war casualties (Alvarez, 2009). Between January and May 2010, the military documented 163 suicides. Forty-six percent of veterans in a recent study reported having experienced suicidal thoughts or behaviors in the month prior to seeking care. Three percent of those veterans reported an actual suicide attempt (Jakupcak et al., 2009). Despite the shocking statistics from the Iraq and Afghanistan wars, it should be noted that suicide among veterans is not a new phenomenon. More than 100,000 Vietnam veterans had killed themselves as of 1998, roughly twice the number lost in the war itself (Capps, 1982; Hallock, 1998; Tick, 2005).

An analysis of the demographic data of those who commit or attempt suicide revealed that veterans who killed themselves were more likely to be young, white, and in lower enlisted ranks. Ninety-five percent of completed suicides were by male veterans. Forty-four percent of veterans who killed themselves and 55 percent of those who attempted suicide had a history that included at least one psychiatric diagnosis of mood disorder, anxiety disorder, or SUD (substance use disorder). Sixty-one percent of those soldiers who killed themselves had served in either Iraq or Afghanistan (Geppert, 2009).

NEWS MEDIA BLAME MILITARY CULTURE AND PENTAGON

A *Dayton Daily News* report (DeBrosse & Srivastava, 2010) identified twenty-one soldiers who served in Iraq and committed suicide after coming home. Although the military does not officially collect data on suicide among returning soldiers, several studies by the Government Accountability Office of Congress and the Army point to the failure of the Pentagon to prepare for the inevitable psychological toll of the nation's first sustained ground combat since the Vietnam War. In recent combat, the suffering of the soldiers has been excessive, which can result in a higher incidence of stress, trauma, and PTSD. For example, of those in Middle East combats, more than 90 percent reported being shot at as well as firing at the enemy (DeBrosse & Srivastava, 2010). In WW II, only 18 percent of the military personnel were involved in direct combat.

The report revealed that almost 60 percent of soldiers felt that seeking help, especially psychological help, might make them seem weak and feared their superiors would then treat them differently or deny them promotions. Nearly half of those interviewed maintained that their superiors would blame them if they reported a psychological problem (DeBrosse & Srivastava, 2010).

Beside the news media, family members are also blaming the military for lack of support. In addition, some believe that a side effect of certain medications (e.g. mefloquine HCl [Lariam®] an antimalaria drug) may have contributed to multiple medical and psychiatric problems, including suicide.

Dr. Michael Blumenfield, in an article in *Psychiatric Times*, criticized the Army's inaccuracies with regard to veteran suicide. He cites an Army review that concludes, "Simply stated, we are often more dangerous to ourselves than the enemy" (Blumenfield, 2010, p. 2). Dr. Blumenfield challenges this notion and finds fault with the Army's explanation for soldier's suicides. He believes the VA is minimizing the fact that these soldiers are psychological casualties of combat and victims of the reality of war. The Army review also states that commanders have failed to identify and monitor soldiers prone to risk-taking behaviors, and, as a result, the number of suicides among soldiers has soared. Dr. Blumenfield believes this to be a misguided view, giving the impression that if we did the right things we could prevent suicide in soldiers. He reported that there were 250 recommendations in a recent report and that the Army has already implemented 240 of them. He explained that, although these are positive actions to provide good mental health care, they do not prevent PTSD and will not eliminate suicide among veterans.

Blumenfield notes that, unlike physically wounded soldiers, those with psychiatric damages do not receive the Purple Heart medal. Likewise, for those soldiers who commit suicide, there is no letter of condolence from the President to the family. Many share Blumenfield's opinion that this is outrageous, and that there is no basis for treating these veterans as if they made the deliberate choice to become psychological casualties of the war (Blumenfield, 2010).

PREVENTION OF SUICIDE

Sher (2009) suggests that suicide prevention in war veterans with PTMD should focus on a number of elements, including: (a) improvement in recognizing PTMD; (b) treating symptoms of PTMD; (c) preventing a relapse when the individual is in remission; (d) treating suicidal ideation; (e) treating co-morbid psychiatric conditions, including addiction; (f) treating medical and neurological disorders, including TBI; and (g) social support.

Sher's ideas provide a foundation to which the following provisions should be added: (a) decrease the frequency of tours of combat; (b) do not return TBI or PTSD patients to combat; (c) identify soldiers who have rage or homicidal ideas and measure the amount of their helplessness, as well as the strength of their connection with significant others; (d) identify any unstable family situations, financial problems, or other significant life stressors in depressed veterans; and (e) diagnose any medical or psychiatric disorders. In any of these cases, treatment should be very aggressive, especially in the case of substance abuse problems. Identify any family history of suicide, losses, and mood disorder, as well as the veteran's own losses in early childhood. These are all elements that increase the risk of suicide.

Treatment and prevention may require hospitalization, and treatment of sleep disorder is very important. Clinicians should determine if any side effects of medication may include sleep problems, nightmares, akathisia (restless leg syndrome) or increase in anxiety and possibility of suicide. Although many antidepressive and mood stabilizing medications carry warnings about causing suicide, there is some indication that lithium carbonate may decrease suicide.

DILEMMA OF COMBAT CLINICIANS: TO EVACUATE OR NOT TO EVACUATE?

Any suicidal statement should be considered seriously and receive immediate and comprehensive evaluation. A chart review of 425 deployed soldiers seen for psychiatric reasons indicated that nearly 30 percent, or 127 soldiers, had considered killing themselves, and nearly 16 percent, or 67 soldiers, had considered killing someone else (not the enemy) within the prior month. Of these soldiers, 75 were considered severe enough to arrange for immediate intervention, which could include unit watch, comprehensive treatment, or medical evacuation to a hospital. Of the 75 dangerous soldiers, 5 were evacuated out of combat. The rest were returned to duty (Hill, Johnson & Barton, 2006).

Hill and colleagues (2006), explain that clinicians in the combat zone are faced with a dilemma in regard to making the decision to evacuate. From one viewpoint, the duty of the clinician is to establish safety and treatment for soldiers who are mentally ill. On the other hand, combat clinicians are aware that they need to conserve the fighting force and may hesitate to evacuate the patient because it would mean that the unit would lose a soldier, resulting in a decrease of fighting ability. Given the necessity of maintaining the strength of the unit, the dilemma for the deployed clinician is whether to evacuate the soldier or to attempt to rehabilitate him or her on site (Ritchie, 2004). Treating such soldiers in the combat zone is always a risky venture and may result in a poor outcome. Additionally, the emotional impact on the provider of taking such a risk is not insignificant (Hill et al., 2006).

In these situations, the job description and assignment of the clinicians, as well as their boundaries, need to be considered. We must remember that a clinician is still a clinician at all times, whether in the combat zone or out, and cannot be a politician, commander, or colonel with the added responsibility of preparing or supplying the troops for combat. Crossing the boundary from being the clinician who cares for a patient to one who worries about a unit's capacity to fight is possibly unethical. After all, there are many politicians, generals, and military personnel who are not clinicians and whose responsibility is to designate the number of soldiers needed and to maintain a reserve of substitutes for those who are evacuated.

CONCLUSION

Suicide in combat veterans may be considered a "state-related" or "state-dependent" phenomenon that can be precipitated by the condition of combat experiences or military milieu. In regard to combat experience, there is enough evidence that the trauma of killing the enemy or civilians, or of being shot at, may cause PTSD and that PTSD may be a mediator, or link, to suicide. As for "military milieu," it seems evident that multiple elements are present in military culture that may contribute to suicide. This may be one explanation for suicide among soldiers who have not yet been deployed.

These include (a) hypermasculine attitudes (which deny feelings or emotions and reward robot-like personnel), (b) systematic conditioning and desensitizing to the taking of human life, (c) familiarity with and possession of arms and weapons and the training to use them with no hesitation, and (d) authoritarianism and lack of empathy. In general, the value of life in the military is decreased and survival is not the priority. Instead, it is the mission that is most important. In regard to suicidal soldiers unfortunately, the mission is suicide.

Suicide is a serious consequence of many elements combined; however, the elements of combat trauma, exhaustion, and the development of psychiatric disorders, such as PTSD and depression, are significant. To prevent suicide, the military needs to be aware of the warning signs and identify vulnerable soldiers and evacuate them immediately.

From a military standpoint, an invasion may need to be postponed until there are enough fresh military personnel in the first line. Cities cannot be attacked with exhausted soldiers who have PTSD, TBI, or depression and are taking multiple medications in order to be able to sleep or follow commands and not fall apart.

REFERENCES

Alvarez, L. (2009, January 29). Suicides of soldiers reach high of nearly 3 decades. *New York Times*, p. A19.

Appell, J.W., and Beebe, G.W. (1946, August 31). Preventive psychiatry: An epidemiologic approach. *Journal of the American Medical Association, 131*(18), 1468–1471.

Bilton, M., and Sim, K. (1992). *Four Hours at My Lai.* New York: Penguin Books.

Bullman, T.A., and Kang, H.K. (1996). Risk of suicide among wounded Vietnam veterans. *American Journal of Public Health, 86*, 662–667.

Bumiller, E. (2010, July 29). Pentagon Report Places Blame for Suicides. *The New York Times.* p A10.

Capps, W.H. (1982). *The unfinished war: Vietnam and the American conscience.* Boston: Beacon Press.

Conesa, M.D.B. (2010). Loss, trauma and suicide in war survivors. *Internet and Psychiatry.* Retrieved from http://www.internetandpsychiatry.com/joomla/home-page/editorials-and-commentaries/418-loss-trauma-and-suicide-in-war-survivors.html

DeBrosse, J., and Srivastava, M. (2010). For some, battle goes on long after the shooting stops. *Dayton Daily News.* Retrieved on November 5, 2011, http://www.daytondailynews.com/project/content/project/suicide/daily/1010suicide.html

Dell'Osso, L., Carmassi, C., Rucci, P., Ciaparelli, A., Paggini, R., Ramacciotti, C.E. and et al. (2009, May). Lifetime subthreshold mania is related to suicidality in posttraumatic stress disorder. *CNS Spectrums, 14*(5), 262–266.

Desai, R.A. (2008). Suicide. In G. Reyes, J.D. Elhai, and J.D. Ford (Eds.), *The Encyclopedia of Psychological Trauma* (pp. 637–639). Hoboken, NJ: Wiley.

Dreazen, Y.J. (2009, November 3). Suicide toll fuels worry the Army is strained. *The Wall Street Journal,* p. A4.

Dripchak. L. (2008). Suicide and self-destructive behaviors: Learning from clinical population. In J.A. Marvasti (Ed.), *Psycho-Political Aspects of Suicide Warriors, Terrorism and Martyrdom* (pp. 121–135). Springfield, IL: Charles C Thomas

Fuchsman, K. (2008). Traumatized soldiers. *The Journal of Psychohistory, 36*(1), 72–84.

Geppert, C.M.A. (2009, October 2). From war to home: Psychiatric emergencies of returning veterans. *Psychiatric Times, 26*(10), 1–5.

Glantz, A. (2010, November 11). Suicide rates soar among WW II vets, records show older veterans twice as likely to take their own lives as those returning from Iraq and Afghanistan. *The Bay Citizen.* Retrieved November 5, 2011 from http://www.baycitizen.org/veterans/story/suicide-rates-soar-among-wwii-vets/.

Gutierrez, P.M., Brenner, L.A., and Huggins, J.A. (2008). A preliminary investigation of suicidality in psychiatrically hospitalized veterans with traumatic brain injury. *Archives of Suicide Research, 12,* 336–343.

Hallock, D.W. (1998). *Hell, healing and resistance.* Farmington, PA: Plough Publishing.

Hendin, H., and Haas, A.P. (1991). Suicide and guilt as manifestations of PTSD in Vietnam combat veterans. *American Journal of Psychiatry, 148,* 586–591. Retrieved from http://ajp.psychiatryonline.org/cgi/content/abstract/148/5/586

Herman, J.L. (1992). Trauma and recovery: *The aftermath of violence–from domestic abuse to political terror.* New York: Basic Books.

Hill, J., Johnson, R.C., and Barton, R.A. (2006, March). Suicidal and homicidal soldiers in deployment environments. *Military Medicine, 171,* 228–232.

Hoge, C.W., Castro, C.A., Messer, S.C., McGurk, D., Thomas, J.L., Cotting, D.I., and Koffman, R.L. (2004). Combat duty in Iraq and Afghanistan, mental health problems, and barriers to care. *New England Journal of Medicine, 351*(1), 13–22.

Jakupcak, M., Cook, J.W., Imel, Z.E., Fontana, A.F., Rosenheck, R.A., and Mcfall, M. E. (2009, August). Posttraumatic stress disorder as a risk factor for suicidal ideation in Iraq and Afghanistan War veterans. *Journal of Traumatic Stress, 22,* 303–306.

Kaplan, A. (2006, January). Hidden combat wounds: Extensive, deadly, costly. *Psychiatric Times, 23*(1), 1–8.

Kors, J. (2010, 8 April). Disposable soldiers. *The Nation.* Retrieved from http://www.thenation.com/print/article/disposable-soldiers.

Kreitman, N. (1977). *Parasuicide.* Chichester, UK: Wiley.

Levin, A. (2009, December 4). Army trying to solve puzzle of rising suicide rates. *Psychiatric News, 44*(23), 1, 45.

Lyke, M.L. (2004, August 13). The war comes home: Rifleman couldn't take any more. *Seattle Post-Intelligencer.* Retrieved from http://www.seattlepi.com/local186127_warsuicide13.html

Marvasti, J.A. (2008). *Psycho-political aspects of suicide warriors, terrorism and martyrdom.* Springfield, IL: Charles C Thomas.

Marvasti, J.A. (2009). It takes two villages to raise a terrorist: Psycho-political aspects of suicide bombers. *American Journal of Forensic Psychiatry, 30*(3), 1–16.

Matsakis, A. (2007). *Back from the Front: Combat Trauma, Love, and the Family.* Baltimore, MD: Sidran Institute Press.

Maze, R. (2010, April 23). 18 veterans commit suicide each day. *Army Times.* Retrieved from http://www.armytimes.com/news/2010/04/military_veterans_ suicide_042210w/>

McNamara, D. (2010, June). Preventing Army suicides: A call for help. *Clinical Psychiatry News, 38*(6), 1–3.

Meagher, I. (2007). Moving a nation to care. *Post-traumatic stress disorders and America's returning troops.* New York: IG Publishing.

Mental Health Advisory Team (MHAT) IV. (2006, November 17). Operation Iraqi Freedom 05-07, "Final Report." Retrieved from http://www.armymedicine.army. mil/news/mhat/mhat_iv/MHAT_IV_Report_17NOV06.pdf,.

Miles, D. (2010, April 23). VA officials strive to prevent veteran suicides. *American Forces Press Service.* Retrieved from http://www.af.mil/news/story.asp?id= 123201368

Notte, J. (2009, March 13). Military suicides continue to increase–sad truth. *The Phoenix.* Retrieved from http://blogs.courierpostonline.com/veteranvoices/2009/ 03/13/military-suicides-continue-to-increase-sad-truth/

Olson, J., and Roberts, R. (1998). *My Lai: A brief history with documents.* Boston: Bedford/St. Martin's

Priest, D., and Hull, A. (2007 June 12). *The war inside. Washington Post.* Retrieved from http://www.washingtonpost.com/wp-dyn/content/article/2007/06/16/AR200 7061600866_pf.html.

Reinberg, S. (2007, June 12). Male U.S. veterans more likely to commit suicide. *Washington Post.* Retrieved from http://www.washingtonpost.com/wp-dyn/con- tent/article/2007/06/12/ AR2007061200711_pf.html.

Ritchie, E.C. (2004). Military issues. *Psychiatric Clinics of North America, 27,* 459–471.

Roberts, A.R. (1991). *Contemporary perspectives on crisis intervention and prevention.* Englewood Cliffs, NJ: Prentice-Hall.

Science Daily. (2009, August 26). Post-traumatic stress disorder primary suicide risk factor for veterans. *Science Daily.* Retrieved November 4, 2011 from http:// www.sciencedaily.com/releases/2009/08/090825151341.htm.

Sher, L. (2009). A model of suicidal behavior in war veterans with posttraumatic mood disorder. *Medical Hypotheses, 73*(2), 215–219.

Smith, D. (Producer). (2009, November 25). Talk Nation Radio: *Chuck Luther, Dis- posable Warrior, Has Thanksgiving Message for President Obama.* Retrieved from http://talknationradio.com/?p=799

Srivastava, M. (2004). Swallowed by pain. *Dayton Daily News.* Retrieved from www. daytondailynews.com/project/content/project/suicide/daily/1011lucey.html

Tick, E. (2005). *War and the Soul: Healing Our Nation's Veterans from Post-traumatic Stress Disorder.* Wheaton, IL: Quest Books.

Walker, M. (2010, May 8). *Moral injury as a wound of war.* Retrieved from http:// www.marin-corps-news.com/2010/05/moralinjuryasawoundofwar.htm

Zahn, P. (2007, July 25). Treating America's Wounded Warriors. *CNN.* Retrieved from http://transcripts. cnn.com/TRANSCRIPTS/0707/25/pzn.01.html.

Chapter 17

PTSD IN ASIAN CULTURES: CAN WE LEARN FROM HOW OTHER SOCIETIES HANDLE TRAUMA IN NATURAL DISASTER?

ALAN R. TEO AND ROBERT LERRIGO

INTRODUCTION

Within the young field of disaster mental health, natural disasters have been a primary focus among researchers and scholars, perhaps even more so than war and civil conflict. Three billion people were affected by natural disasters over a twenty-four year period from 1967 to 1991 in one review by the Red Cross (Kokai, Fujii, Shinfuku, & Edwards, 2004). Given this scale and scope, the growth of disaster psychiatry studying natural disasters is understandable, and the lessons learned are in many ways applicable to the healing of war trauma. Both natural disaster and war can create mass casualties and similar mental and physical trauma and often leave survivors with comparable psychopathological profiles. Earthquakes and tsunamis may be as devastating as the nuclear bombing of Hiroshima. Asia, among all regions of the world, is an excellent forum for learning about natural disaster psychiatry for the unfortunate reason that it is the most disaster prone. From 1995 to 2004, 79 percent of all deaths associated with natural and technological disasters occurred in the Asia-Pacific region (Udomratn, 2008).

In this chapter, we focus on the lessons learned from a review of recent major natural disasters in Asia, including the 1995 Kobe earthquake in Japan, the 2004 Southeast Asian tsunami, the 2008 Nargis cyclone in Myanmar, and the 2008 Sichuan earthquake in China. The chapter identifies risk and resiliency factors for natural disasters; reviews the frequency of mental health problems; reveals methods for detection and diagnosis; explores health services issues; and, finally, considers treatment options, including factors of both efficacy and cultural sensitivity.

RISK AND RESILIENCY FACTORS IN NATURAL DISASTERS

Although the manifestations of PTSD across a population affected by a common disaster may be similar, demographic, clinical, psychosocial, and disaster risk factors, as well as counteracting resiliency factors, play an important role in determining who among the exposed will develop long-term psychological sequelae. Well-defined demographic risk factors for PTSD following natural disasters include the extremes of age (children and the elderly), female gender, lower education, and lack of income.

Risk Factors of Age and Gender

With regard to age, it has been suggested that those under twelve and over sixty years old have impaired psychological buffering capacities to cognitively manage traumatic events and possess other risk factors that make them more prone to developing PTSD. In a study of the 2008 Sichuan earthquake, Jia and colleagues felt the reason the elderly were at high risk for PTSD was a combination of prevalent medical comorbidities with physical impairment, decreased sensory awareness, and common socioeconomic limitations (2010). In a study of the mental health status of Indian children exposed to the 2004 tsunami, Vijayakumar, Kannan, and Daniel felt that a child's developmental level, exposure to the responses of family members, and a family history of psychopathology conferred vulnerability to PTSD (2006).

A number of studies have also identified females as a significant high-risk group. Among the more interesting speculations as to the reason are physiological differences between genders (e.g. the ability to swim during a tsunami) and female efforts to physically protect their children (Frankenberg et al., 2008). Cultural norms in traditionally patriarchal Asian societies also left women who lost their husbands in disasters with more economic losses than men had, which may add to the burden of stress and make PTSD more likely (Ghodse & Galea, 2006).

Among females in a coastal village in Tamil Nadu, India, affected by the tsunami, the odds ratio for developing PTSD was 2.83 (95% confidence interval [CI]: 1.36–5.91) (Kumar et al., 2007). Finally, although there is conflicting evidence whether socioeconomic status (determined through standard indicators of education and predisaster levels of economic resources) is a risk factor for PTSD, loss of income and lower levels of education, independently, may increase the risk (Frankenberg et al., 2008; Kumar et al., 2007; Wang et al., 2009). In a study of the 2008 Sichuan earthquake survivors, Kun and associates write that loss of income due to the disaster was an additional stressor and risk factor for PTSD (Kun et al., 2009). A separate investigation into the mental health status of the Sichuan earthquake survivors identified lower levels of education as a PTSD risk factor (Wang et al., 2009).

Preexisting Medical and Psychological Disorders

Preexisting health conditions and other clinical risk factors also may explain why only some people in a natural disaster develop PTSD. For instance, a personal history of trauma, including exposure to war and sexual trauma, was a PTSD risk factor among tsunami survivors in Thailand, and this was especially true for those under age twelve (Thavichachart et al., 2009). Any physical illness or injury surrounding the time of the disaster also increases the likelihood of developing PTSD (Kuwabara et al., 2008). Preexisting mental health disorders, including substance use and a family history of suicide (attempted or completed) or mental disorder also correlate with worse affective and somatic PTSD-related problems, especially in children eleven to fourteen years old (Vijayakumar et al., 2006).

Due to the disruption of primary care health services and the distribution of psychotropic medications, many mentally ill survivors of natural disasters acutely decompensate. This, coupled with a baseline scarcity of mental health workers in Asia and the fact that trauma can trigger relapses of mental disorders, makes the mentally ill especially vulnerable to developing PTSD (Ghodse & Galea, 2006).

Lack of Social Support

Although inherent factors such as physical and mental health status affect one's risk for developing PTSD, external psychosocial factors and lack of support also contribute and cannot be ignored. The chaos and breakdown of social order associated with sudden and traumatic civil disasters not only contribute to the psychological trauma but also erode protective factors such as social support. Survivors of the Niigata-Chuetsu earthquake in Japan who stayed with unfamiliar people the night after or who were forced to live in temporary shelters in camps demonstrated impaired psychological recovery five months after the disaster (Kuwabara et al., 2008). Furthermore, the death of a family member in the disaster nearly doubled the odds of developing

PTSD (95% CI: 1.05–4.01) (Kumar et al., 2007), with the deaths of closer family members and witnessed deaths having a more profound effect than more distant family members or unwitnessed deaths (Frankenberg et al., 2008).

Cultural factors and a high degree of community support are also considered resiliency factors following natural disasters. In their study of the people in Tamil Nadu affected by the tsunami, Rajkumar, Premkumar, and Tharyan (2008) noted that culturally grounded coping mechanisms existed to incorporate survivors in the community in a process of shared healing. The community rallied to return to normalcy, widowers were wed to other survivors to preserve the family unit, and ritual customs were created to honor the loss of loved ones.

Severity of Events

Psychosocial and clinical risk factors for PTSD are influenced by the nature and severity of the inciting disaster itself. The more "severe" the natural disaster, the more likely survivors will accumulate psychologically destabilizing risk factors. In a study of adult survivors of the Sichuan earthquake, the most important predictor of PTSD severity was the degree of disaster exposure determined by the intensity of the initial fear and the proximity of the survivors to the epicenter of the earthquake (Wang et al., 2009). In the study by Frankenberg and associates of the mental health effects of the tsunami in Sumatra, his team used remotely sensed satellite data to determine the degree of environmental and infrastructural damage caused by the tsunami, which directly correlated with the prevalence of PTSD (2008).

Children are especially vulnerable to the effects of intense trauma in natural disasters. Of those hit directly by the tsunami in Thailand, up to 27.3 percent developed PTSD, versus 3.1 percent of children indirectly affected by the tsunami (Piyasil et al., 2007). This trend may be related to the degree of physical harm caused by the traumatic event, however, which, as in other civil disasters, is also a strong predictor of PTSD in all age groups (Wang et al., 2009). Other PTSD risk factors in the context of disasters include household and property damage (Frankenberg et al., 2008; Kuwabara et al., 2008), which were by far the most common types of trauma suffered after the Asian tsunami (John, Russell & Russell, 2007).

Proximity to the Disaster

As discussed in the section on risk factors, the severity of a disaster affects the likelihood of developing PTSD. In a similar vein, the proximity of indi-

viduals to a disaster is also closely and positively correlated with rates of
PTSD. A *primary* survivor is one directly exposed to the physical effects of
the natural disaster, a *secondary* survivor is one with close family and personal ties to primary survivors, and a *tertiary* survivor is an individual from a
community beyond the physical impact area of the disaster (Math, Tandon,
et al., 2008). In a study of children six weeks after the 2004 Asian tsunami,
27 percent of primary survivors had PTSD compared with 3 percent of secondary survivors, with a relative risk of 5.2 (95% CI, 4.0–6.6) (Piyasil et al.,
2007).

HUMOR AND DRUGS AS COPING DEVICES

The incidence and severity of PTSD among the survivors of natural disasters is modified not only by the risk factors mentioned but also by protective factors, including humor, substance use, and social support. In the study
by Thavichachart and colleagues of Thai tsunami survivors, humor was
found to be an effective coping tool for developing psychological resiliency,
and the authors suggest the reciprocal inhibition theory that two antagonis-
tic responses–humor and anxiety–cannot coexist within the same organism
at a given time (2009). Moreover, the use of psychoactive substances and
alcohol allowed some tsunami survivors to improve their mood and escape
adverse emotions and memories of the trauma. Substance use and PTSD
lead to a poorer clinical course due to substance dependence and its psychiatric and physical health sequelae, however (Thavichachart et al., 2009).

EPIDEMIOLOGY OF MENTAL HEALTH PROBLEMS
AFTER DISASTER

Within the context of any disaster–natural or man-made–trauma can take
multiple forms, and it is often the indiscernible mental health trauma that has
the most severe long-term consequences. Given that disaster psychiatry is a
relatively recent field in Asia and that cultural and language barriers have
prevented a single, universally agreed-upon PTSD screening and diagnostic
tool from emerging, it is no surprise that prevalence data vary widely. The
data are also difficult to compare across studies, given different follow-up
periods and the difficulty in controlling for the level of trauma exposure of
the different subjects across studies. Nevertheless, several articles noted
alarmingly high PTSD rates. Among youths exposed to the 2004 tsunami,

upward of 71 percent have been diagnosed with PTSD, and among adults, the prevalence is as high as 33 percent. Importantly, however, the rate of PTSD symptomatology steadily decreases with the passage of time, consistent with the case of other forms of trauma, such as civil conflict. Researchers in Thailand, for instance, surveyed children in the 2004 tsunami disaster area at six weeks, six months, one year, and two years post disaster. Rates of PTSD trended down over these time points from a high of 57 percent to 7.6 percent (Piyasil et al., 2007). This suggests that post-disaster PTSD symptoms are common shortly after a major natural disaster but are fortunately transient, and this pattern is consistent with the biological model of anxiety as an acute stress response.

Partial PTSD

Symptoms are much more common than full-blown *diagnoses*, and the former can be part of a normal response. Redwood-Campbell and Riddez (2006) found 24 percent of outpatients in a Red Cross hospital had at least four symptoms of depression or PTSD yet only a much smaller fraction—1.4 percent of the study population—suffered from a clear mental disorder. Moreover, the trauma literature has demonstrated that perhaps less than half of those who develop PTSD met criteria for acute stress disorder during the first six months post trauma (Bryant, 2006). Depression, in contrast, does not peak until months after the disaster, when effects such as unemployment and financial problems become more apparent. Psychiatric comorbidity studies support these contrasting peaks in PTSD versus depression (Kokai et al., 2004). Thus, for PTSD at least, experts have recommended ongoing surveillance after a period of normal grief (Rajkumar et al., 2008).

Predisaster Resources and Infrastructures

Response to a natural disaster relies on resources, plans, and infrastructure already in place before the disaster. Having an able and ready workforce to address mental health issues after the disaster is crucial. In Thailand, a Mental Health Crisis Center—a mobile mental health team—was established within three days after the 2004 tsunami (Visanuyothin, Somchai Chakrabhand & Bhugra, 2006). Training programs to assess and treat mental health needs were implemented successfully in Indonesia too. "Refresher" courses for more than 100 general practitioners were conducted by mental health professionals and focused on diagnosis and management of common mental disorders seen in primary care (Prasetiyawan, Viora, Maramis & Keliat, 2006). A couple hundred physicians with this training is hardly sufficient to care for the larger population, however. Therefore, Indonesia also developed and implemented a community mental health nurse training program. This program has three levels from basic to more advanced. Although the numbers trained were still in the hundreds (Prasetiyawan et al., 2006), the approach of using "physician-extenders" to reach a much wider patient population is an effective one.

WHO Guidelines

The World Health Organization (WHO) has set out guidelines for mental health management in natural disasters. The guidelines emphasize the following eight tenets (Ghodse & Galea, 2006):

1. Preparation—systems should be in place before disasters occur.
2. Assessment—needs, urgency, and resource availability should be examined quantitatively and qualitatively.
3. Collaboration—different government branches and nongovernmental organizations should work together.
4. Integration—to decrease mental health stigma, integration of mental health services into primary health-care systems is helpful.
5. Access—wide availability across the population is important.
6. Training and supervision—mental health professionals should conduct training and organize supervision to ensure sustainability.
7. Long-term perspective—effective mental health response cannot occur with immediate postdisaster response alone.
8. Monitoring—ongoing evaluation with clear indicators of progress towards goals should occur.

TREATMENT APPROACHES AND THEIR EFFICACY

A review of the literature suggests the following basic principles for mental health interventions in natural disasters. First, comprehensive interventions should be multitiered. That is, care should occur at multiple levels, from the local community to public health centers to specialty-care hospitals. Interventions will certainly vary based on the tier, and the combined effect is not just additive but multiplicative. Second, interventions should be temporally staged. Short-, medium-, and long-term time frames are all necessary for an effective response. Third, wherever possible, interventions should be evidence based. Fourth, cultural sensitivity and appropriateness must guide implementation and choice of intervention for a particular locale.

The multiple stages of mental health response are integrally related to the multiple stages of natural disaster response. Chakrabhand and colleagues describe three phases of a disaster response. Phase I is the emergency and crisis phase (the first two weeks). Phase II is the post impact phase (two weeks to three months) where the focus of mental health services is on primary survivors and those with risk factors for mental illness (e.g. children and those with preexisting psychiatric illness). During this phase, activities such as interview-based needs assessments and surveys of the community population may be conducted. Finally, Phase III is the rehabilitation and recovery phase (beyond three months), in which prevention and psychoeducation efforts at the community level are areas of focus (Chakrabhand et al., 2006). For instance, stigma-reduction initiatives might occur in this phase.

Treatment Interventions

Immediate treatment interventions during phase I include provision of food, water, housing, sanitation, and other practical requirements. Other priorities that take precedence include reuniting families and attending to physical health problems. Attending to these needs could also indirectly improve mental health outcomes post disaster because psychosocial stressors such as lack of housing are well-known risk factors for mental illness among disaster survivors. Perhaps the most consistently recommended early mental health intervention is "psychological first-aid," which was described in detail as early as the 1950s (American Psychiatric Association, 1954). Core elements include providing basic psychoeducation, offering comfort and support, and facilitating access to further care (Everly & Flynn, 2006). The affected are specifically not probed regarding their reactions to the disaster, however. That is, "debriefing" about the disaster is not recommended. Instead, psychological first aid is designed to foster an environment that promotes psychological recovery. It assumes resiliency among individuals—rather than the inevitable development of psychiatric disorder—and reinforces positive coping mechanisms.

Later, mental health treatment interventions in phases II and III include psychosocial, group, and community-based interventions. A comprehensive psychosocial care model that includes normalizing emotional reaction to disasters, removing clinical labels, creating support groups organized by trained community workers, and group activities (e.g. shelter construction) has been shown to significantly reduce PTSD symptoms as measured by the Impact of Events Scale in a group of women survivors of the 2004 tsunami in India (Becker, 2009). Although the study can be criticized for its comparisons to a control group that received no intervention, it is still among the best available in terms of specific evidence.

Part of the Thai long-term response was establishing and maintaining a mental health recovery center in the disaster area. Also, keeping this in operation for one to two years after the crisis provided help, since the prevalence of mental health problems was notably higher than baseline existing local resources alone would have been able to cope with (Panyayong & Pengjuntr, 2006).

Group-level interventions used for Indian children after the 2004 tsunami included art therapy and group discussion in school classrooms, but no data on efficacy were obtained (Math, Tandon, et al., 2008). A brief group cognitive-behavioral therapy approach was efficacious but only in children categorized as high risk for PTSD, and they were only evaluated two weeks after the intervention, so durability of effect remains questionable (Pityaratstian et al., 2007). Evidence-based individual interventions that have been tested specifically in natural disaster populations are lacking.

ENSURING CULTURALLY APPROPRIATE CARE

The cultural diversity between and within different Asian countries creates a unique anthropological and psychiatric dilemma when creating culturally appropriate disaster mental health responses. Just as investigators in different countries have used different tools to screen for and diagnose PTSD among the survivors of natural disasters, so too is there great variability in the choice of treatment. As Math and colleagues point out, "'off-the-shelf' interventions are difficult to use in diverse settings of developing countries because they are unknowingly embedded with religious and cultural expectations. These diversities may influence the need for help, availability of help, comfort in seeking help, and appropriateness of that help" (Math, John et al., 2008).

Finding New Life: No One Should Suffer Alone

In Tamil Nadu, India, the community was empowered in a different way by taking responsibility for finding new wives for the widowed men under the principle that "no one should suffer alone" (Rajkumar et al., 2008).

The reason community action is an important aspect of community healing is because it employs culturally grounded coping mechanisms to overcome adversity, such as the use of spirituality and family unity (Rajkumar et al., 2008). In the same community of Tamil Nadu, tsunami survivors adopted a custom created by the local district administration. If a survivor had lost a child, he or she would plant and care for coconut saplings, ritually offering food favored by his or her child to the saplings and sit under its shadow as a sign of reverence (Rajkumar et al., 2008).

In Thailand following the tsunami, emergency health services recruited volunteers from the different affected communities; each was trained to recognize, assess, and report common mental health problems in ten families within their community (Visanuyothin et al., 2006).

In order to gain people's trust, especially when it comes to expressing psychiatric problems, mental health responses must take into account local traditions, cultures, languages, livelihood, and power structures (Choudhury, Quraishi & Haque, 2006). If necessary, disaster mental health teams must be comfortable with rebranding their image to suit local customs and to win the trust of an already shaken population. Kokai and colleagues (2004) cite an example in which Japanese mental health workers hung up the traditional white coat and instead began outreach to a volcanic eruption–affected community by organizing nonstigmatizing recreational activities such as baseball games.

An important component of culturally integrated mental health care is the ability to involve the community in shared decision-making processes, which is especially important when the trauma is a shared community experience. Detection is achieved by recruiting community leaders and teachers as valuable conduits of information and using schools as familiar, community-based sites for care and monitoring (Visanuyothin et al., 2006). At the heart of sustaining this community-based model of care is a "train-the-trainer" system in which health personnel, teachers, and community health volunteers were trained not only to screen for and refer mental health cases but also to teach their skills to others and in doing so tailor existing mental health programs to recognize the culture and diversity of the affected community (Chakrabhand et al., 2006).

Applicability to War Trauma

Despite limited evidence, there are some lessons from natural disasters that are applicable to situations of war trauma. First, negative consequences of PTSD following natural disaster parallel those of war (e.g. loss of life, loss of property, proximity to the epicenter of conflict). Second, the unpredictable nature and large scale of trauma for both civil disaster and war trauma demands that a refined system and plan for response be developed in advance. Thus, infrastructure and logistic lessons from natural disaster preparation and response can be applied to war situations. Third, the concept of primary, secondary, and tertiary survivors readily adapts to those in war environments; likewise, the triaging of response based on survivor type seems useful for those exposed to war trauma. Fourth, cultural sensitivity and community-based approaches are equally important for those suffering from war trauma.

Certainly there are differences too. Health problems and medical needs differ from those in conflict zones (Redwood-Campbell & Riddez, 2006). A multistaged response to war trauma is more complicated because the stages can simultaneously exist when war persists over an extended period of time, and soldiers are often exposed to repeated trauma rather than a single event like a natural disaster. Nonetheless, civil and war trauma have more similarities than differences. It makes sense to pool collective knowledge about PTSD and natural disaster to enhance our approaches to the same disorder in war.

REFERENCES

American Psychiatric Association. (1954). *Psychological First Aid in Community Disasters.* Washington, DC: American Psychiatric Association.

Becker, S.M. (2009). Psychosocial care for women survivors of the tsunami disaster in India. *American Journal of Public Health, 99*(4), 654–658.

Bryant, R.A. (2006). Recovery after the tsunami: Timeline for rehabilitation. *Journal of Clinical Psychiatry, 67* (Suppl 2), 50–55.

Chakrabhand, S., Panyayong, B., & Sirivech, P., (2006). Mental health and psychosocial support after the tsunami in Thailand, I*nternational Review of Psychiatry, 18* (6), 599–605.

Choudhury, W.A., Quraishi, F.A., and Haque, Z. (2006). Mental health and psychosocial aspects of disaster preparedness in Bangladesh. *International Review of Psychiatry, 18*(6), 529–535.

Everly, G.S., Jr., and Flynn, B.W. (2006). Principles and practical procedures for acute psychological first aid training for personnel without mental health experience. *International Journal of Emergency Mental Health, 8*(2), 93–100.

Frankenberg, E., Friedman, J., Gillespie, T., Ingwersen, N., Pynoos, R., Rifai, I.U., et al. (2008). Mental health in Sumatra after the tsunami. *American Journal of Public Health, 98*(9), 1671–1677.

Ghodse, H., and Galea, S. (2006). Tsunami: Understanding mental health consequences and the unprecedented response. *International Review of Psychiatry, 18*(3), 289–297.

Jia, Z., Tian, W., Liu, W., Cao, Y., Yan, J., and Shun, Z. (2010). Are the elderly more vulnerable to psychological impact of natural disaster? A population-based survey of adult survivors of the 2008 Sichuan earthquake. *BMC Public Health, 10*(1), 172.

John, P.B., Russell, S., and Russell, P.S. (2007). The prevalence of posttraumatic stress disorder among children and adolescents affected by tsunami disaster in Tamil Nadu. *Disaster Management of Response, 5*(1), 3–7.

Kokai, M., Fujii, S., Shinfuku, N., and Edwards, G. (2004). Natural disaster and mental health in Asia. *Psychiatry and Clinical Neurosciences, 58*(2), 110–116.

Kumar, M.S., Murhekar, M.V., Hutin, Y., Subramanian, T., Ramachandran, V., and Gupte, M.D. (2007). Prevalence of posttraumatic stress disorder in a coastal fishing village in Tamil Nadu, India, after the December 2004 tsunami. *American Journal of Public Health, 97*(1), 99–101.

Kun, P., Chen, X., Han, S., Gong, X., Chen, M., Zhang, W., et al. (2009). Prevalence of post-traumatic stress disorder in Sichuan Province, China after the 2008 Wenchuan earthquake. *Public Health, 123*(11), 703–707.

Kuwabara, H., Shioiri, T., Toyabe, S., Kawamura, T., Koizumi, M., Ito-Sawamura, M., et al. (2008). Factors impacting on psychological distress and recovery after the 2004 Niigata-Chuetsu earthquake, Japan: Community-based study. *Psychiatry and Clinical Neurosciences, 62*(5), 503–507.

Math, S.B., John, J.P., Girimaji, S.C., Benegal, V., Sunny, B., Krishnakanth, K., et al. (2008). Comparative study of psychiatric morbidity among the displaced and non-displaced populations in the Andaman and Nicobar Islands following the tsunami. *Prehospital and Disaster Medicine, 23*(1), 29–34; discussion 35.

Math, S.B., Tandon, S., Girimaji, S.C., Benegal, V., Kumar, U., Hamza, A., et al. (2008). Psychological impact of the tsunami on children and adolescents from the Andaman and Nicobar Islands. *Primary Care Companion to Journal of Clinical Psychiatry, 10*(1), 31–37.

Panyayong, B., and Pengjuntr, W. (2006). Mental health and psychosocial aspects of disaster preparedness in Thailand. *International Review of Psychiatry, 18*(6), 607–614.

Pityaratstian, N., Liamwanich, K., Ngamsamut, N., Narkpongphun, A., Chinajitphant, N., Burapakajornpong, N., et al. (2007). Cognitive-behavioral intervention for young tsunami victims. *Journal of the Medical Association of Thailand, 90*(3), 518–523.

Piyasil, V., Ketuman, P., Plubrukarn, R., Jotipanut, V., Tanprasert, S., Aowjinda, S., et al. (2007). Post traumatic stress disorder in children after tsunami disaster in Thailand: 2 years follow-up. *Journal of the Medical Association of Thailand, 90*(11), 2370–2376.

Prasetiyawan, Viora, E., Maramis, A., and Keliat, B.A. (2006). Mental health model of care programmes after the tsunami in Aceh, Indonesia. *International Review of Psychiatry, 18*(6), 559–562.

Rajkumar, A.P., Premkumar, T.S., and Tharyan, P. (2008). Coping with the Asian tsunami: Perspectives from Tamil Nadu, India on the determinants of resilience in the face of adversity. *Social Science and Medicine, 67*(5), 844–853.

Redwood-Campbell, L.J., and Riddez, L. (2006). Post-tsunami medical care: Health problems encountered in the International Committee of the Red Cross Hospital in Banda Aceh, Indonesia. *Prehospital and Disaster Medicine, 21*(1), s1–s7.

Thavichachart, N., Tangwongchai, S., Worakul, P., Kanchanatawan, B., Suppapitiporn, S., Pattalung, A.S., et al. (2009). Posttraumatic mental health establishment of the Tsunami survivors in Thailand. *Clinical Practice and Epidemiology in Mental Health, 5*, 11.

Udomratn, P. (2008). Mental health and the psychosocial consequences of natural disasters in Asia. *International Review of Psychiatry, 20*(5), 441–444.

Vijayakumar, L., Kannan, G.K., and Daniel, S.J. (2006). Mental health status in children exposed to tsunami. *International Review of Psychiatry, 18*(6), 507–513.

Visanuyothin, T., Somchai Chakrabhand, M.L., & Bhugra, D. (2006). Tsunami and mental health in Thailand. *International Review of Psychiatry, 18*(3), 271–273.

Wang, L., Zhang, Y., Wang, W., Shi, Z., Shen, J., Li, M., et al. (2009). Symptoms of posttraumatic stress disorder among adult survivors three months after the Sichuan earthquake in China. *Journal of Traumatic Stress, 22*(5), 444–450.

Part II

WITNESSES TO WAR

Chapter 18

WARRIOR VALUES IN MODERN TIMES: MY EXPERIENCE IN THE IRAQ WAR

ROBERT J. CAFFREY

Soldiers are not as other men . . . . They are those of a world apart, a very ancient world which exists in parallel with the everyday world but does not belong to it . . . . The distance can never be closed, for the culture of the warrior can never be that of civilization itself.

John Keegan (1993)

It is only the dead who have seen the end of war.

Plato

MY EXPERIENCE AS A CITIZEN-SOLDIER

As a lifelong student of the martial arts and an Army Reserve officer who has studied both warfare and warrior cultures for decades, I have been struck by the consistent appearance of certain rules of conduct that underpin almost all warrior traditions. These are (a) discernment, (b) restraint, (c) mercy, (d) adaptability, and (e) honor.

My interest and experience in these issues does not stem from mere academic or philosophical curiosity; for fourteen years I served as a citizen soldier for this country. As an Army Reserve officer in the branch of the special operations community known as Civil Affairs, my duties often confronted me with the seeming contradiction that is a warrior's sometimes exquisite dilemma. Although I was a "war fighter" dedicated to the defeat or destruction of my enemy, I was also inextricably bound to a warrior code of ethics and morality ruled by these values.

My specific mission as a special operations warrior was to help protect civilians from the ravages of combat and, after the guns fell silent, to maintain or rebuild essential human services for both our enemies' and our allies' population. I last performed this mission in eastern Baghdad with the First and Second Squadrons of the Second Armored Cavalry Regiment (2ACR) from the beginning of the Iraq War in 2003 until March 2004.

Unfortunately, the gunfire never did quite fall silent. In fact, it often seemed to be coming our way.

Before Iraq, I served as a "peacekeeper" in Haiti in 1995, where the armed forces of several countries tried to rebuild that tragic nation and its government. In 1996, I served in Bosnia as a "peacemaker" where, along with my brother and sister warriors, I stood between ancient enemies fueled by historic hatreds and saw the effects of genocide firsthand.

WAR, WARRIORS, AND LEADERS OF ENDLESS WAR

We are a nation at war. Perhaps we always have been. As we enter the tenth year of America's longest armed struggle, we are forced to confront a harsh reality that is our unmistakable heritage. Ours is a nation born in war, it has grown larger through war, preserved its freedom and the freedom of others by war, and suffered horribly through participating in ill-advised and misguided wars.

A gulf has always existed in America between those who bear the burden of war and the rest of our citizenry. Unlike many societies where the burden of war is shared by almost all, America is composed of a small minority that accepts the obligation of fighting, thereby subjecting themselves and their loved ones to this unique form of human trauma, and a majority that decides when others will fight, kill, and die for the nation.

More importantly, fewer and fewer of the decision makers who are our national leaders have ever experienced the burden of warriorhood. This creates the paradoxical situation that *we are a people at war, often led into war by nonwarriors.*

Our nation is thus comprised of two distinct and separate cultures when the issue of war becomes an element of our national dialogue. Furthermore, those who know the least about war and what it is to be a warrior often do little to remedy their level of ignorance. Given our democratic structure, America participates in its wars through its citizen's collective decisions. To decide wisely, one must have knowledge. To have knowledge, one must listen to those who know. To listen to those who know, one must be humble and acknowledge one's own ignorance. One also must be willing to endure the discomfort that comes with hearing hard truths about a different and often frightening world, where violence and hatred walk side by side with courage and self-sacrifice.

To decide wisely about war, we must learn what a warrior knows. We must listen to their tales of what one must cling to so that a soul can survive intact in the cauldron of human conflict. We must let go of what we "think" we know, and listen to what they have to teach us.

This is an obligation that all those who send others to fight and die must undertake if they seek to act as responsible citizens. Wars fought in the wrong way or for unworthy goals damage us all as citizens and particularly threaten the souls of our warriors. To address the challenge to protect our nation and those who fight for it from unwarranted moral and psychological harm, an understanding of both the realities of war and the values that guide a warrior in his or her calling is essential. Those who live in the culture of peace that is everyday life in America must have an honest conversation with the men and women from our warrior culture. This conversation can often be difficult because warriors are members of a unique and often misunderstood world (Keegan, 1993). Over the centuries, however, this culture has developed certain values that guide warriors in the exercise of their duties. Ultimately, these values enable them to preserve their souls in the crucible of violence that is human conflict.

Over the years of my service, I have come to appreciate the difficulty that citizens are confronted with in trying to understand war and the code of a warrior. In my experience it is this lack of understanding that has, at times, allowed our country to be led astray from principled warrior values by our leaders, our own fears, or both. As with any other moral or ethical lapse, these have proved incredibly costly to both our nation's soul and our own.

In a time-honored warrior tradition, I would like to share with you a different aspect of human conflict, another side of the face of war. I would like to tell you of the opportunities I had to actually see and to live these warrior values in action. A precept of warriorhood is that we only truly learn those lessons that we live. These are the lessons I have lived and seen others live. I hope I do them justice in their retelling.

THE ELEMENT OF WARRIOR DISCERNMENT

Discernment is the ability to discriminate, an acuteness of judgment and understanding that is at the foundation of a warrior's applied wisdom. Warriors understand that the "great dividing line between words and results is courageous action" (Greitens, 20110, p. 58).

Discernment: The Raid in Garmah, September 5, 2003

The heat was stifling. It was after midnight, but it still felt as if we were inside a blast furnace. We waited outside of the town of Garmah in the darkness. Silent. Calm. Poised. Ready. Garmah was in western Iraq, at the tip of what was known as the Sunni Triangle. We were there as part of Operation Longstreet, an attempt to interdict the flow of insurgents into Baghdad that had begun over a week earlier. "We" were elements of the First Squadron of the 2ACR, known as the "War Eagles," and we had left our home base in eastern Baghdad to hunt and be hunted by the enemy. We had been in a running fight with bands of insurgents, what we euphemistically called "contact," since our arrival.

On this night we were poised to descend on eight insurgent leaders reported to be hiding in the city and take them into custody. Garmah was a city of several thousand. We numbered less than one-hundred. As we waited, bad news began to filter to us over our radios. Our staging area had been mortared shortly after we left the base. Reports of units coming into contact with insurgent elements were increasing.

We were relying on surprise, but it appeared the enemy knew we were coming. If the insurgent numbers were sizable and they had prepared ambushes, getting in and out of the city would be a nightmare. Tension mounted, as visions of the movie *Black Hawk Down,* which recounted the ambush and the day-long fight for survival of a unit of army rangers in Mogadishu, Somalia in 1993, replayed in my mind. Suddenly, the radio crackled with a report from the helicopters flying over the city. They had observed hundreds of Iraqis in groups on the roofs of the buildings, exactly where insurgent fighters would position themselves to trap us in the narrow streets below. Time was running out, and a decision needed to be made. Some men would have simply stuck to the time schedule, the element of tactical surprise being all important. When cobbled together, the mortar attacks on the base, the earlier contact with insurgent elements, and now the presence of Iraqis on the roofs could only mean one thing: our mission was compromised. Given that risk, many would say it was best to "go in hard" rather than risk the success of our mission or increase the risk of our suffering casualties. But what if we were wrong?

The commander of the First Squadron chose to do something critically important. He applied his combat-tested judgment to the facts to give them context. He knew that Iraqis often slept on their roofs to try to counter the oppressive heat of the summer nights. It was just as likely that these were families, innocent men, women, and children, sleeping in the dark, unaware of our presence.

He ordered the helicopter pilots to sweep the area again and to ascertain two vital pieces of information: if the people on the roofs were moving and if there was any evidence that they were armed. He told all the units to "stand fast" to give the pilots a chance for another over flight.

The pilots confirmed there was no evidence of weapons. More importantly, it appeared most of the people were sleeping or smoking. The commander ordered the units to move to their appointed positions and the raid began as planned; the potential tragedy of an over-reaction by the helicopter gunships or our units was averted. The insurgents were captured. There were no civilian casualties. The commander's discernment had allowed him to accomplish the mission and avert tragedy.

In this case, the commander's combat instincts were informed by his experience as well as his humanity. The timing of the mission was critical, but not so critical that he would tolerate injury to potentially innocent civilians for the sake of expedience.[1]

Leaders, War, and Discernment

As citizens of this country, we must apply the same discernment to national decisions about war and peace. "Gut instincts," chest pounding, and hubris-laden pronouncements about how "clean" or "quick" a war will be by our political leaders must be considered with great caution.

This caution must ever remain in the forefront of our minds, because discernment is most often lacking in those making decisions about war who have never seen war. They tend, as the Greek philosopher Pindar of Thebes said, to "see war as so 'sweet,' while the experienced are frightened at the heart to see it advancing" (Tick, 2005, pp. 261–262). When those leaders attempt to argue that war is, or should be, a first choice/preemptive strike as opposed to a last resort, we should see their lack of experience, discernment, and immaturity for what it is. We would then do well to consider the counsel of the Greek philosopher Posidonius who said that "swords should never be placed in the hands of children" (Holland, 2003, p. 78).

THE ELEMENT OF WARRIOR RESTRAINT

Restraint is understood as the act of holding back, of controlling or checking. It is a quality that is especially required in the crucible of war, where life and death are the consequences of the choices a warrior makes, often under incredible duress.

Restraint: The Drunk at Squaretown, October 2003

Dignitaries, both military and civilian, love tours of a battlefield, as long as the battle is over, that is. Iraq in October 2003 was no different. A general from our higher headquarters wanted a tour of some of the reconstruction projects we were conducting in our zone of operation. The First Squadron had managed to blunt the insurgency by winning the trust and support of local Iraqis and part of that was due to the reconstruction projects my six-man team was supervising.

We were in what we called "Squaretown," an abysmally poor neighborhood in Baghdad located to the southeast of Sadr City. It appeared as an almost perfect square on our maps, hence the name. It was late afternoon and our column of ten Humvees was positioned in a line in the center of Squaretown. The general met with local leaders, who enthused about our clean water delivery project to the neighborhood. All seemed right with our world. We stood at staggered distances around our vehicles pulling security, observing the adjacent buildings and crowd to ensure no insurgent attacks took place. To my left, approximately 25 meters away, two Iraqi women screamed at the top of their lungs through the window of a house at its occuanpt. I looked toward our translator, Dhia, who said they were castigating their neighbor who apparently, against the principles of Islam, had gone on a "bender" and was sleeping off his drinking binge.

Out of the corner of my eye I saw a blur then heard the unmistakable sound of AK-47 rounds being fired. The next think I knew, I was looking into the eyes of a terrified Iraqi man who had a red dot on the center of his forehead.

It took me a second to process the fact that the reason I could see his face so clearly was because I was looking at him through the optical AimPoint lens on my M-16. The red dot was the designation of where the bullet would go, but it hadn't.

In the next seconds, I heard my voice, and the voice of other troopers yelling, "Hold your fire! Hold your fire!" The drunk and now totally terrified Iraqi had staggered out of his home and fired his AK-47 into the ground in an attempt to drive away his screeching neighbors, all the while not realizing that 25 meters away 50 heavily armed cavalry troopers were monitoring the street. He threw his rifle down, raised his hands, and bolted into his house. None of the troopers, including myself, in the split second between his shot and our response, could have known that the warrior value of restraint was guiding our actions and, ultimately, preserving our souls and his life.

As we took custody of the drunk, we all recognized that each of us, in the split second we heard the shots, had acquired our target (the shooter), assessed the risk (identified that he was standing near two innocent women and that he was firing at the ground), and held our fire. Had that individual swiveled his rifle in our direction, it was clear that all fifty troopers would have fired at him and obliterated him.

The truth we recognized from that split second was that a result of our training and our commitment to protect civilians if at all possible was that the drunkard was not a threat to us. He did not have to die. More importantly we would not have to carry the burden of having killed an undoubtedly reckless, but ultimately harmless, drunk, either that day or, more importantly, for the rest of our lives.

Most people think of warriors as destroyers, but a warrior's ultimate responsibility is to preserve life if at all possible (Tick, 2005). The blood-thirsty madness of a celluloid "Rambo," destroying all he encounters in a vengeful rage, bears a stronger resemblance to the legends about the "ber-serker" than to the warrior (Shay, 1994). In warrior tradition, a berserker was a man undone by so much killing that he was literally driven to madness by the desire to destroy (Shay, 1994).

Given this very real possibility of bloodlust, a warrior's actions must be governed by restraint. A warrior will seek to do what is necessary to end a conflict, but nothing more or less than is necessary to resolve hostilities (Spencer, 1993). For warriors, our humanity must always serve as a constraint on our actions, and one of the indispensable lessons warriors learn is that "vengeful violence is self-abuse as well as the abuse of others" (Sherman, 2005, p. 178).

Counselors who work with Vietnam veterans suffering from PTSD have documented that, in many cases, it was the heedless destruction and killing that often went along with that war that continues to haunts many veterans and seems to serve as the cause of their suffering (Shay, 1994). The violation of the warrior's code, especially at the direction or orders of others in positions of legitimate authority, appears to have a particularly searing and damaging impact on these men (Shay, 1994). A recent study of Operation Iraqi Freedom and Enduring Freedom veterans has also confirmed that the taking of the lives of combatants or noncombatants "was associated with PTSD symptoms, peritraumatic dissociation, functional impairment, and violent behaviors after controlling for exposure to general combat" (Maguen et al., 2009, p. 443).

Leaders and the Principle of Restraint

As citizens, we must hold our leaders accountable when they suggest that our warriors must violate the time-honored principle of restraint. Nothing less than soul wounding occurs when men are obligated to visit greater violence than is required in the service of politicians' vanity (Tick, 2005). In this respect, we should remain mindful of the fact that the desire to appear "tough" and the admonition that we need to "take the gloves off" against particular enemies, are often the words of an uninformed coward.

As set forth in a samurai maxim, "A true warrior would never prey on weaker individuals or act as a bully, and one who does so is not a true warrior, but an absolute coward" (Yuzan, 2003, p. 19). Perhaps it is because they are called upon to contend with darkness, often on its terms, that warriors understand that darkness cannot kill darkness, and it is light and wisdom, not hatred and cruelty, that will ultimately "banish shadows from this world" (Millman, 2005, p. 235).

THE ELEMENT OF WARRIOR MERCY

Mercy is the compassionate or kindly forbearance shown toward someone who is your enemy. It is compassion or forgiveness shown toward someone whom it is within one's power to punish or harm. The power of a warrior is often felt to be found in their skills in the taking of life to those unfamiliar with the warrior's code. The truth I have learned, however, is that a warrior's true power lies in his ability to spare or give life, especially to an enemy.

Mercy: The Prisoners in Garmah, September 2003

"Sir, would you head over to the police station and meet me. We got a problem."

We were in the first days of reconnaissance in Operation Longstreet, and I'd received a radio call from the captain commanding "DAWG" Troop of the First Squadron, Second Cavalry. I arrived with my team and entered a walled complex that was the newly built police station and jail, a gift from Saddam Hussein to his supporters in the Sunni triangle. I met the captain, who simply said, "Major, you better take a look at the prisoners they got here." Even the face of a hated enemy conveys the shared human experience of despair, hopelessness, fear, and misery if you look for it. The cells held seven or eight prisoners, broiling in the afternoon temperatures that now exceeded 120 degrees. They were terrified but listless. The police officer who accompanied us shifted uncomfortably from one foot to the other.

"When were these men last given food and water?" I asked.

"They are terrorists," he replied, as if that answered my question.

"Open the cell."

"I have no orders . . . " his voice trailed off.

"Open the cell, right now."

My translator, Dhia, the captain, and the rest of our team entered the cell along with me. The men were obviously dehydrated.

"Sergeant, get some water bottles from the Humvee and some MREs for these men. Get the medical kit and check and make sure we don't need to give them IVs to rehydrate them."

My translator spoke to the prisoners.

"Dhia, what's going on?"

"Sir, they admit they are thieves, but they say they aren't terrorists."

"How long have they been here?"

"About two days, sir."

"How long without food and water?"

"Two days, sir."

The captain and I left the cell with Dhia to find the police commander, a colonel who was also a relative of the town's mayor.

"Dhia, why are they being treated this way?"

"Sir. Those men are Shia."

We found the police colonel who commanded the station in his air-conditioned office. He refused to feed the men or give them water without orders from the mayor. They were terrorists, after all, he said. He made it a point to inform us he had friends in Baghdad—important men who worked with Ambassador Bremer. He suggested we mind our own business. These were his people, our enemies, terrorists. Perhaps they plotted to kill Americans. Why should we care about their well-being? He was both puzzled and indignant at our concern for the prisoners.

"Dhia," I said, "translate for me, word for word."

"Colonel, here is how this works. The captain and I will be back tomorrow at 12 noon. Those men had better have received food and water, and you better have a plan to keep doing that until they are sent to Baghdad for trial."

"I won't," he said with the sound of a man who was accustomed to intimidating others. "Not unless the mayor orders it. You have no authority here."

"Fair enough," I said. "But if I come back tomorrow and these men haven't been taken care of, you and the mayor are both going to be locked in the same cell as the prisoners, and then you two can explain the lack of appropriate dining arrangements to them personally."

The colonel blanched. I'd gotten his attention.

"You cannot do that."

"Watch me, pal! Food and water, or you and your mayor both go into the cell with them."

The colonel spoke anxiously to Dhia, whose voice took on the same edge as mine had when he answered the question the colonel had posed to him.

"What's up, Dhia?"

"He asked me if you and the captain are crazy enough to do that, sir."

"What'd you tell him?"

Dhia smiled, "I tell him, crazy, scary, and mean, sir."

We returned the next day as promised. The police colonel was nowhere to be found, but the prisoners reported they'd been fed and received water. The colonel's aide, a major, explained that the colonel had been "unavoidably called away," but showed Dhia an official order, signed by the mayor himself no less, specifying the times the prisoners would be fed and what they would receive. Dhia advised me that the colonel was sufficiently frightened of the "crazy American major and captain" that the men would be taken care of. That night, the translator for the squadron commander approached me at our campsite. Dhia had told all the translators of what we had done. To the translators, many of whom were Shia who had been oppressed by Hussein for decades, the captain, my team, and I became celebrities of a sort.

He asked, "Sir, is it true? Did you and the captain do that, even though they may have been terrorists, even though they were Shia?"

"Yes," I said.

"Why, sir? Why risk the trouble?"

"Because, we don't' allow things like that to go on when we can stop it."

He took both my hands and gave me the traditional Iraqi kiss on each of my cheeks which is shared in that country and many others in the Middle East as a symbol of recognized brotherhood.

"God bless you, sir." He walked off back to the other translators.

Mercy to one's enemy is a sign of strength, not weakness. Mercy is a value and a quality of the strong. Those of us who are warriors are not in the calling simply because we are strong, but because we choose to apply that strength for a good purpose (Greitens, 2011). True warriors understand that our fierceness in battle, and our prowess in the art of war, does not require disdain or contempt for our enemy.[2] As Cicero aptly put it, "We must exercise respectfulness towards men, both towards the best of them and also towards the rest" (Sherman, 2005, p. 171).

THE ELEMENT OF WARRIOR ADAPTABILITY

Adaptability is the quality of adjusting oneself readily to different and changing conditions. It is based on the warrior admonition that we must see the world, reality, as it is and not as we wish it to be.

Adaptability: The War Eagle Water Company, July 2003–April, 2004

The commander of the War Eagles, First Squadron of the 2ACR, stood in the doorway of our team's operations center. He was wearing more than 60 pounds of ammunition, water, and body armor. He was covered with dirt and sweat after a daylong patrol in the 120 degree heat.

"Major," he said, "with the electricity down the way it is, these people can't get any clean water." Our area of operation had 1.25 million Iraqis in it, and many of them could not get clean water due to the fact that Baghdad's electricity grid was in tatters. The purification plants could not get enough electricity to properly filter the water.

Unclean water is the largest cause of infant mortality in third-world countries, and Iraqi children would start to die unless some way was found to get clean water to these poorest of neighborhoods. He continued, "Bob, I saw a family with kids getting water out of the canal because they can't get any drinking water at all. The canal has raw sewage in it." He stopped and a smile lit his face. "Bob, you, me, and the War Eagles are going into the water business. You're now the president of the War Eagle Water Company, and I'm the chairman of the board." He paused for a second, and then the weight of what we faced seemed to physically settle on his shoulders. "Bob, kids aren't going to die in my area 'cause they can't get clean water. Let's fix this."

"Yes, sir," I said, and as the newly minted president of the "War Eagle Water Company," I realized that I had absolutely no idea how I was going to make water deliveries happen. For the next 48 hours my team and I went to the Red Cross, the Coalition Provisional Authority, the United Nations, Doctors Without Borders, and every aid organization we could think of. No one was able or willing to handle the problem.

We tried to get an answer or help from our Army support units; no luck again. We were going through all the right channels, following all the right rules, and failing miserably. If you spend any amount of time in the Army, you learn that some of the most brilliant men in the service are noncommissioned officers, traditionally known as NCOs or simply sergeants. They often have an uncanny ability to cut through established ways of doing things and adjust to the situation, to find better answers by thinking "outside the box." I was blessed to have three such men on my team.

After 48 fruitless hours of trying to get things done through proper Army channels, my sergeants had what turned out to be a brilliant idea. They spotted one of the water trucks that brought clean water to one of eastern Baghdad's richer neighborhoods and followed it to its staging area.

"How much do you guys get paid for a tanker of full water," they asked.

"Twelve U.S. dollars per truck," they were told.

"How'd you like to make eighteen?"

We had no trucks, but what we did have was access to money in the form of reconstruction funds. Haggling is an NCO virtue and by a couple of hours later, for $18 a tanker, we had an entire fleet of tankers courtesy of my sergeants, the new "assistant vice presidents" of our rapidly growing company. Soon the "War Eagle Water Company" was delivering tens of thousands of liters of clean water to Baghdad's poorest neighborhoods. While violence began to spike in other areas of Baghdad, and Iraq began to spiral into internecine war during that long, hot summer, the War Eagle's zone remained remarkably quiet. It was said that the Iraqis never forgot the Americans who brought them and their children water. Upon our departure from Iraq in 2004, the local leaders who saw us off and wished us a safe journey home simply said, "We will never forget you. You brought us hope...you brought us water."

The essence of warrior skill is to notice what is happening in the environment and then respond accordingly.[3] Thus, as asserted by the Chinese philosopher Liu Ji, "The essence of the principles of warriors is responding to change" (Fields, 1991, p. 129).

THE ELEMENT OF WARRIOR HONOR

Honor pertains to fairness, honesty, or integrity in one's beliefs and actions. It may be considered an inherent component of the human condition, along the lines of character and dignity.

Honor: The Schoolhouse in Amin, April 2003

At the war's outset in March 2003, Saddam Hussein moved tons of his military's munitions (artillery shells, mortar shells, land mines, bullets, hand grenades, etc.) into schools situated throughout the city of Baghdad. He knew that the U.S. would not bomb schools with children in them to destroy munitions. Now, with him defeated, we had literally tons of dangerous ordnance that had to be cleared from schools and quickly or the education of virtually all children in Baghdad would come to a screeching halt.

Hussein had made sure that most of the munitions went into schools in poor Shia neighborhoods, such as Baghdad, where we had been stationed for barely a week. I stood with the commander of Ghost troop as the principal of the Amin elementary school pointed to more than a half dozen tractor trailers stuck in 3 feet of mud and garbage inside the school's walled complex. Each was fully loaded with explosive ordnance. Dozens of schoolrooms contained crates of ammunition as well.

The school was useless for education, a danger to the entire neighborhood surrounding it, and a target of opportunity for insurgents. A single explosion would set off a chain reaction that would flatten a city block. We needed to move the ordnance quickly, but had no trucks to do so. As often happens in war, time was not our friend.

The commander and I listened to the principal's plea for help. As his subordinates supplied input, Ghost troop's commander, a father of three, simply said to our translator, "Tell the principal we'll handle it right away." Over the next 24 hours we searched for a solution, coming up empty one time after another. At one point, when one of his subordinates suggested we might have to advise the principal we could not help him, the commander's response was both simple and direct.

"Can't do that, fellas. I gave my word. Once any of us do that to these people, we got to do what we said we'll do. No exceptions." He paused for a second.

"They've been told enough lies. We're not gonna do that to 'em, too."

As fate would have it, an army vehicle designed to free tanks and trucks that had become stuck or broken down happened to be stationed at our base camp. With a little "gentle persuasion," the crew agreed to remove the tractor trailers from the compound.

A search by my team enabled us to find day laborers who would load the ammunition from the classrooms into the now free trucks and hire drivers to bring tractors to take our now fully loaded trailers to the ammo collection point that had been created to handle the ammunition that Hussein had spread throughout the city.

The school reopened and the principal and his staff completed the school year on time. The community, in those early days, rallied behind us and our efforts to rebuild Iraq (although that support would vanish after we left in 2004).

Nonetheless, what I will always remember is the positive impact our commitment to do what we said we would had on those people and that community. For all of us, a simple lesson in honor and how one lives that warrior value had been given.

Simply put, you give your word, you keep it, especially when it is difficult to do so. That is what gives your word value. That is why it is called your "word of honor."

For a warrior, there may be no more important value than honor. Honor, and adhering to the moral rectitude that is implicit in possessing a code of honor, must underpin a warrior's every word and deed.[4]

CONCLUSION

War and warrior values cannot and must not be the province only of our nation's warriors. It is incumbent upon us as a nation, a government, and a people to know and understand these values so that we may know when the sacrifices we ask of our warriors are those that are worthy and noble. We must also know and see truthfully when what they are being asked to do dishonors the foundational values of warriorhood.

We know that requiring warriors to dishonor their code at the behest of misguided authority figures has corrosive and, sometimes, cataclysmic consequences on the hearts and souls of our warriors (Shay, 1994). It wounds the souls and spirits of those who send them as well. Care must be taken in fighting an enemy that seemingly has no code, however; as Friedrich Nietzsche warned, if we do what they do, no matter how justified we believe we are, we will ultimately become what they are (Hobart, 2003, p. 130). As a warrior, I have and always will pray for peace. As a warrior, however, I am also required to be a realist. War will be with us for a long time to come.

To know what wars need to be fought and what wars should not be fought, we must know what war truly is and what it means to fight in one. Some may feel that there are times when this final of all possible options must be undertaken to avert greater tragedy. We would do well at these times to remember the admonition of Mary Malmros as we struggle with our yearning for peace, that "An unwillingness to deal forcibly with violence does not equate with moral rectitude." (www.mvkarate.com).

Not all warriors are willing to share their stories, but for those who are, we must ask ourselves if we have the courage to listen. I hope the answer is "yes."

NOTES

1. Warriors know only too well that, as H.A.L. Fisher once wrote, "War is the parent of illusion." Simply assuming that one's preconceived notions or beliefs can serve as sufficient foundation to make the critical life and death decisions that war requires is unacceptable. War is and always will be merciless with untruth (Parker, 2005). Warriors, as are we all, are servants of both creation and destruction, requiring their acts to be governed by wisdom, restraint, and compassion (Tick, 2005).

2. I have often been startled by the seeming bloodthirstiness of those who have never seen battle. Perhaps it is easiest for those who will not have to "do" violence, or live with its aftermath, to most forcefully advocate for its use. As informed citizens, however, seeking to have the force that we use remain consonant with our warrior values, we should view with great caution those who advance the clarion call for the total destruction of our enemies by any means available. As one warrior so eloquently put it, "what distinguishes a warrior from a thug . . . . ultimately, we're distinguished by our values . . . . any act of wanton brutality is not only counterproductive . . . . but on a personal level it degrades the warrior and turns him into a thug" (Greitens, 2011, p. 228).

3. Warriors are not hide-bound traditionalists. Warriors understand that the level of thinking that created our problems is not sufficient to help us solve them. When confronted with intractable stubbornness in our leaders and their stated positions, warriors and citizens would do well to follow the admonition of the philosopher Sophocles that "stubbornness and stupidity are twins."

4. The warrior profession requires one to make an unflinching commitment to "see" reality and a similar commitment to say what one sees as well. This obligation must also be placed on those who would send our warriors into battle, and all of us as citizens must hold our leaders to this obligation.

REFERENCES

Fields, R. (1991). *The code of the warrior: In history, myth, and everyday life.* New York: Harper Perennial.

Greitens, E. (2011). *The heart and the fist: The education of a humanitarian, the making of a navy seal.* New York: Houghton Mifflin Harcourt.

Hobart, P. (2003). *Kishido: The way of the western warrior.* Prescott, AZ: Hohm Press.

Holland, T. (2003). *Rubicon: The last years of the roman republic.* New York: Anchor.

Keegan, J. (1993). A History of Warfare. New York: Vintage Books.

Maguen, S., Metzler, T.J., Litz, B.T., Seal, K.H., Knight, S.J., and Marmar, C.R. (2009). The impact of killing in war on mental health symptoms and related functioning. *Journal of Traumatic Stress, 22*(5), 435–443.

Millman, D. (2005). *The journeys of socrates.* New York: Harper Collins.

Parker, G., (2005). *The assassin's gate: America In Iraq.* New York: Farrar, Straus & Giroux.

Shay, J., (1994). *Achilles in Vietnam: Combat trauma and the undoing of character.* New York: Scribner.

Sherman, N. (2005). *Stoic warriors: The ancient philosophy behind the military mind.* New York: Oxford University Press.

Spencer, R. (1993). *The craft of the warrior.* Berkeley, CA: Prog. Ltd.

Tick, E., (2005). *War and the soul: Healing our nation's veterans from post-traumatic stress disorder.* Wheaton: Quest Books.

www.MVKarate.com, (nd), retrieved on Nov. 11, 2011 from http://www.MVKarate.com/library/insights/martial_arts_quotes_collection.htm

Yuzan, D. (2003). *The Code of the Warrior.* (Trans. by D.E. Tarver). Lincoln, NE: Writers Club Press.

Chapter 19

MY EXPERIENCES AS A MEDICAL OPERATIONS OFFICER IN AFGHANISTAN

Seth Mastrocola

INTRODUCTION

In this chapter, I recount my experience as a Medical Operations Officer (MEDO) in Afghanistan in 2010, and the path that led me to that place of duty. I joined the Army Reserve in 2004 after I graduated high school and reported to boot camp that summer. At first, our basic combat training simply seemed like an extension of my boyhood adventures.[1] I was engaged in training opportunities and experiences such as rifle marksmanship, first aid, obstacle courses, and combatives. What I did not fully realize at the time was that I was being trained to serve in one of the most austere, dangerous, and life-changing places in the world–Afghanistan.

In 2007, I received my commission as a second lieutenant in the Medical Service Corps. I was trained in emergency management and medical operations at Fort Sam Houston, Texas, the home of the U.S. Army Medical Command. I was immediately assigned to an infantry battalion of more than 700 soldiers who were already alerted for an upcoming deployment in support of Operation Enduring Freedom. I was put in charge of a combat medic platoon, responsible for deploying thirty-three men, some as young as seventeen years of age, to a combat zone 9000 miles away. I was twenty-two at the time, and suddenly I was being saluted and addressed as "Sir." The days of being accountable only to myself were over. I was catalyzed into a leadership experience that is unrivaled in the civilian sector. I was not scared; I was confident. Admittedly, however, I was also inexperienced and perhaps naïve. I reminded myself that in the history of conflict, boys as young as 16

271

had stormed the beaches of Normandy in World War II and fought valiantly in massive combat operations such as Iwo Jima. I found comfort in the fact that so many people had served our country before me, and my duty as an officer suddenly became less personal and more profound.

PREPARING FOR WAR

The methods used by the military to train and mobilize new recruits have changed drastically over the last decade. When I joined the Army in 2004, boot camp predominantly consisted of learning conventional warfare techniques, such as the use of a claymore mine system or moving in a platoon wedge formation through dense terrain. A small amount of our instruction was designed specifically for military operations in an urban environment. At the time, Operation Iraqi Freedom was the focus of the Bush Administration's "War on Terror."[2] Casualties rose into the thousands as a result of attacks with IEDs, and the military began training new recruits in the recognition and mitigation of these homemade bombs.

By the time I received my commission as a second lieutenant in 2007, the Department of Defense had completely transformed the way it approached the training of both new enlisted recruits and junior officers. The focus of training was specifically designed for counterinsurgency (COIN) operations, and included SWAT-style room clearing procedures, IED awareness, female engagement teams, and civil medical engagement training.

The intent of this training is to breed out an ideology of hate and violence through community partnerships and positive interaction with the citizens of the occupied country. These interactions are referred to by the military as "key leader engagements" (KLE). By the Afghans, they are called *shuras*, which is the Arabic word for "consultation." It is not uncommon for an infantry platoon leader to have tea with a district governor and discuss the security of a polling site for an upcoming election, versus planning and executing an ambush on an enemy stronghold.[3] These *shuras* have become a strategic priority in Afghanistan, whether the Department of Defense will admit to it or not. For some, this fact produces a professional cognitive dissonance between serving as a soldier and serving as a diplomat.

The strategic COIN objectives in Afghanistan are much more fluid and broad than those seen in any other conflict in U.S. history. This war is not against a country with a well-defined, structured, and uniformed military. It is against a group of insurgents of unspecified number, strength, capabilities, location, financing, and motives. For these reasons, the current U.S. military activities in Iraq and Afghanistan are being called counterinsurgency. One of the central theses of military doctrine on COIN strategy is the idea of winning the hearts and minds of the people. In order to do this, we must invest time, money, and resources to bolster the infrastructure of the country. This is accomplished through initiatives such as building schools and hospitals or digging wells. To achieve these objectives, military leaders must have an extensive supply of resources and technical expertise at their command.[4]

MILITARY OCCUPATION OF AFGHANISTAN

The military bases in Afghanistan are far more developed than most people may think. Almost all of the bases have hardstand concrete structures, running water, electricity, and either a military-operated or civilian-contracted dining facility. Every base has a morale, welfare, and recreation (MWR) facility, but they vary in size, connectivity, and recreational assets, such as pool tables and television sets. At most bases, service members are afforded the opportunity to call home through the defense services network, telephone lines that are set up specifically for personal and professional use; the majority of military members, however, purchase cellular phones from local Afghans. These come preconfigured to call or text the United States. Additionally, personnel have civilian contracted or self-use laundry services available to them. For example, on Forward Operating Base (FOB) Mehtar Lam, where my battalion was first stationed, a group of Bosnian civilians were contracted to operate our dining and laundry facilities. Both the Bosnian workers and the military command recognize that these accommodations are implemented with the intent of mitigating some of the incidental stressors that are put on troops on a daily basis. In doing this, the military essentially maintains a focus on the mission, instead of on the activities of daily living that are built into civilian life.

The interactions occurring between military and civilian workers on these bases can range from card playing to physical altercations or sexual intercourse.[5] Some interactions can be quite pleasant and platonic. I remember one Bosnian woman who sought me out on the base every day, insisting that I give her my dirty clothes, even when I did not have any. I found it strange that she was so persistent about washing my clothes. I am used to taking care of myself and almost feel guilty when others assist me in my activities of daily living. After months of this constant accommodation, I finally asked the woman why she was so passionate about doing my laundry. She gave me a big hug and said, "You saved my life." Needless to say I was surprised to hear this, and had no idea what she was referring to. She went on to explain that during the Serbian invasion of Bosnia in the 1990s, two of her four siblings were executed by the Serbian Army. She and her remaining family members were set to meet the same fate approximately one week later. She explained that their names had been placed on an execution list. Three days before the execution date, the U.S. Army along with Coalition Forces liberated Bosnia from the Serbian invasion. She looked up at me with a humble tear in her eye and repeated her words, "You saved my life."[6]

COMBAT HEALTH SUPPORT OVERVIEW

Any unit that is doctrinally responsible for carrying out direct combat missions in a warzone requires a very detailed plan in order to mitigate both the risks of the mission to coalition forces and collateral damage. The primary military occupational specialists responsible for executing direct combat operations are infantry men and women. Each infantry regiment has one MEDO who is responsible for the combat health support of the entire battalion. Combat Health Support (CHS) is also commonly referred to as "force health protection." CHS has many facets that MEDOs are responsible for, and they must constantly adapt to the changes on the battlefield. The primary responsibilities of a MEDO in CHS are (a) preventive medicine, (b) medical evacuation, (c) tactical combat casualty care (TC3), and (d) tracking and forecasting of injuries and ailments.

Preventive Medicine

Preventive medicine involves measures to prevent diseases or injuries, such as providing every soldier with antimalarial prophylaxis. The primary malaria prophylaxis in Afghanistan is doxycycline, given the contraindication of antimalarial drugs such as mefloquine (Lariam®) and primaquine (Leoprime®, Malirid, Primacip®), due to their severe behavioral health side effects, which can include vivid dreams and suicidal ideation.

Medical Evacuation

There are five echelons of care in the military medical evacuation system. **Echelon I** provides basic to mid level care at the point of injury or a local base but does not have any surgical capability. Most bases and outposts are able to provide this echelon of care. **Echelon II** care consists of midlevel and physician providers with surgical capability and often serves as the initial evacuation point for stabilization of potentially life-threatening traumatic injuries, such as tension pneumothorax (collapsed lung) or severe loss of blood. In northeast Afghanistan, the primary Echelon II facility is located on FOB Fenty in Jalalabad. **Echelon III** provides physician-level care with comprehensive surgical, laboratory, and analysis capabilities. Once an individual is stabilized at an Echelon II facility, he or she may be transferred to the only Echelon III hospital in Afghanistan, located on Bagram Air Field. **Echelon IV** care involves full-spectrum medical, laboratory, and testing capabilities with the exception of rehabilitative or convalescent care assets. In Afghanistan, the primary Echelon IV facility for soldiers being medically evacuated from theater is Landstuhl Regional Medical Center. **Echelon V** care is also administered at full-spectrum medical facilities with long-term rehabilitative and convalescent care, such as Walter Reed Medical Center.

Tactical Combat Casualty Care

TC3 refers to the care of service members injured in direct combat operations with the enemy. It is typically administered through the application of basic life-saving measures, such as the use of a combat application tourniquet, or a needle chest decompression when a pneumothorax is suspected. This care is considered Echelon I in the medical evacuation system but requires specific attention and planning by medical operations officers because the injury and treatment are taking place in a dangerous kinetic situation. In these situations, a medical evacuation (MEDEVAC) helicopter may not be able to fly into the landing zone to remove the casualty because of the volatility or severity of the combat scenario. It is therefore the responsibility of the MEDO to be sure there is enough Echelon I medical personnel on every combat mission to ensure TC3 treatment until an evacuation can take place to a higher level of care.

Tracking and Forecasting of Injuries and Ailments

This includes administrative tracking, trending, and forecasting of any and all injuries and ailments in a combat zone. A MEDO will typically supervise approximately thirty combat medics, one physician's assistant, and one physician. It is important to note that MEDOs do not supervise clinical operations or treatment of patients. MEDOs officers serve as direct advisors to the unit or battalion commander on all components of combat health support. They plan grid coordinates for landing zones and coordinate immunizations against endemic diseases such as anthrax, influenza, and hepatitis. Additionally, they coordinate behavioral health assets across all five echelons of care to deal with the inherent mental health conditions that affect soldiers in a combat zone.

STRESS IN A COMBAT ZONE IN AFGHANISTAN

There are significant amounts of situational and environmental stressors incumbent to military service in Afghanistan. The degree and variability of the effects of these stressors is the topic of many studies, both in the military and in the private sector. It may be difficult for a civilian to envision going to war even once, let alone multiple times, yet, the average active duty service member is deployed to Iraq or Afghanistan at least twice in his or her career. When catalyzed into a theater of operation in the Middle East and/or Southwest Asia, there are environmental conditions to which a soldier must acclimate.[7] The average temperature in Afghanistan, depending on the season, can range from 19 to 91°F. Soldiers operating in higher elevations have the added difficulty of maneuvering in less-dense air, opening them to the possibility of medical complications such as altitude sickness or pulmonary edema. An additional environmental concern is the exposure to endemic diseases such as malaria, tuberculosis, and hepatitis.

Commanders' Responsibilities to Subordinates

Financial, personal, and occupational stressors can be exacerbated if they are not dealt with, and for soldiers these situations can worsen as the duration of the deployment lengthens. One medic in my platoon exhibited a pronounced change in his demeanor and work performance. When I asked him if there was something bothering him, he proceeded to tell me that he and his wife were having financial difficulties, which were causing significant tension within their marriage. The credit card companies were making phone calls and sending letters to his residence in attempt to collect their debts. I told him that, as his platoon leader, I could assist in deconflicting this problem. I drafted an official memorandum that cited the Service Members Civil Relief Act of 2003, specifically requiring credit card companies and other lenders to lower their annual interest rates to a minimum of 6 percent, and defer debt payments until after a soldier returns from a military deployment. Two weeks later the harassing letters and phone calls had stopped and the tension was relieved from the marriage. The soldier's demeanor and job performance climbed back up to exceptional.

This incident highlights a unique and rewarding experience in the military. We, as leaders, own every single problem a subordinate has in a combat zone. In the civilian labor force, if you called your boss at 2 AM to tell him or her that you were having trouble sleeping, you might not get such an empathetic response. However, in Afghanistan, if your soldier can not sleep and he is the driver of a lead vehicle on a highly dangerous mission at 5 AM the next day, it becomes your problem as a leader. We do not have the luxury of telling our subordinates "that is not my problem." If a soldier has financial burdens back home that are so stressful that he or she can not focus on the mission in combat, then they become our problems as leaders. This is the most challenging, but rewarding, leadership experience a person could ever ask for. The idea that there is no excuse to ever turn your back on someone is an overwhelming concept that, at times in war, can create a pendulum of emotions.

Responsibility for the Care of Injured Civilians

The responsibility to help those in need is not limited to the ranks of the coalition forces. As a medical officer, I am compelled to assist those in need, whether they are local workers, injured enemy personnel, or American forces.

I recall a particular incident when the military police platoon assigned to our task force was on a mounted combat patrol in a dangerous village in our province. As they were passing through the village, which was a known Taliban haven, a grandmother holding her three-year-old grandson was, reportedly, pushed out in front of one of the military police vehicles. According to the medic on the ground, the vehicle struck her, split her body in half, and threw the boy approximately twenty feet down the road. The medic in the unit immediately dismounted the vehicle and ran to the boy, who was unconscious with a suspected closed head injury. As she attempted to assess the boy's vital signs, villagers surrounded her and prevented her from treating the boy. Locals dragged the boy off by his hands as he hung unconscious in their arms. Our operations officer, who was monitoring the situation from the tactical operations center on the base, gave the order to bring the MP unit back to the base without the boy because he feared retaliation from the civilians. When the unit returned to the base the medic approached me, visibly distraught as she explained what had happened. As the MEDO of the battalion, I was the expert on the Geneva Convention medical requirements for treating civilian casualties. I knew that the right thing to do would be to care for this young boy and try to save his life. I walked over to our intelligence section, where we were able to ascertain the boy's location at a nearby provincial hospital. I gave the order to secure the boy and bring him back to the base for treatment.[8] This order was to an extent, a form of kidnapping. I never spoke with the boy's parents to obtain permission to treat their injured child.

When the boy arrived, he was unconscious with multiple cranial and orbital fractures and presumptive trauma to his brain. We stabilized his injuries and flew him to Bagram Air Field Hospital, where he remained in the intensive care unit for three weeks. He eventually came out of his coma and made a full recovery. Months later, he was back in the village, smiling and riding his bike.

Managing Combat Stress Casualties

The military deploys behavioral health specialists to execute various support roles and intervention across the area of operation. These specialists include military trained mental health technicians, social workers, licensed psychologists, and psychiatrists. They work in two-person teams called combat stress teams (CSTs) and are further assigned in support of their own task force or region in Afghanistan. Their job is to provide resiliency training, tobacco cessation counseling, crisis intervention, and emergency psychiatric recommendations for higher echelon care. They must also be prepared to recognize and treat acute stress reactions. In the combat zone, these manifest themselves in many different ways.[9] The classic symptoms seem to include anxiety, lack of sleep, loss of appetite, and melancholia. If a soldier is diagnosed with an acute stress reaction by a CST, he or she may be given a period of bed rest, commonly referred to in the military as "quarters." These soldiers may also begin systematic counseling sessions during which clinicians employ different techniques, including prolonged exposure therapy. One resource in Afghanistan is a facility called the Freedom Restoration Center, located at the heavily fortified Bagram Air Field. This center provides soldiers with seventy-two hours of physical fitness, rest, nourishment, and counseling before returning to combat duty.

Suicide and Self-Destructive Behavior

If a soldier is deemed an immediate threat to himself or others, his weapon is immediately secured, and he may be emergency evacuated to Echelon III care in Bagram for a psychiatric evaluation. Afghanistan does not have inpatient psychiatric care; therefore, more often than not, patients suffering from acute psychosis are flown to Germany. The CSTs and MEDOs, through telephone consultations with licensed medical providers, coordinate the best course of action in handling mental health conditions on a case-by-case basis. Sadly, even with all the previously mentioned mitigation techniques and procedures, four completed suicides took place in our higher task force within an eight-month period of time. Out of the twenty-six service members that we emergency evacuated out of Afghanistan, four of them were psychiatric evacuations. Unfortunately, there were instances in which we could not coordinate care for psychologically distressed soldiers before it was too late.

One soldier allegedly detonated a grenade, intentionally, and bled to death on our aid station table. When the grenade detonated, everyone presumed the base was under attack, and we implemented defense procedures. A few moments later, witnesses clarified the explosion was friendly and that they needed medical assistance for the unconscious victim. The soldier was nineteen years old and was brought into our aid station with small puncture wounds to his back. He had agonal respirations, with fixed and dilated pupils. We immediately began CPR and when we administered bag valve resuscitation, the soldier spewed a massive amount of blood all over us. Our physician ordered a surgical cricothyroidotomy, but after twenty minutes of intensive resuscitative efforts, he was pronounced dead. By this time a medical helicopter was en route to transport the patient, and I notified them to change the status of the evacuation to a *hero flight*. This is the term used when a fallen service member is placed in a human remains bag and flown to the nearest mortuary affairs location in Afghanistan. It was one of the most difficult tasks I had to perform in Afghanistan.[10]

No matter how difficult this situation was, I still had the responsibility of ensuring that my junior medics were coping with the atrocity of seeing a "suicide by grenade." I coordinated multiple critical incident stress debriefings (CISD) with our task force psychologist, but ultimately, I question the efficacy of such interventions. It is imperative that service members lean on each other for moral, professional, and spiritual support. This is why the military has relied on chaplains, embedded with combat arms units, to provide spiritual and moral support for soldiers without stigmatizing them with clinical referrals. Furthermore, it is argued that CISD intervention may impede or completely circumvent a soldier's typical support system. Barboza contests that "the very act of implementing CISD intervention may 'medicalize' stress symptoms" (Barboza, 2005). Similarly, I question how these psychological debriefings can be efficacious if the participants are immediately thrown back into the environment that produced the stress in the first place.

I recount one such circumstance. One of the medics who performed CPR on the alleged suicide victim went through a stress debriefing immediately following the incident. This medic returned from the intervention and had no desire to speak further about the incident with his peers or myself. Months later when we returned to the United States, I received a call in the middle of the night from the soldier, stating that he wanted to hurt himself. I had him committed to a hospital as an emergency. One of his most distressful memories was his "failed" efforts to perform CPR on a fellow soldier. I consequently ask the question of how the CISD mitigated this soldier's psychological distress in Afghanistan.

Quality of War: Resilience

It was not long before I arrived at the conclusion that the days of an enemy front and classic war are gone. We fight in an asymmetric battlefield where the enemy is indistinguishable from the innocent, and where every turn of the road can mean an IED attack. There are no more "safe" places on the battlefield. Whenever a soldier lands in Afghanistan, he or she is on the front lines. Similarly, Colonel Young, of the Connecticut Army National Guard, explains that Iraq is a "360 degree" battlefront as well, and that due to the constant fear that this environment produces, 60 percent of combat troops in Iraq had symptoms of ASD (Young, Gillan, Dingmann, Casinalli & Taylor, 2008). This presents a unique new stressor to soldiers in combat, and it highlights the importance of resiliency training during the mobilization process. It is understood that some soldiers cope with stress better than others. Some have better support structures than others do, and it is hoped that resiliency training for service members going to war will build upon these protective factors prior to deployment.[11]

Furthermore, there is the issue of cognitive dissonance among soldiers serving in today's military. The change of military strategy from combat operations to COIN has produced a professional dissonance between what our military occupational specialties are and what duties we actually perform in Afghanistan. Paul Bartone (2006), of the National Defense University, asserts that certain categories of stressors such as ambiguity and powerlessness affect the resiliency of service members. He further explains that the current rules of engagement often prevent coalition forces from engaging the enemy and that mission objectives are often unclear (Bartone, 2006). Our infantry soldiers are trained to engage in kinetic operations with an opposing force, but instead they wind up securing polling sites and engaging in *shuras*. I can imagine how my fellow infantrymen feel about the U.S. commando raid on Osama Bin Laden's compound in Pakistan and would guess that it leaves those who are fighting in Afghanistan feeling the same powerlessness and confusion that Bartone talks about. One group of service members is granted full authorization to proceed into a sovereign nation (Pakistan), with the direct guidance to capture or kill a single person, whereas the other is restricted because the focus is on winning the hearts and minds of the people. For this reason, the fundamentals of being a soldier in a time of war have been modified almost arbitrarily to fit the COIN strategy. This may leave a junior soldier with a lack of confidence in his or her training, and leadership and, ultimately, in himself or herself. This, of course, produces high levels of combat stress casualties and deserves extensive research in the years to come. For now, I am glad I am home, and the only stress I am under is in knowing that others are still there.

NOTES

1. I can remember being fearless as a child. I would come home with cuts on my arms and legs from climbing trees in the woods. My mother would clean them and apply the most masculine Band-Aids® she could find, realizing full well that a few days later she would be applying calamine lotion to the poison ivy rash that was surely developing. Somewhere along the line of adolescent development I began to realize that the boundaries I was authorized to play in as a child were expanding. My neighborhood became wherever I could find to go hiking, swimming, driving, smoking, drinking, and chasing the older girls. However, I came to discover that I was never satisfied. I always wanted something more. I wanted to lose myself in a cause bigger than I am.

2. The term war on terror was coined by President Bush in a September 20, 2001 address to a joint session of Congress. The President stated that, "Our war on terror begins with Al Qaeda but it does not end there. It will not end until every terrorist group of global reach has been found, stopped and defeated. They (terrorists) hate what they see right here in this chamber: a democratically elected government. Their leaders are self-appointed. They hate our freedoms: our freedom of religion, our freedom of speech, our freedom to vote and assemble and disagree with each other." The President seemed to have correlated terrorist ideology to a hatred of democracy. I do not feel that all Afghans hate democracy, and if they do, then in their opinions, it does not in and of itself make them terrorists. Afghans, for this reason, may misconstrue the strategic and military intent of United States in its "war on terror." It is, in my opinion, to end terror, not cultivate a worldwide love of democracy. (*See* http://articles.cnn.com/2001-09-20/us/gen.bush.tra nscript_1_joint-session-national-anthem-citizens?_s=PM:US).

3. I can remember traveling to a provincial hospital and meeting with the director, who insisted that our provincial reconstruction team allocate over $7 million to build a new hospital. He pointed out that the war had produced growing amounts of civilian casualties, and the demand for health care had exceeded the capabilities of his hospital. I began to generalize the proverbs of Confucius to the situation and realized that building them a massive new hospital without the ability for them to staff it or sustain it over a long period of time would be counterproductive to the overarching strategy that General Petraeus outlined when he assumed command in Afghanistan. Both myself and the PRT Medical Advisor left the meeting without endorsing any extravagant requests for more money, and I think we made the right decision.

4. These resources include the U.S. Department of Agriculture, the State Department, the Federal Bureau of Investigation, the Drug Enforcement Agen-

cy, provincial reconstruction teams, lawyers, doctors, and, of course, the strongest fighting force in the world.

5. In one instance in December 2009, there was a murder at FOB Mehtar Lam. This homicide remained under investigation during our entire deployment in Afghanistan, earning our base the nickname "FOB Murder Lam."

6. Who would have thought that one of the days I felt most proud of my service in Afghanistan was at the laundry facility on the base? I do not typically find myself at a loss for words, but in this instance I truly I had no idea what to say to this woman. It reminded me of my childhood desire to lose myself in a cause, and it felt good.

7. When we first boarded the C17 airplane from Kyrgyzstan bound for the combat zone, I had no idea what to expect. The anticipation about what was awaiting us when we got off the airplane was very anxiety producing. When we landed at Bagram Air Field in Afghanistan, it was intensely cold, and the noise from the F-15 fighter jets scrambling every hour for close-air support missions was deafening. I remember asking myself "What the hell did I get myself into?"

8. To "secure" means to go into a location with full force. In this case it meant to enter the hospital and take the boy, possibly against his parents' or the hospital's agreement.

9. One night our base was attacked with multiple 107-millimeter rockets. The rockets were fired a great distance from the base, approximately 2000 meters away. They were fired with such velocity that fragments would detach and fall on the roofs of structures on our base. This fragmentation sounded like hard rain or hail. Immediately following this sound the rocket impacted and shook the base remarkably. After returning to the United States, the sounds of strong rain falling on the roof of my house reinvigorate the memories of being in Afghanistan.

10. I could not escape the idea that our treatment was not good enough. We could not save this young soldier. Still covered in his blood, we continued the mission. We packaged his immediate belongings, placed his body onto a litter, and moved him up to the flight line. There is a specific procedure for loading a fallen soldier onto a hero flight. Everyone stands at the position of attention and renders multiple salutes as the body is loaded onto the aircraft it takes off. At this point I was faced with the second most difficult order I have had to give. As the tears ran down my medic's faces, I ordered them to clean and re-stock the aid station. I gave them no time to cry or talk about what happened. We were in a combat zone, and at any point we could receive more casualties or an attack on our base. We needed to continue the mission and prepare for the care of others. A few hours later I coordinated a CISD for my medics with a military psychologist. As a group, we recounted the incident and discussed what we did well, both operationally and clini-

cally, and what we needed to improve. There was guilt then, and there is still guilt to this day. It was senseless and tragic, and I feel remorse. Maybe I could have scrambled the MEDEVAC quicker, or maybe I could have known that this soldier was experiencing psychological distress and coordinated care for him. Ultimately, however, history has shown us that suicide is an inevitable reality in a war zone. As a veteran MEDO after any suicide action, I ask myself, can something be done to prevent it?

11. Currently, there is no specifically mandated resiliency training by the DoD as part of the mobilization process. In 2009, the Army began pilot programs and integrating the Comprehensive Soldier Fitness Master Resilience program. This program focused on five dimensions of strength: emotional, social, spiritual, family, and physical. However, it is not compulsory education or training for soldiers in the pipeline to deploy overseas. In addition, I believe the idea of utilizing prolonged exposure therapy or CID while the individual is still in a combat zone is counterintuitive. I disagreed with our behavioral health team's implementation of this therapy in Afghanistan, and I still disagree. Desensitization should be implemented in a systematic and controlled way, neither of which can be guaranteed in a combat zone.

REFERENCES

Barboza, K. (2005). Critical incident stress debriefing (CISD): Efficacy in question. *The New School Psychology Bulletin, 3*(2), 49–70.

Bartone, P.T,. (2006). Resilience under military operational stress: Can leaders influence hardiness? *Military Psychology, 18*(Suppl), S131–S148.

Young, R.S.K., Gillan, E., Dingmann, P., Casinalli, P., and Taylor, C. (2009, January). Army Health Care Operations in Iraq. *Connecticut Medicine, 72*(1), 13–17.

Chapter 20

GUIDED MISSILES AND MISGUIDED LEADERS: CIVILIANS IN WAR ZONES AS OBSERVED BY A CHRISTIAN ACTIVIST

CHRISTOPHER J. DOUCOT

They sow the wind and reap the whirlwind.

Hosea 8:7

In America, references to war-related PTSD exclusively conjure up images of emotionally and psychologically wounded veterans. Oftentimes these psychic injuries are the only ones borne by the soldier, especially if the wounded combatant performed his duties from afar. Perhaps it is only natural for us to be concerned about the repercussions of war as they affect fellow Americans, and so we focus our attention on returning soldiers and sailors, pilots, and marines. Left untreated, the effects of PTSD will reverberate beyond the wounded veteran and have the potential to harm his family via domestic violence and society at large via substance abuse, unemployment, and homelessness.

What of the repercussions on the receiving end of the action(s) that induced the PTSD to begin with? If the action in question had the potential to induce PTSD in the soldier then how much more trauma was experienced by the wounded civilian? Missiles and rockets, grenades and rounds are not simply lethal but also trauma-inducing implements that tether warrior and civilian, ally or enemy in suffering. The percussion waves of our weapons extend beyond the ragged borders of blast capacity marked by blood and limb. The waves of calamity released by our munitions are confined by neither time nor space; rather, they undulate across cultures and down generations-like a tsunami across an ocean—until they come ashore, seemingly out of nowhere, with devastating impact.

THREE WOUNDED CHILDREN

Every war is a war against children.

Howard Zinn (Ortiz-Leff, 2010)

Consider the experiences of three children wounded in war. Extending the tsunami metaphor, the trauma endured by these children would be the equivalent of a tsunami-triggering earthquake–whether you think their traumas have unleashed tidal waves depends, I guess, on how close you are to the shore.

Six-Year-Old Ali

In late July 1999 I was travelling through Najaf, Iraq, on a fact-finding mission. Two days prior to my arrival our warplanes had bombed the area. According to *The New York Times*, "precision guided munitions" were used to strike a "missile battery" and a "military communications site." What I saw was an unscathed antiquated piece of antiaircraft artillery and some small businesses with minor damage consistent with what a cluster bomb would do. Looking at shrapnel I had recovered at one of the bomb sites, a British Special Forces commander concurred that it was likely from a cluster bomb. A cluster bomb is an antipersonnel weapon, meaning it is designed to maximize injury to the enemy while minimizing damage to infrastructure (buildings, roads, artillery, and the like). A cluster bomb is composed of dozens, and sometimes hundreds, of smaller bomblets, that scatter just before impact to maximize their effective radius. A percentage of the bomblets, upward of 30 percent, typically fail to detonate on impact, withholding their fury until disturbed by the elements, an animal, and sometimes a child; farmers in Cambodia and Vietnam are still losing legs to cluster bombs dropped thirty-five years ago. The initial toll of the bombs dropped on Najaf that July day were thirteen civilians killed and eighteen seriously injured. Among the injured was a six-year-old boy, Ali, whose right arm was blown off at the shoulder. Standing by his bedside his father asked me: *"Why does America bomb us? We are not criminals."* There were no soldiers among the dead or wounded.

Whereas cluster bombs are intentionally indiscriminate, the AGM-130 missile, made by Boeing, is among the "smartest" weapons in the Pentagon's repertoire. Precision, however, is not a guarantee of accuracy.

Haider and Mustafa

My closest Iraqi friend is Iqbal F. She is a middle-aged schoolteacher and a mother. On January 25, 1999, she had just shooed her four- and five-year-old sons out the door of her humble concrete home in the southern Iraqi city of Basra. They had been bickering, and in anger she hollered at them to go outside. A few moments later she heard what she thought was a truck rumble down her rutted dirt street. The blast that quickly followed kicked her in the gut. Clinging to her flowing black abaya she bolted down the street in the direction of the blast. On the corner she found five-year-old Haider bloody and motionless, the pale pall of death formed instantly by the concrete dust that filled his hair and covered his face. Next to him four-year-old Mustafa wailed; his left hand had been partially severed. Um Haider, (i.e. "the mother of Haider"), as she is now known, gathered Mustafa's broken body and ran toward a busy thoroughfare where a passing taxi sped her to the hospital. Much of Mustafa's hand was lost, but his life was saved. The missile involved in this attack was an AGM-130. A Pentagon spokesman told me that ground coordinates of the intended target are programmed into the missile before launch. As this so-called "smart weapon" actually more of an "idiot-savant" in our arsenal, approaches its target, the "weapon's system operator" takes manual control of the missile. An onboard video monitor broadcasts a live video feed of the target so that using a "joystick" the weapons system operator can *"choose the window pane or door knob"* of his liking. This particular missile landed in the middle of a sprawling and poor residential neighborhood killing eleven civilians, four of them were in grade school, and injuring another fifty-nine. A dozen times over the last decade Um Haider has asked me *"What did I do to deserve this?"*

Is there any justice for civilians who are being hurt in urban wars? In another part of the Middle East the status of civilians is apparently denied. In a court hearing in Israel concerning the murder of American citizen Rachel Corrie, an officer from the Israeli Defense Forces (IDF) testified that "During war, there are no civilians."[1] He added, "When you write a [protocol] manual, the manual is for war" (Barrows-Friedman, 2010).

Nine-year-old Marwa With A Bullet in Her Head

Marwa Al-Sharif was a precocious 9 year old Palestinian girl in 2001 who was lucky enough to have her own bedroom with an expansive view that included a hill not too far off. Marwa was too young to know why the IDF (Israel Defense Forces) took possession of that hilltop, but she did know when they commandeered it because it coincided with her sleeping in the hallway. With an IDF military base outside her window providing a clear shot into her bedroom, the family decided it was no longer safe for Marwa to sleep in her own bed. A few weeks before her tenth birthday Marwa's skull was pierced by a sniper's round that was shot into her window. The copper and lead slug hit the metal bars outside the window and ricocheted into the hallway before coming to rest in Marwa's brain. When I met her in August she was confined to the family couch with the bullet still lodged in her brain because her family was not able to get surgery in the West Bank and did not trust an Israeli hospital to cut open the girl's head. A team of humanitarian workers jumped through hoops with the Palestinian Authority, the Israeli government, the U.S. State Department, British Airways, and an American children's hospital to get Marwa and her mother Sahar to Connecticut to have the bullet safely removed. Marwa was recovering in my north Hartford home on September 11 when all television and radio stations interrupted regular broadcasts to inform us that America was under attack.

Sahar's family, friends, and neighbors were (and continue to be) themselves ordinary people who had been subjected to the trauma of war. They had seen the bodies of loved ones torn apart by the instruments of war and the minds of "survivors" likewise torn by the grief and guilt of surviving; they had no desire for others to be likewise traumatized. Marwa and Sahar watched television pictures of 9/11 atrocities and wept.

FOLLOW-UP OF WOUNDED CHILDREN

Today, Marwa is a nineteen-year-old university student studying fashion, "traveling" the world on the Internet and building community on Facebook. Aside from a scar hidden by hair and a hijab and occasional headaches, Marwa's body has healed amazingly well. As far as I can tell her psyche has experienced an encouraging recovery. What of others innocently traumatized by war? What of Marwa's brother, who fled the house in the dark of night covered in his sister's blood? What of Mustafa in Basra or Ali in Najaf, with their damaged and visibly mangled bodies? What if their psyches are not as resilient as Marwa's? Their opportunities may be more limited. Where will their trauma ultimately take them? Is there any research being done on their conditions of PTSD?

I think about the exchange I had with the mother of Ali. While she held his remaining hand and stroked his face I apologized in broken Arabic: "Asif, asif." Through an interpreter Um Ali responded: "You do not need to apologize, I do not hold you responsible. You did not do this to my son; your government did." I was left speechless by the generosity of her pardon, a pardon that in all fairness was not fully warranted. Our nation is, after all, a society governed of people, by people, and for people, as Lincoln suggested, and it was "we the people" who purchased with our tax dollars the cluster bomb that maimed Ali, it was "we the people" who elected our president and endorsed his policy of bombings with our silence. In a democracy we bear responsibility for the actions of our government–but Ali? He was just a child. How could he be responsible for the actions of his government or held accountable for the actions of a dictator we had armed for a decade?

Ali and Mustafa are now young men missing limbs living in a land occupied by the same military forces that maimed them. What is their place in occupied Iraq? How do they react when a U.S. Humvee full of soldiers passes in front of them? Do they wish to pick up a rock with the hand that is left for them and throw it at the Humvee as a form of symbolic revenge? Is there meaningful employment available to those physically wounded by war? Has their disfigurement isolated them socially, romantically, or even spiritually? I fear that the trauma-induced existential pain of isolation and alienation has made them more vulnerable to becoming recruits for groups that deploy suicide bombers as a misguided means to their liberation.

REACTIONARY POLICIES AFTER THE TRAGEDY
OF SEPTEMBER 11, 2001

The White House and U.S. military encouraged Americans to make certain assumptions about their "enemies" in Iraq and Afghanistan in a post-9/11 world. They also cultivated certain assumptions about the way U.S. soldiers viewed the command to war. Ultimately, those who deployed to Afghanistan and Iraq were forced to return to war time and time again by a military that is short on personnel for its long wars. Thousands of U.S. soldiers have had to endure repeated exposure to the horrors of war. America's ongoing response to the attacks of September 11 has evolved over the decade of its prosecution. Our current policy is dissonant by design: tens of thousands of battle clad American soldiers have daily personal contact with civilians in Iraq and Afghanistan via military occupation; meanwhile coterie of khaki-clad soldiers launch and control deadly drones from thousands of miles away. Although the distance between soldier and casualty has increased over the decade from the pilot at 30,000 feet dropping a cluster bomb to the drone operator guiding missiles into Pakistan from a base 5000 miles away, the impact remains the same: civilians, very often children, are losing limbs, lives, and families.

What do our veterans and pilots feel when they are exposed to the result of their shooting, bombing, and exploding? Research on veterans with PTSD reveals the element of guilt and shame as a contributing factor to their PTSD development. Some resort to suicide to alleviate their suffering and punishing superego, as the images of dead civilians are chasing them in nightmares at night and flashbacks and hallucinations in daytime. "Misguided" leaders and commanders placed them in the circumstances that they have to kill, or get killed—as Edward Tick explained skillfully in his book, "Many soldiers' most devastating lesson is the discovery that we are not, after all, the good cavalry led by John Wayne to save the helpless settlers from savages; nor are we the blessed crusaders slaying the turbaned barbarians from Evil Empires. Instead, what soldiers often discover is that those we are trying to save see us as the savage invaders, needing to be stopped by their own painful, heroic sacrifices" (Tick, 2005, p. 160).

The tragic irony of America's response to the tragedy of September 11 is that in seeking to protect Americans from future trauma, a cadre of traumatized civilians has been created across the Middle East. When a wave is met by another wave traveling with the same amplitude, they merge into a single more powerful wave, but when a wave is met by another wave traveling with the opposite amplitude, they cancel each other and disappear. So it is with violence. By responding to the violent attacks of September 11 with violence of our own we have created a more powerful wave of violence that continues to circle our planet gathering strength and leaving destruction and trauma wherever it crashes onshore. As Gandhi mentioned, an eye for an eye makes the whole world blind.

The treatment of those traumatized—soldier and civilian alike—may be within the purview of clinicians and therapists, but to rid our world of war-induced trauma, an opposite force of equal strength must be unleashed. The ultimate and only remedy to trauma will be a coordinated effort by the civilians of this planet to practice works of understanding, empathy, and mercy.

Our air-to-ground missiles and daisy cutter bombs (weighing 15,000 pounds), our cluster munitions and drones, are leaving in their wake a legion who are disabled, disturbed, and traumatized, some of whom will be propelled by their wounds to seek vengeance. As Edward Tick mentioned, "When women and children are willing to die to stop us, and an entire population resists us, then our soldiers' belief in our goodness cracks-and so does their spirit" (2005, 161).

WORK OF MERCY VERSUS WORK OF WAR

In the Catholic tradition, the Works of Mercy are a list of ways to care for body and soul. The corporeal works of mercy are to *feed the hungry, clothe the naked, house the homeless, give drink to the thirsty, liberate captives, comfort those who are ill, and bury the dead. The spiritual works of mercy are to teach the unknowing, counsel those in doubt, admonish those who do wrong, comfort those who are sorrowful, bear wrongs patiently, forgive injuries, and pray for the living and the dead.* The Works of Mercy are the opposite of the Works of War, which destroy crops and contaminate water. War burns homes and occupation holds a nation captive; war makes people sorrowful; it is impatient and inimical to forgiveness. Modern war is fought from a distance; enemies and strangers are killed but never met. The Works of Mercy are best performed on a daily basis and in a personal manner and can turn enemies and strangers into neighbors and friends. This has been my experience with Um Haider and Sahar. The practice of mercy is transformative for both parties. Practicing mercy creates an opening for the traumatized to be heard and healed; the ensuing conversation(s) results in dialectics with a restorative brand of justice that is the foundation for the peace we all seek.

Our response to the 9/11 attacks set off trauma waves in Pakistan, Iraq, and Afghanistan that have landed in Madrid (2004) and London (2005) and almost in Time Square (2010), as well as many other places. Tragically, we have not seen the last of these attacks. New waves of trauma continue to emanate from the epicenter of every drone attack, rocket barrage, and car bombing. We have become the world leader in arms exports and military expenditures. What if we led the world in the export of mercy instead? As the Persian prophet Zarathustra said thousands of years ago, "When I go to fight the darkness, I carry a torch, not a sword."

NOTES

1. Nora Barrows-Friedman: "During War there are No Civilians" (Al Jazeera, OPED, September 8, 2010). An American woman named Rachel Corrie was standing in front of the home of a Palestinian, trying to prevent its demolition, when a tank ran over her, backed up, and ran over her again, breaking her back. At a 2010 court proceeding on the death held in Haifi District Court, in Israel, Israeli Military Force training unit leader "Yossi" answered a question from the defense by saying, "During war there are no civilians." For further information: http://english.aljazeera.net/indepth/opinion/2010/09/201098123618465366.html

REFERENCES

Barrows-Friedman, N. (2010, September 8). During war there are no civilians. *Aljazeera. Net.*

Ortiz-Leff, D., (2010, Feb 1). Every war is a war against a child, Cal Coast news.Com. Retrieved on Nov 13, 2011 from http://calcoastnews.com/2010/02/every-war-is-a-war-against-a-child/

Tick, E. (2005). *War and the soul: Healing our nation's veterans from post-traumatic stress disorder.* Wheaton, IL: Quest Books.

Chapter 21

FAR FROM BEING A HERO: MY LIFE AS A WWII PILOT

SIDNEY GITLIN

I once read that anyone who writes his own autobiography becomes the hero of his tale. I hope that it is not true in my case, because I feel far from being a hero. I am a retired psychologist, but during WWII, I flew a bomber plane. I have a Ph.D. and consider my career to have been a success; however, 60 years after the war, I still cry, have nightmares, and suffer from the effects of PTSD. In the war, my crew's motto was, "We don't want a liar on the crew because we could never trust him. We don't want a coward on the crew because he would crack up just when we needed him to function. Most of all, we don't want someone who wants to be a hero, because he will surely endanger all of us just so he can win himself a stupid medal."

MY FAMILY BACKGROUND

I came from a working-class family. When he was a young man, my father was a seaman—a stoker on steamships. Unlike most Jewish men, he had a tattoo on his left shoulder of a Liberty head, even though tattoos were considered a desecration of one's body and therefore against Jewish tradition. Although he came from an Orthodox family, he was an atheist, because he believed that rabbis and priests were hypocrites. I was never bar mitzvahed, nor did I receive a Jewish education.

My father was keenly aware of the existence of anti-Semitism and racism and often said to me, "Remember that you are Jewish, because if you forget they will make you remember.

My sister, who is eight years older than I am, was also influenced by our parents' willingness to fight for what they believed was "right." Because she was a voracious reader, when she went to the library I went along with her to help her carry home her load of books. When I was about five years old, I was with her when one librarian refused to allow her to take out the adult books she requested, because, she told us, they were for adults only. My sister looked at her and told her she had read all of the books in the children's section, but the librarian refused to believe that this slim thirteen-year-old could possibly have done such a thing. My sister turned away, took my hand, and marched us to another library, where the librarian offered to help her find the adult books she wanted.

My dad, mother, and sister taught me to stand up for what I knew was right instead of being afraid of authority. To this day, at the age of ninety-four, my sister continues to challenge authority and fight for the welfare of others.

MY FIRST BOMBING MISSION

My first mission was to Blechhammer, Germany, which the air crews called the Black Hammer because of its heavy fortifications and the losses we sustained. Because it was a major industrial center and produced synthetic oil and ball bearings, it was bombed frequently. The Germans employed numerous antiaircraft guns to protect Blechhammer, but their principal weapon was the notorious 88-mm FlaK antiaircraft artillery gun. The Fifteenth Air Force dropped something like 300,000 tons or more of bombs on this target and lost many airplanes and crews. The thirty-second squadron was awarded a unit commendation for its actions and heavy losses.

Once we took off and were at our stations, the experienced crew would ask me to turn on the radio so they could hear some music. If the pilot agreed, I would tune into Axis Sally on German radio, even though she played rather sad songs and told us how the war was the result of the Jews. She also liked to name the targets we were scheduled to hit. Much of her comments were met with derision, but the music was welcome because we could not get Allied stations.

When we started our bomb run I could feel the plane lurch, but I could not hear any explosions—just popping sounds. However, once I looked outside from my small window I could see black puffs of smoke. That carpet of black smoke made me feel like I was watching a movie, which is why the danger we were in did not completely register until the bombardier called out that he was opening the bomb bay doors and taking control of the aircraft. He jolted me out of my reverie, and I started to perform my job. I grabbed boxes of chaff, aluminum strips, and dropped them out the bomb bay door, with the hope that the aluminum strips would create false readings on German radar. My next job was to tune the radar-jamming devices, watch the bombs drop, and ascertain whether we had hit our target.

BOMBING BLECHHAMMER

I believe it was on this mission that we spotted a group of German fighters. One of our crew began to curse and shout out vile racial slurs because he did not see our fighter coverage, the Tuskegee Airmen. The Red Tails, the ninety-ninth fighter squadron, generally flew cover for us and usually were a few thousand feet above us. They flew the vaunted P51. Our pilot did not stop the guy from interfering with the intercom system or reprimand him for his racist comments, because all of our guns were pointed in the direction of the German fighters and our anxiety was high. I felt compelled to say something, but this time I could not because the fighters were coming after us. Then, the Red Tails came roaring down from above and chased them away, and I believe they may have shot one or two down.

On one mission to Berlin we were attacked by German jets. This encounter was extremely frightening to me, because if we were attacked by a regular fighter plane we at least felt some control because we had powerful 50 calibers to aim and shoot at it. You may not have hit a damn thing, but at least there was some feeling of fighting back. When that jet came after us, however, we could not do a thing. For years I remembered it as a bad dream, or thought I had confabulated an incident where a jet was shot down or badly damaged by four P51s that came straight down shooting in front of that jet. In essence, I watched as the jet ran through a hail of bullets.

After I was discharged, I mentally replayed this image many times, until I read in the Rutherford, NJ, newspaper about one of the Tuskegee Airmen, a Captain Spann. I called him to thank him for his fighter coverage and asked him about this incident. He confirmed that it had occurred and told me the name of the pilot who received credit for the "kill."

I CRIED THEN, AND I CRY NOW

On the way back to my base after my R&R, the truck broke down and I did not get back until late in the afternoon. I reported to the squadron officer of the day and learned that I had been scheduled to fly with my crew on a mission. The planes should have returned from the mission, but my friend Abe told me that my crew had been shot down and all aboard were presumed dead. I can not recall my reaction, or maybe it is buried in my deep unconscious, but later, Abe told me I cried like a baby.

I am not ashamed of being told that I cried. In fact, the pain of losing ten comrades is so painful that as I write this the tears have returned. For a long time I could not recall if I slept in the tent alone or if a replacement crew took their place. Only as I write about it do the feelings of loss and loneliness now make themselves evident, as does the long-forgotten reappearance of that empty tent.

DEFUSING A BOMB WHILE FLYING: A BRAVERY IGNORED BY MILITARY OFFICIALS

In addition to facing antiaircraft fire, other situations were also frightening to me. On one mission our bombardier released a bomb load, but one bomb on the lower rack was hung up and would not release. The armament specialist tried everything to get it released, but all of his efforts failed. The bomb bay doors could not be closed; if they did, they would set the bomb off. We could not land with a loaded bomb because the bomb could shake loose as a result of the impact in landing and blow us up. The only solution was to defuse the bomb. Since the bomb bay doors were open, we were not able to maneuver easily and were sitting ducks for German fighters.

Our armament specialist decided that the tail gunner and I should hold him by the ankles and lower him until he could reach the fuse of the bomb. The pilot agreed and took the plane to an altitude where we did not need oxygen. He had to keep the plane from bouncing too much and tried not to hit an air pocket that could jostle us and cause us to lose our grip on the armament specialist. We had to stand on a catwalk that was only six inches wide. We held our breath, lowered him, and gently swung him into position. He was able to defuse the bomb, and when we closed the doors it was with deep relief. He should have been awarded a medal, because he did this task without a parachute. If we had lost our grip, he would have been killed. Unfortunately, our recommendation to the pilot that he be recommended for a medal was ignored. The crew felt badly that his bravery had been ignored, but he said that he never looked for a medal, because he was just doing his "job." He never complained about our pilot's dismissive attitude.

Other situations also made me very anxious. After one bomb run the pilot checked each position to see if any of us had been wounded, but when he asked the ball turret gunner to reply, there was no answer. He directed me to see if he was wounded or dead, and I grabbed an oxygen canister, plugged it into my oxygen tube, grabbed another for the silent ball turret gunner, opened the turret, and dragged him out to the radio space. I worked on his oxygen mask to break the ice that had formed until he opened his eyes and nodded thanks. At that moment I passed out, because I had been so busy taking care of him that I had not cracked my own oxygen mask. He cracked my mask, and we sat in the radio area, exhausted but relieved to be alive. We began to laugh in relief and laughed until we reached home base.

THE MOST DIFFICULT EVENTS TO TALK ABOUT

I think that the most difficult event to talk about is when I watched a plane blow up upon landing at home base. When we returned safely from a run, we would often stay by the landing area to count the planes coming in or wait hopefully for friends to return. There were times when a seriously damaged plane radioed in to ask to have the runway cleared, because the pilot knew that he might have trouble landing safely. We would watch as those skilled pilots landed their crippled ships safely. There was also more than one occasion when the plane had been so badly damaged that it collapsed and blew up with men on board. I witnessed this and can never forget it.

MY LAST FLY

My last mission was over northern Italy in support of the ground forces. When the weather cleared, I believe that every airplane that could fly was put into service and sent to support the GIs surrounded at the Battle of the Bulge. I must admit to a great deal of pride at seeing hundreds and hundreds of planes in the air at the same time, flying with the intention of destroying the German ground forces.

WAR IS OVER: WHY NOT SOONER?

After I landed my last mission, a jubilant gang informed me that the war was now over and we were going to go home. I was pleased but perplexed. Even though we had just dropped bombs on German troop concentrations, somehow in that short space of time between the action of killing people and coming back to the base, peace had been declared? Why now? Why not sooner? Had all that killing really been necessary? What was its purpose? Was my tail gunner right when he said that the people who really control things would never change? Would we be facing another world war later or sooner?

SEGREGATED AFRICAN-AMERICAN TROOPS

At night we were taken to a local movie theater along with some African-American troops. What was unacceptable to me, and others who had been saved by the Tuskegee Airmen, was that the German prisoners were seated with all of us, while the African-American troops were segregated to the balcony. This was not what we had fought for, so some of us issued complaints. We were told that this was the South and that the Army had no control over local policies. We should have remembered: the armed services were segregated and racist to the core. Not until 1948 did President Truman issue the order as Commander-in-Chief that the armed services become desegregated.

CIVILIAN LIFE

Because I had no idea what to do with my life, I ended up drifting from one job to another, until I was pressured by my family to go to college. I went to night school to take some refresher courses and met my future wife, who not only loved school but also seemed much smarter than I.

When my son was two-and-a-half years old he contracted childhood nephrosis, and the next seven years put terrible stress on all of us. We almost lost our son several times, but I still worked and completed school. If there is a hero in this story, it is my wife, because she held the family together and sacrificed her own needs and ambitions for the welfare of our daughter, son, and me. If they handed out medals for real-life combat, my wife, daughter, and son would receive the highest awards.

CANCER AND RETIREMENT

In 1972, I was diagnosed with lymphoma and required intensive chemotherapy and radiation. I was busy with family, school, work, teaching, supervising younger psychologists, and taking care of my health, which might be why my nightmares, tears, and thoughts of the war stopped. In 2004, I experienced a recurrence of my cancer. This cancer was virulent, and I was unable to withstand the assault of the chemotherapy. I had to spend a lot of time in the hospital, and I could no longer work. Because I was unable to sustain my concentration or guarantee my presence for a therapy session, I reluctantly retired.

RELIVING WWII, SIXTY YEARS LATER

Once I retired, the memories of my combat experiences came flooding back. At first I thought that they were symbolic of the threat of having cancer and possibly dying from my ailment. I did not understand why after a sixty-year hiatus my nightmares and anxiety reactions to past memories of my friends and crew had returned. By chance I tuned into my local PBS station and heard an interview conducted with two bomber pilots who spoke of their war experiences. As they talked, both became teary and sad, and I realized, hey, I am not alone. I also learned that after the film *Saving Private Ryan* came out, many WWII vets ended up going to their local VAs for counseling. This gave me a feeling of connection with my fellow veterans that civilians rarely understand and helped me deal with my now-recurring memories of my war traumas.

When I needed expensive medication for my cancer, as well as a new hearing aid, I went to my nearest VA facility, where I saw vets from WW II, Korea, and Vietnam. Some were without arms or legs, and all were in some way impaired. Looking at them, I found myself frozen in the middle of the floor. I again experienced an overwhelming sense of grief and sadness–this time for these walking wounded vets. All I wanted to do was leave. Just as I was walking toward the door, a nurse gently placed her hand on my shoulder and said, "Having some flashbacks, like you're back in the service?" I shook my head yes, and she told me that a lot of WWII vets do. She helped me sit down and slowly went over the bureaucratic procedures I would need to follow.

Even though I had wanted to be a pilot, those childhood dreams of flying turned into a constant state of alert as I struggled to stay alive during WWII. War damages us permanently, and its horrors are lasting, which is why I now believe only a few things are worth fighting for: peace and an end to racism and bigotry. Because war challenged my most basic sense of humanity and beliefs and made me question its purpose, I can no longer accept any rationale for going to war. Instead, I protest our involvement in it, even though some people promote it, hiding behind patriotism as a weapon that will keep America safe. I am guessing they were not combat veterans, or they would not be so ignorant of the trauma their fantasy of war produces.

I recently start wearing a cap that says *I am an Air Force Veteran*, because it allows me to instantly reconnect with other veterans. My story is pretty much their story. I have yet to find a combat vet who is eager to see us go to war again, because they do not want their children or grandchildren to go to war. Those who are eager to fight a war have no concept of the trauma that war causes to veterans and civilians alike, even though they spout patriotic slogans and are eager to have others fight for them. I agree with Samuel Johnson, who in 1775, claimed that "Patriotism is the last refuge of a scoundrel."

Appendix

12-STEP SELF-HELP PRINCIPLES FOR COMBAT VETERANS WITH PTSD

Jamshid A. Marvasti

As part of a treatment protocol, the editor of this book has also designed a 12-step self-help program for combat veterans with PTSD, inspired by addiction self-help and support groups. The author believes there are similarities among these disorders. This is an experimental plan that has thus far helped a number of warriors, but requires further research to confirm its benefits. To the best of the author's knowledge this is the first 12-step program that has been developed specifically for war trauma soldiers.

DR. MARVASTI'S 12-STEP SELF-HELP PRINCIPLES FOR VETERANS WITH WAR TRAUMA

1. We came to accept that we are, and always will be, veterans of war, but that we did not create the war, and when we deployed we were people who would have chosen to prevent the suffering of others, of ourselves, and of our families.
2. We entered the hell of war, and witnessed many horrors no human should ever have to witness; upon our return, we left a part of ourselves in those areas of conflict, trapped and helpless to impact our surroundings.
3. Those of us who possess spiritual faith believe our faith will save us; still others believe that a healing power exists within each of us.
4. We do not expect any civilian to understand what we have endured in combat, and we often are unable to put our experiences into words, because there are not enough words to explain.

5. We were placed in circumstances where we witnessed and undertook activities that go against our conscience, ethics, and morals.

6. Although "there is no atheist in a foxhole," some of us, having escaped the foxhole, have lost our faith. We ask ourselves, "Where was God when we were exposed to massacres and atrocities of war?"

7. We hope to make a searching and fearless moral inventory of ourselves. We want to make amends for our errors and those actions that we committed out of fear or necessity.

8. We confess our actions in order to lessen the burden of guilt and emotional pain, and we take full responsibility for our actions during combat–including those that inflict pain upon their reflection.

9. We were strong warriors but return home with great suffering. Some of us have become involved in self-destructive behavior–among them homelessness, substance abuse, and rage.

10. We believe that by helping others who suffer from the similar disorders we will help ourselves and we will start a new life with a new code of behavior.

11. Humbly, we ask those we violated, and the spirits of those we annihilated, to forgive us, so that we may forgive ourselves.

12. One may redeem the self by rehabilitating and renovating the damage done to others–one can reconstruct the building that was bombed, and heal the innocents that were harmed.

GLOSSARY AND TERMINOLOGY

Jennifer Bordonaro Mastrocola

Active Duty (AD): refers to service members who serve full-time in the armed forces, not to be confused with reservists or National Guardsmen.

Activities of Daily Living (ADL): term used in health care in reference to basic daily self-care activities. The ability or inability to perform these tasks is often used as a measurement of a person's functional status.

Acute Stress Disorder (ASD): one of the DSM-IV (2000) diagnoses, resulting from experiencing or witnessing a traumatic event. Patient may present with dissociative symptoms, increased arousal/anxiety, reexperiencing, and/or avoidance, resulting in significant impairment. Generally occurs within four weeks of the event and lasts between two days and one month after the experience.

Altruistic suicide: taking of one's own life for the benefit of a greater good such as honor, society, and so on.

Amygdala: an almond-shaped group of nerve cells located in the temporal lobes of the brain involved in the fear response. It is speculated the amygdala stimulates the secretion of corticotropin releasing hormone (CRH) and consequently stimulates the rest of the hypothalamic-pituitary-adrenal (HPA) axis.

Anhedonia: inability to experience pleasure from usual activities that are pleasurable.

Anniversary Reactions: experiencing increased symptoms of grief, reexperiencing, or distress on or around a particular date or time relating to an emotionally stressful event.

Battered Child Syndrome: In 1962, Dr. Kempe and Dr. Brandt F. Steele published their important paper, "The Battered Child Syndrome." Publishing this paper led to the identification and recognition of child abuse within the medical community. This syndrome is a clinical condition in children who have received physical abuse.

Battered Soldier Syndrome: the editor of this book developed this terminology, prompted by "battered child" "and "battered wife" syndromes. Factors such as multiple deployments, stop-loss procedures, and the nature of "urban warfare," which requires fighting in civilian areas, contribute to psychological and physical battering of our veterans.

Battered Wife Syndrome: psychological condition often thought of as a subcategory of PTSD, now renamed as battered *person* syndrome, where the person is a victim of domestic violence but often is unable to leave the abuser despite the long-term physical and psychological damage experienced.

Betrayal Trauma: psychological trauma resulting from a breach of a presumed trust or confidence between individuals or organizations and individuals.

Brainwashing: attempt to manipulate or change one's thoughts, beliefs, and behaviors against one's will to those of the manipulator, also known as "mind control."

Cognitive Impairment: limited mental functioning, especially in regard to judgment, learning, memory, or speech; may lead to difficulty with tasks that require such functions.

Collateral damage: unintended or incidental injuries, damages, or deaths, to people or objects that were not intended targets, usually in reference to a military offensive strategy.

Combat Stress Team (CST): military term for an interdisciplinary team that provides behavioral health support to Coalition Forces in a Combat Zone.

Comorbidity: presence of two or more physical or psychiatric conditions in a person. Often these multiple conditions have large implications on one another, including a person's presentation, treatment, and prognosis. PTSD is often found in conjunction with other conditions.

Complex PTSD: diagnosis suggested by Dr. Judith Herman of Harvard University for those who meet the criteria for PTSD but, in contrast to the acute traumatic experience of most PTSD sufferers, these individuals have experienced chronic or prolonged trauma, usually associated with a state of captivity, which holds particular implications for treatment.

Compulsive Reexposure: a drive to reexperience situations that resemble or cause similar feelings experienced during the initial traumatic experience. Freud believed this is in attempt to achieve a form of mastery. Examples include soldiers choosing careers in law enforcement, children who were sexually abused becoming prostitutes, and so on.

Cortisol (hydrocortisone): one of the glucocorticoids produced by the adrenal cortex in humans; a stress response hormone.

Dehumanization: to deprive one of humanistic qualities such as individuality, personality, or compassion; often occurs in environments that produce emotional trauma. In combat, this is indicated by placing the enemy in a "nonhuman" category, as to facilitate killing.

Depersonalization: altered perception of self, feeling of being detached from one's body and mind; often described by patients as a dreamlike state or a state of being an outside observer of oneself.

Derealization: altered perception of the external world; feeling the environment seems unreal or unfamiliar, lacks color, is two-dimensional, and so on.

Dichotomy of us versus them: creation and perpetuation of a mentality where a supposed "enemy" is distinct from us, and possibly dehumanized, and we are exceptional and glorified. Used by cultures or governments to create an enemy and potentially a war against that enemy.

Dissociation: disruption or detachment of awareness or consciousness due to psychological trauma.

Emotional Numbing: one of the avoidance symptoms of PTSD; includes decreased interest in activities, feeling distant from others, and difficulty experiencing positive emotions. Numbing behaviors lead to a progressive avoidance of any stimulation in an attempt to feel nothing.

Euphemism: an inoffensive or indirect term or expression substituted for one that is offensive, e.g. "collateral damage" for civilian death and injuries in war.

Geneva Conventions: four treaties and three protocols that are a part of international humanitarian law and set the standards for the treatment of persons not involved in the hostilities of war, e.g. Abu Ghraib was a direct violation of the Geneva Conventions.

Hague International Conference: also Hague Conventions or First and Second Peace Conferences at The Hague, Netherlands; addressed the use of weapons of war and banned use of some warfare, including hollow point bullets and air bombing. The Geneva Protocol to Hague Convention specifically banned the use of chemical and biological warfare.

Hypothalamic-pituitary-adrenal (HPA) axis: This axis includes the hypothalamus, a section of the brain, and the pituitary and adrenal glands. The hypothalamus secretes corticotropin releasing hormone (CRH) and arginine vasopressin (AVP) which in turn stimulates the secretion of corticotropin (ACTH) from the pituitary gland and through the bloodstream causes the production of glucocorticoid by the adrenal gland.

Improvised Explosive Device (IED): military term for a homemade bomb, constructed and employed in methods other than conventional military warfare.

Intrusive Symptoms: one group of PTSD symptoms that includes flashbacks, daydreams, nightmares, and sudden onset of thoughts or emotions associated with the trauma that makes a person feel as if he or she is reliving the traumatic event.

Laws of War: part of international law pertaining to war, includes *jus ad bellum*–laws pertaining to justify war and criteria to ensure a "just war," the *why* war is fought–and *jus in bello*–laws pertaining to actions during a war, the *how* war is fought. These laws include conventions and treaties such as the Geneva Conventions and Hague Conventions.

Medical Operations Officer (MEDO)/Medical Service Corps (MSC) Officers: military term for an officer who serves as the direct advisor to the unit or battalion commander on all components of combat health support and is responsible for supervising medical personnel, and planning and coordinating all support services.

Medical Rules of Engagement (MROE): military term for the guidelines established and used in determining what, if any, care is authorized for civilian casualties in a combat zone.

Morale, Welfare, Recreation (MWR): military term for the network of support and leisure services designed for use by military personnel both current and retired, their families, and eligible civilian employees.

Neurotransmitters: chemicals that act in the brain to transmit signals from neuron to neuron, electrical messages are transformed to chemical messages and vice versa, e.g. serotonin, norepinephrine, dopamine.

Opioid Agonists: morphine-like medications that work on opioid receptors; administration results in analgesia, sedation, respiratory depression, and constipation; use of these drugs has a risk of dependence.

Panic Disorder: an anxiety disorder characterized by recurrent panic attacks usually without an obvious trigger. Symptoms include increased heart rate, increased blood pressure, sweating, palpitations, shortness of breath, extreme anxiety and fear; often patients confuse these episodes with a heart attack. Patients also experience significant anxiety regarding the possibility of future episodes that can, at times, lead to a limitation in a person's activities.

Parasuicidal Acts: nonlethal self-harm behaviors, including suicide attempts and self-mutilation; also referred to as "suicidal gesture." There is some controversy as to whether or not intent is critical in the definition of these acts.

Reenactment of Trauma: aspects of a trauma incorporated into everyday life through various behaviors where a patient can take on role of either victim or victimizer; believed to be an attempt to achieve mastery over the trauma or to relieve some of the anxiety of the trauma.

Reserve Component (RC): military term for armed forces that are not active duty; typical training includes approximately forty days per calendar year.

Rules of Engagement (ROE): military term for the directives that govern when and how enemy forces may be engaged with lethal force in a combat zone.

Survival Guilt: feelings experienced by those who remain after others die or are killed.

Tactical Combat Casualty Care (TC3): military term for the care of service members injured in direct combat operations with the enemy, e.g. application of combat application tourniquet (CAT), antihemolytic fluids, emergency needle chest decompression.

Trauma: "experiencing an event that is outside the range of usual human experience" (from DSM-IV-TR, 2000).

Traumatic Stressor: "experiencing, witnessing, or confronting events that involve actual or threatened death or serious injury, or a threat to the physical integrity of self or others" (from DSM-IV-TR, 2000, criterion A.1.).

Vicarious Traumatization: process that occurs in those who work with trauma victims in which providers experience inner changes secondary to the experiences that are shared with them, which can affect their spirituality, identity, interactions with patients and others, and worldview.

Vietnam Syndrome: form of PTSD experienced by Vietnam veterans; also refers to America's reluctance to become involved in combat oversees to prevent another war such as that in Vietnam, which caused significant psychological trauma to soldiers and the country as a whole.

War Crimes: violations of the laws of war as described in Hague and Geneva Conventions and in subsequent updates and amendments, punishable by fines, imprisonment, or death (*see also* Geneva Convention).

War propaganda: messages and communication provided in attempt to affect opinions, emotions, and actions during a war, often used to justify war and cause opposition to be perceived as true enemies to be hated and acted against.

SELECTED REFERENCES

Corsini, R. (2002). *The dictionary of psychology.* New York: Brunner/Routledge.
Department of Defense. (2010 Nov 8). *Dictionary of Military and Associated Terms.* Retrieved from http://www.dtic.mil/doctrine/dod_dictionary/
DSM-IV-TR (2000). *Diagnostic Statistical Manual of Mental Disorders* (4th ed., text revision. Washington, DC: American Psychiatric Association.
Reber, A., Reber, E., and Allen, R. (2009). *The penguin dictionary of psychology* (4th ed.). New York: Penguin.
Wikipedia. *Glossary of Psychiatry.* Retrieved from http://en.wikipedia.org/wiki/Glossary_of_psychiatry

INDEX

ABOUT THE EDITOR

Jamshid A. Marvasti, M.D. is a child and adult psychiatrist who grew up in a military family in Iran and has been practicing psychiatry in the United States for the last thirty years. He is a specialist in psychological trauma, terrorism, and child maltreatment, topics on which he has published articles and books including *Psycho-Political Aspects of Suicide Warriors, Terrorism and Martyrdom* (2008). Dr. Marvasti may be contacted at Manchester Memorial Hospital in Manchester, Connecticut 06040, USA.